Treatment of Chronic Pain by Medical Approaches

Timothy R. Deer
Editor-in-chief

Michael S. Leong
Associate Editor-in-chief

Vitaly Gordin
Associate Editor

Treatment of Chronic Pain by Medical Approaches

the AMERICAN ACADEMY *of* PAIN MEDICINE
Textbook on Patient Management

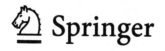 Springer

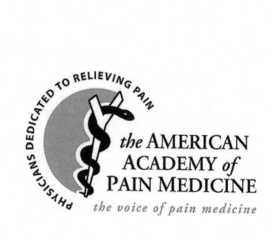

Editor-in-chief
Timothy R. Deer, M.D.
President and CEO
The Center for Pain Relief
Clinical Professor of Anesthesiology
West Virginia University School of Medicine
Charleston, WV, USA

Associate Editor
Vitaly Gordin, M.D.
Associate Professor
Associate Vice Chair of Pain Management
Department of Anesthesiology
Pennsylvania State University
College of Medicine
Director
Pain Medicine
Milton S. Hershey Medical Center
Hershey, PA, USA

Associate Editor-in-chief
Michael S. Leong, M.D.
Clinic Chief
Stanford Pain Medicine Center
Redwood City, CA, USA

Clinical Associate Professor
Department of Anesthesiology
Stanford University School of Medicine
Stanford, CA, USA

ISBN 978-1-4939-1817-1   ISBN 978-1-4939-1818-8 (eBook)
DOI 10.1007/978-1-4939-1818-8
Springer New York Heidelberg Dordrecht London

Library of Congress Control Number: 2014952895

Printed on acid-free paper

Springer is part of Springer Science+Business Media (www.springer.com)

To my wonderful wife, Missy, and the blessings I have been given in my children Morgan, Taylor, Reed, and Bailie.
I also want to thank my team for their awesome, continued support: Chris Kim, Rick Bowman, Doug Stewart, Matt Ranson, Jeff Peterson, Michelle Miller, Wil Tolentino, and Brian Yee.

Timothy R. Deer, M.D.

To all of my mentors, colleagues, and patients who have taught me about pain medicine. I would also like to acknowledge the patience and love of my family, particularly my children, Isabelle and Adam, as well as Brad, PFP, and little Mia. I have discovered more about myself during my short career than I thought possible and hope to help many more people cope with pain in the exciting future.

Michael S. Leong, M.D.

To Maria, Yuri, and Jacob for their patience and understanding, and to my fellows for choosing the field of pain management.

Vitaly Gordin, M.D.

Foreword to *Comprehensive Treatment of Chronic Pain by Medical, Interventional, and Integrative Approaches*

A brand new textbook is a testament to many things—an editor's vision, many authors' individual and collective expertise, the publisher's commitment, and all told, thousands of hours of hard work. This book encapsulates all of this, and with its compendium of up-to-date information covering the full spectrum of the field of pain medicine, it stands as an authoritative and highly practical reference for specialists and primary care clinicians alike. These attributes would be ample, in and of themselves, yet this important addition to the growing pain medicine library represents a rather novel attribute. It is a tangible embodiment of a professional medical society's fidelity to its avowed mission. With its commission of this text, under the editorial stewardship of highly dedicated and seasoned pain medicine specialists, the American Academy of Pain Medicine has made an important incremental step forward to realizing its ambitious mission, "to optimize the health of patients in pain and eliminate the major public health problem of pain by advancing the practice and specialty of pain medicine."

This last year, the Institute of Medicine (IOM) of the National Academies undertook the first comprehensive evaluation of the state of pain care in the United States. This seminal work culminated in a report and recommendations entitled "Relieving Pain in America: A Blueprint for Transforming Prevention, Care, Education, and Research." Clearly, as a nation, we have much work to do in order to meet the extraordinary public health needs revealed by the IOM committee. This comprehensive textbook is both timely and relevant as a resource for clinicians, educators, and researchers to ensure that the converging goals of the American Academy of Pain Medicine and the Institute of Medicine are realized. This book has been written; it is now all of ours to read and implement. Godspeed!

Salt Lake City, UT, USA

Perry G. Fine, M.D.

Foreword to *Comprehensive Treatment of Chronic Pain by Medical, Interventional, and Integrative Approaches*

The maturation of a medical specialty rests on both its ability to project its values, science, and mission into the medical academy and the salience of its mission to the public health. The arrival of the American Academy of Pain Medicine (AAPM)'s *Comprehensive Treatment of Chronic Pain by Medical, Interventional, and Integrative Approaches: the American Academy of Pain Medicine Textbook on Patient Management* is another accomplishment that signals AAPM's emergence as the premier medical organization solely dedicated to the development of pain medicine as a specialty in the service of patients in pain and the public health.

Allow me the privilege of brief comment on our progress leading to this accomplishment. The problem of pain as both a neurophysiological event and as human suffering has been a core dialectic of the physician-healer experience over the millennia, driving scientific and religious inquiry in all cultures and civilizations. The sentinel concepts and historical developments in pain medicine science and practice are well outlined in this and other volumes. Our history, like all of medicine's, is replete with examples of sociopolitical forces fostering environments in which individuals with vision and character initiated major advances in medical care. Thus the challenge of managing chronic pain and suffering born of injuries to troops in WWII galvanized John Bonica and other pioneers, representing several specialties, into action. They refused to consider that their duty to these soldiers, and by extension their brethren in chronic pain of all causes, was finished once pain was controlled after an acute injury or during a surgical procedure. They and other clinicians joined scientists in forming the IASP (International Association for the Study of Pain) in 1974, and the APS (American Pain Society) was ratified as its American chapter in 1978. Shortly thereafter, APS physicians with a primary interest in the development of pain management as a distinct medical practice began discussing the need for an organizational home for physicians dedicated to pain treatment; in 1984, they formally chartered AAPM. We soon obtained a seat in the AMA (American Medical Association). Since then, we have provided over two decades of leadership to the "House of Medicine," culminating in leadership of the AMA's Pain and Palliative Medicine Specialty Section Council that sponsored and conducted the first Pain Medicine Summit in 2009. The summit, whose participants represented all specialties caring for pain, made specific recommendations to improve pain education for all medical students and pain medicine training of residents in all specialties and to lengthen and strengthen the training of pain medicine specialists who would assume responsibility for the standards of pain education and care and help guide research.

Other organizational accomplishments have also marked our maturation as a specialty. AAPM developed a code of ethics for practice, delineated training and certification requirements, and formed a certifying body (American Board of Pain Medicine, ABPM) whose examination was based on the science and practice of our several parent specialties coalesced into one. We applied for specialty recognition in ABMS (American Board of Medical Specialties), and we continue to pursue this goal in coordination with other specialty organizations to assure the public and our medical colleagues of adequate training for pain medicine specialists. We have become a recognized and effective voice in medical policy. The AAPM, APS, and AHA (American Hospital Association) established the Pain Care Coalition (PCC), recently joined by the ASA (American Society of Anesthesiologists). Once again, by garnering sociopolitical support galvanized by concern for the care of our wounded warriors, the PCC was able to partner with the American Pain Foundation (APF) and other organizations to pass three new laws requiring the Veterans Administration and the military to report yearly on advances in pain management, training, and research and requiring the NIH (National Institute of Health) to examine its pain research portfolio and undertake the recently completed IOM report on pain.

AAPM has developed a robust scientific presence in medicine. We publish our own journal, *Pain Medicine*, which has grown from a small quarterly journal to a respected monthly publication that represents the full scope of pain medicine science and practice. Annually, we conduct the only medical conference that is dedicated to coverage of the full scope of pain medicine science and practice and present a robust and scientific poster session that represents our latest progress. Yet, year to year, we lament that the incredible clinical wisdom displayed at this conference, born out of years of specialty practice in our field, is lost between meetings. Now comes a remedy, our textbook—*Comprehensive Treatment of Chronic Pain by Medical, Interventional, and Integrative Approaches*.

Several years ago, Editor Tim Deer, who co-chaired an Annual Meeting Program Committee with Todd Sitzman, recognized the special nature of our annual conference and proposed that the AAPM engages the considerable expertise of our membership in producing a textbook specifically focused on the concepts and practice of our specialty. Under the visionary and vigorous leadership of Tim as Editor-in-Chief and his editorial group, *Comprehensive Treatment of Chronic Pain by Medical, Interventional, and Integrative Approaches* has arrived. Kudos to Tim, his Associate Editor-in-Chief Michael Leong, Associate Editors Asokumar Buvanendran, Vitaly Gordin, Philip Kim, Sunil Panchal, and Albert Ray for guiding our busy authors to the finish line. The expertise herein represents the best of our specialty and its practice. And finally, a specialty organization of physician volunteers needs a steady and resourceful professional staff to successfully complete its projects in the service of its mission. Ms. Susie Flynn, AAPM's Director of Education, worked behind-the-scenes with our capable Springer publishers and Tim and his editors to assure our book's timely publication. Truly, this many-faceted effort signals that the academy has achieved yet another developmental milestone as a medical organization inexorably destined to achieve specialty status in the American medical pantheon.

Philadelphia, PA, USA   Rollin M. Gallagher, M.D., M.P.H.

Preface to *Treatment of Chronic Pain by Medical Approaches*

We are grateful for the positive reception of **Comprehensive Treatment of Chronic Pain by Medical, Interventional, and Integrative Approaches: The AMERICAN ACADEMY OF PAIN MEDICINE Textbook on Patient Management** following its publication last year. The book was conceived as an all-encompassing clinical reference covering the entire spectrum of approaches to pain management: medical, interventional, and integrative. Discussions with pain medicine physicians and health professionals since then have persuaded us that the book could serve even more readers if sections on each of the major approaches were made available as individual volumes – while some readers want a comprehensive resource, others may need only a certain slice. We are pleased that these "spin-off" volumes are now available. I would like to take this opportunity to acknowledge once more the outstanding efforts and hard work of the Associate Editors responsible for the sections:

Treatment of Chronic Pain by Medical Approaches:
The American Academy of Pain Medicine *Textbook on Patient Management*
Associate Editor: Vitaly Gordin, MD

Treatment of Chronic Pain by Interventional Approaches:
The American Academy of Pain Medicine *Textbook on Patient Management*
Associate Editors: Asokumar Buvanendran, MD, Sunil J. Panchal, MD, Philip S. Kim, MD

Treatment of Chronic Pain by Integrative Approaches:
The American Academy of Pain Medicine *Textbook on Patient Management*
Associate Editor: Albert L. Ray, MD

We greatly appreciate the feedback of our readers and strive to continue to improve our educational materials as we educate each other. Please send me your input and thoughts to improve future volumes.

Our main goal is to improve patient safety and outcomes. We are hopeful that the content of these materials accomplishes this mission for you and for the patients to whom you offer care and compassion.

Charleston, WV, USA
Timothy R. Deer, M.D.

Preface to *Comprehensive Treatment of Chronic Pain by Medical, Interventional, and Integrative Approaches*

In recent years, I have found that the need for guidance in treating those suffering from chronic pain has increased, as the burden for those patients has become a very difficult issue in daily life. Our task has been overwhelming at times, when we consider the lack of knowledge that many of us found when considering issues that are not part of our personal repertoire and training. We must be mentors of others and elevate our practice, while at the same time maintain our patient-centric target. Not only do we need to train and nurture the medical student, but also those in postgraduate training and those in private and academic practice who are long separated from their training. We are burdened with complex issues such as the cost of chronic pain, loss of functional individuals to society, abuse, addiction, and diversion of controlled substances, complicated and high-risk spinal procedures, the increase in successful but expensive technology, and the humanistic morose that are part of the heavy load that we must strive to summit.

In this maze of difficulties, we find ourselves branded as "interventionalist" and "non-interventionalist." In shaping this book, it was my goal to overcome these labels and give a diverse overview of the specialty. Separated into five sections, the contents of this book give balance to the disciplines that make up our field. There is a very complete overview of interventions, medication management, and the important areas of rehabilitation, psychological support, and the personal side of suffering. We have tried to give a thorough overview while striving to make this book practical for the physician who needs insight into the daily care of pain patients. This book was created as one of the many tools from the American Academy of Pain Medicine to shape the proper practice of those who strive to do the right things for the chronic pain patient focusing on ethics and medical necessity issues in each section. You will find that the authors, Associate Editor-in-chief, Associate Editors, and I have given rise to a project that will be all encompassing in its goals.

With this text, the American Academy of Pain Medicine has set down the gauntlet for the mission of educating our members, friends, and concerned parties regarding the intricacies of our specialty. I wish you the best as you read this material and offer you my grandest hope that it will change the lives of your patients for the better.

We must remember that chronic pain treatment, like that of diabetes and hypertension, needs ongoing effort and ongoing innovation to defeat the limits of our current abilities. These thoughts are critical when you consider the long standing words of Emily Dickinson…

"Pain has an element of blank; it cannot recollect when it began, or if there were a day when it was not. It has no future but itself, its infinite realms contain its past, enlightened to perceive new periods of pain."

Best of luck as we fight our battles together.

Charleston, WV, USA

Timothy R. Deer, M.D.

Contents

Contributors

Charles E. Argoff, M.D. Department of Neurology, Albany Medical College, Albany, NY, USA

Comprehensive Pain Cente, Albany Medical Center, Albany, NY, USA

Iwona Bonney, Ph.D. Department of Anesthesiology, Tufts Medical Center and Tufts University School of Medicine, Boston, MA, USA

Brandi A. Bottiger, M.D. Department of Anesthesiology, Duke University Hospital, Durham, NC, USA

Asokumar Buvanendran, M.D. Department of Anesthesiology, Rush Medical College, Chicago, IL, USA

Orthopedic Anesthesia, Rush University Medical Center, Chicago, IL, USA

Daniel B. Carr, M.D., DABPM, FFPMANZCA (Hon) Departments of Public Health, Anesthesiology, Medicine, and Molecular Physiology and Pharmacology, Tufts University School of Medicine, Boston, MA, USA

Robert I. Cohen, M.D., M.A. (Educ) Department of Anesthesia, Critical Care and Pain Medicine, Beth Israel Deaconess Medical Center, Boston, MA, USA

Timothy R. Deer, M.D. The Center for Pain Relief, Charleston, WV, USA

Department of Anesthesiology, West Virginia University School of Medicine, Charleston, WV, USA

Kelly Donnelly, DO Department of Neurology, Albany Medical Center, Albany, NY, USA

Jill Eckert, DO Pennsylvania State University College of Medicine, Hershey, PA, USA

Department of Anesthesiology, Pennsylvania State Milton S. Hershey Medical Center, Hershey, PA, USA

Scott M. Fishman, M.D. Division of Pain Medicine, Department of Anesthesiology and Pain Medicine, University of California, Davis School of Medicine, Sacramento, CA, USA

David M. Giampetro, M.D. Department of Anesthesiology, Pennsylvania State University College of Medicine, Hershey, PA, USA

Vitaly Gordin, M.D. Department of Anesthesiology, Pennsylvania State Milton S. Hershey Medical Center, Hershey, PA, USA

Andrea G. Hohmann, Ph.D. Department of Psychological and Brain Sciences, Indiana University, Bloomington, IN, USA

Gary L. Horowitz, M.D. Department of Pathology, Beth Israel Deaconess Medical Center, Boston, MA, USA

Harvard Medical School, Boston, MA, USA

Piotr K. Janicki, M.D., Ph.D., DSci, DABA Department of Anesthesiology, Pennsylvania State Milton S. Hershey Medical Center, Hershey, PA, USA

Laboratory of Perioperative Geriatrics, Pennsylvania State University College of Medicine, Hershey, PA, USA

Manpreet Kaur, M.D. Department of Neurology, Albany Medical Center, Albany, NY, USA

Kenneth L. Kirsh, Ph.D. Department of Behavioral Medicine, The Pain Treatment Center of the Bluegrass, Lexington, KY, USA

Michael S. Leong, M.D. Stanford Pain Medicine Center, Redwood City, CA, USA

Department of Anesthesiology, Stanford University School of Medicine, Stanford, CA, USA

Jianren Mao, M.D., Ph.D. Department of Anesthesia, Harvard Medical School, Boston, MA, USA

Department of Anesthesia, Critical Care and Pain Medicine, Massachusetts General Hospital, Boston, MA, USA

Beth B. Murinson, MS, M.D., Ph.D. Department of Neurology, Johns Hopkins University School of Medicine, Baltimore, MD, USA

Bruce D. Nicholson, M.D. Division of Pain Medicine, Department of Anesthesiology, Lehigh Valley Health Network, Allentown, PA, USA

Denny Curtis Orme, DO, MPH Billings Anesthesiology PC, Billings, MT, USA

Steven D. Passik, Ph.D. Professor of Psychiatry and Anesthesiology, Vanderbilt University Medical Center, Psychosomatic Medicine, 1103 Oxford House, Nashville, TN, USA

Selina Read, M.D. Department of Anesthesiology, Penn State College of Medicine, Penn State Milton S. Hershey Medical Center, Hershey, PA, USA

Ethan B. Russo, M.D. GW Pharmaceuticals, Vashon, WA, USA

Pharmaceutical Sciences, University of Montana, Missoula, MT, USA

Saloni Sharma, M.D. Pittsburgh, PA, USA

Naileshni Singh, M.D. Department of Anesthesiology, UC-Davis Medical Center, Sacramento, CA, USA

Howard S. Smith, M.D., FACP, FAAPM, FACNP Department of Anesthesiology, Albany Medical College, Albany Medical Center, Albany, NY, USA

Christopher A. Steel, M.D. Department of Anesthesiology, Pennsylvania State University Milton S. Hershey Medical Center, Hershey, PA, USA

Kyle Tokarz, DO Department of Anesthesiology, Naval Medical Centerm, San Diego, San Diego, CA, USA

Andrea Trescot, M.D. Algone Pain Center, St. Augustine, FL, USA

Yakov Vorobeychik, M.D., Ph.D. Department of Anesthesiology, Pennsylvania State University, Milton S. Hershey Medical Center, Hershey, PA, USA

Carol A. Warfield, M.D. Department of Anesthesia, Harvard Medical School, Boston, MA, USA

Prides Crossing, MA, USA

Ashley J. Wiese, DVM, MS, DACVA Department of Anesthesiology, University of California, San Diego School of Medicine, La Jolla, CA, USA

Channing D. Willoughby, M.D. Department of Anesthesiology, Pennsylvania State University Milton S. Hershey Medical Center, Hershey, PA, USA

Tony L. Yaksh, Ph.D. Department of Anesthesiology, University of California, San Diego School of Medicine, La Jolla, CA, USA

A Survey of Systems Involved in Nociceptive Processing

Tony L. Yaksh and Ashley J. Wiese

Key Points

- A pain state can be generated by high-intensity stimuli, injury and inflammation, and injury to the peripheral nerve.
- Acute stimuli activate small primary afferents through terminal transducer protein that lead to a frequency dependent activation of the second-order dorsal horn neurons which project contralaterally in the ventrolateral tract to (i) the somatosensory thalamus that project to the somatosensory cortex and (ii) into the medial thalamus to project into limbic forebrain.
- With tissue injury, there is the local release of active products that sensitize the peripheral terminal and initiate an ongoing discharge which by its persistency leads to a spinal sensitization that yields an enhanced response to any given stimulus.
- Nerve injury leads to initiation of an ongoing (ectopic) activity which arises from trophic changes generated by the nerve injury at the terminal (neuroma) and in the dorsal root ganglion of the injured axon.
- In addition to the afferent traffic, nerve injury leads to changes in dorsal horn sensory processing such that large afferent input can initiate a strong activation in spinal nociceptive neurons as a result of a loss of local dorsal horn inhibitory control.

T.L. Yaksh, Ph.D. (✉)
Department of Anesthesiology, Anesthesia Research Lab 0818,
UC San Diego, 9500 Gilman Dr (CTF-312), La Jolla,
CA 92093, USA

University of California, San Diego School of Medicine,
La Jolla, CA, USA
e-mail: tyaksh@ucsd.edu

A.J. Wiese, DVM, MS, DACVA
Anesthesia Research Lab 0818, UC San Diego,
9500 Gilman Dr (CTF-312), La Jolla, CA 92093, USA

Department of Anesthesiology, University of California,
San Diego Medical Center, La Jolla, CA, USA
e-mail: ajwiese@ucsd.edu

Background

High-intensity afferent input, tissue injury and inflammation, and injury to the peripheral nerve will initiate pain states with characteristic psychophysical properties. As will be considered below, this information processing can be modified to change the content of the message generated by a given stimulus to enhance the pain state (e.g., produce hyperalgesia), normalize a hyperalgesic state, or produce a decrease in pain sensitivity (e.g., produce analgesia). Management of that pain state is addressed by the use of agents or interventions which though specific targets at the level of the sensory afferent, the spinal dorsal horn or at higher-order levels (supraspinal) modify the contents of the sensory message generated by that physical stimulus. The important advances in the development of pain therapeutics have reflected upon the role played by specific underlying mechanisms which regulate these events. The aim of this overview chapter is to provide a context for the more detailed discussion of analgesics and their actions, which occur in accompanying chapters.

Overview of the Psychophysics of Nociception

Acute Stimulation

Transient thermal or mechanical stimulus of an intensity as to *potentially* yield injury evokes an escape response and an autonomic reaction (increased blood pressure and heart rate). The functional phenotype typically has four characteristics. (i) The response magnitude or pain report covaries with stimulus intensity. (ii) Removal of the stimulus immediately terminates the sensation and/or attendant behaviors. (iii) The sensation/ behavior is referred specifically to the site of stimulation, for example, it is somatotopically delimited,

T.R. Deer et al. (eds.), *Treatment of Chronic Pain by Medical Approaches: the AMERICAN ACADEMY of PAIN MEDICINE Textbook on Patient Management*, DOI 10.1007/978-1-4939-1818-8_1,
© American Academy of Pain Medicine 2015

Pain psychophysics

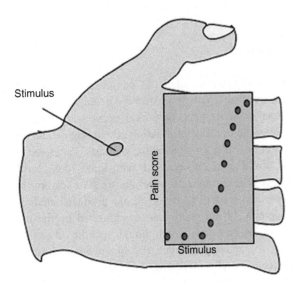
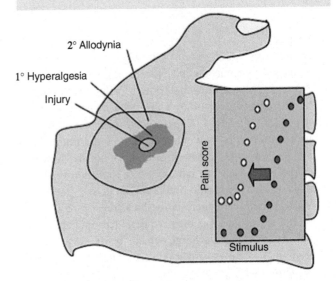

Acute high intensity stimulus

- Coincident with stimulus

- Localized pain referral

- Limited to area of stimulation

- Proportional to stimulus intensity

Tissue injuring stimulus

- Persists after removal of stimulus

- Referred to area of injury (1°) and to area adjacent to injury (2°)

- Initiated by moderately aversive (hyperalgesia) or otherwise innocuous Istimuli (allodynia)

Fig. 1.1 Schematic displays the defining psychophysical properties that characterize the pain report after an acute high-intensity stimulus (*left*) and that after a local tissue injury (*right*). As indicated, in the inset plotting pain score vs. stimulus intensity, with the acute stimulus, the pain report for a given displays a threshold above which there is a monotonic increase in the magnitude of the reported pain state. After a tissue injury, there is an ongoing pain, and a stimulus applied to the injury site reveals that there is a greater pain report for a given stimulus (e.g., a primary hyperalgesia). In addition, it is appreciated that an innocuous mechanical stimuli applied to an adjacent uninjured area yields an enhanced response referred to secondary tactile allodynia

typically to the dermatome to which the stimulus is applied and the response, for example, the stimulated paw is the paw that is withdrawn. (iv) Often with an acute stimulus (such as a thermal probe), there are two perceived components to the aversive sensation: an immediate sharp stinging sensation followed shortly by a dull throbbing sensation (Fig. 1.1).

Tissue Injury

The psychophysics of pain associated with a tissue injury and inflammation has several distinct psychophysical elements that distinguish it from the events initiated by an acute high-intensity stimulus (Fig. 1.1):

(i) With local tissue injury (such as burn, abrasion, or incision or the generation of a focal inflammatory state as in the joint), an acute sensation is generated by the injuring stimulus which is followed by an ongoing dull throbbing aching sensation which typically referred to the injury site—skin, soft tissue, or joint—and which evolves as the local inflammatory state progresses.

(ii) Application of a thermal or mechanical stimulus to the injury sited will initiate a pain state wherein the pain sensation is reported to be more intense than would be expected when that stimulus was applied to a non-injured site. That is to say, as shown in Fig. 1.1, the stimulus response curve is shifted up (e.g., an ongoing pain) and to the left. This lowered threshold of stimulus intensity required to elicit an aversive response to a stimuli applied to the injury site is referred to as primary hyperalgesia. Thus, modest flexion of an inflamed joint or moderate distention of the gastrointestinal (GI) track will lead to behavioral reports of pain.

(iii) Local injury and a low-intensity stimuli applied to regions adjacent to the injury may also produce a pain condition, and this is referred to as 2° hyperalgesia or allodynia. Thus, light touch may be reported as being aversive and is referred to as tactile allodynia.

These examples of "sensitization" secondary to local injury and inflammation are observed in all organ systems. Common examples would be sunburn (skin inflammation) leads to extreme sensitivity to warm water, inflammation of the pleura leads to pain secondary to respiration, and eyelid closure is painful secondary to corneal abrasion [1, 2].

In the case of inflammation of the viscera, the ongoing pain sensations are typically referred to specific somatic dermatomes. Thus, cardiac ischemia is referred to the left arm and shoulder, while inflammation of the bowel is associated with ongoing pain and hypersensitivity to light touch applied to the various quadrants of the abdomen. Such "referred" pain states reflect the convergence of somatic and visceral pain systems [3].

Nerve Injury

As described by Silas Weir Mitchell in 1864, frank trauma leads to two identifying elements: ongoing dysesthetic pain typically referred to the dermatome innervated by the injured nerve and prominent increase in the sensitivity to light touch applied to these regions. Injury to the nerve may be initiated by a wide variety of physical (extruded intervertebral disc compression section), toxic (chemotherapy), viral (postherpetic neuralgia: HIV), and metabolic (diabetes). In most of these syndromes, these two elements are expressed to varying degrees [4].

Encoding of Acute Nociception

As outlined in Fig. 1.2, the systems underlying these effects of acute high-intensity stimulation may be considered in terms of the afferents, the dorsal horn, and projection components. Under normal conditions, activity in sensory afferents is largely absent. However, peripheral mechanical and thermal stimuli will evoke intensity-dependent increases in firing rates of lightly myelinated (A∂) or unmyelinated (C) afferents. Based on differential blockade, these two fiber types, differing markedly in conduction velocity, are thought to underlie the acute sharp pain and subsequent dull throbbing sensation, respectively.

Transduction Channels and Afferent Terminal Activation

The transduction of the physical stimulus is mediated by specific channels which increase their conductance when certain stimulus properties are present. Channels vary in the range of temperatures which activate them, ranging from hot (such as the TRPV1) to cool to cold (TRPM1). The acute response

properties of the afferent are thus defined by the collection of transducer channels that are expressed on its terminals. Activation of these channels increases inward sodium and calcium currents and progressive depolarization of the terminal (Fig. 1.2a) [5, 6].

Chemical Sensitivity of Temperature Channels

An important element regarding these channels is that while they are to varying degrees temperature sensitive, they also show sensitivity to specific chemicals. Thus, the TRPV1 responds to capsaicin, while the TRPM1 responds to menthol. Accordingly, when these agents are applied to the tongue, the sensation associated with their application corresponds with the sensation produced by the fibers which normally activate these fibers, hot and cool, respectively [7].

Action Potential Generation

Peripheral terminal depolarization leads to activation of the voltage-gated sodium channels which then leads to action potentials in the respective afferent. Subtypes of sodium channels (designated as NaV 1.1 through NaV 1.9 channels) have been identified.

These channels differ in terms of their activation properties as well as their pharmacology (e.g., tetrodotoxin sensitive or insensitive) and their distribution. Thus, some channels may be found principally on unmyelinated afferents (Nav 1.7) or distributed widely on all types of excitable membranes ranging from myocytes to brain neurons to a variety of afferents. Importantly, the frequency of afferent discharge is proportional to terminal depolarization which is proportional to stimulus intensity (Fig. 1.2b) [8, 9].

Encoding Properties of Primary Afferents

There are three important properties that define the encoding properties of any given class of primary afferents (Fig. 1.2b) [10]:

(i) Under resting conditions, the primary afferent, whether A or C, shows little or no spontaneous activity.

(ii) Primary afferents typically begin to respond to their respective stimulus modality (e.g., Aβ-tactile or C-thermal/mechanical/chemical) at some minimal intensity (e.g., threshold).

(iii) Above threshold, the frequency of firing evoked in the afferent axon will be proportional to stimulus intensity over a range of intensities. "Low-threshold" afferents will typically discharge at intensities that are considered to be nonnoxious. "High-threshold" or nociceptive afferents will discharge at intensities that are considered to be aversive in character.

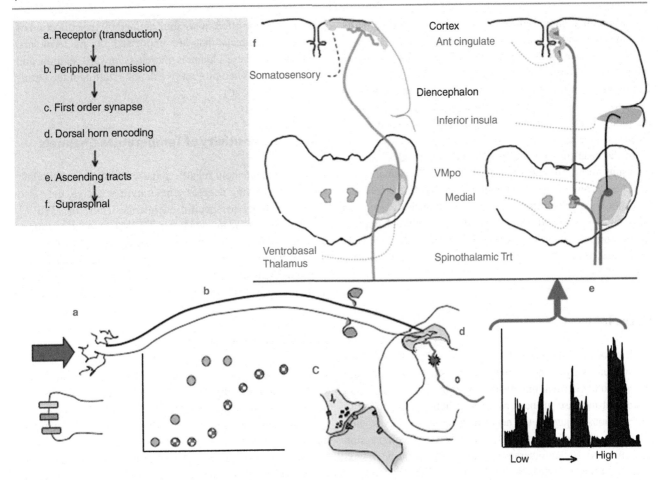

Fig. 1.2 This schematic provides an overview of the organization of events that initiate pain state after an acute high-intensity stimulus applied to the skin. (**a**) A physical stimulus activates channels such as the TRP channels on the terminal of small diameter afferents (*light line*). (**b**) There are two classes of afferents: large low-threshold afferents (**Ab**: *dark line*) and small high-threshold afferents (A∂/C: *light line*). As the stimulus intensity increases, there is a monotonic increase in the discharge rate of each class of afferents with the low-threshold afferents showing an increase at low intensities, whereas the high-intensity afferents show an increase at higher intensities. The low and high threshold afferents project respectively into the deep and superficial dorsal horn. (**c**) The afferent input leads to depolarization of these spinal afferent terminals (**d**) which release excitatory transmitters yielding an (**e**) intensity-dependent depolarization of the second-order neuron. (Shown here is an example of the response of a neuron receiving convergent input from high and low threshold afferents.) Populations of these neurons project into the contralateral ventrolateral pathways to project to higher centers. (**f**) Broadly speaking, there are two classes of outflow. There are those which project into the somatosensory (ventrobasal) thalamus which then sends projection to the somatosensory cortex. A second type of projections goes to more medial thalamic regions and sends projection into areas of the old limbic forebrain (e.g., anterior cingulate/inferior insula)

Afferent Synaptic Transmission

Afferent action potentials invade the spinal terminal and depolarize these terminals. Such activation opens voltage-sensitive calcium channels which activate a variety of synaptic proteins which mediate the mobilization of synaptic vesicles and thereby initiate transmitter release.

Calcium Channels and Afferent Transmitter Release

There are a variety of voltage-sensitive calcium channels that regulate terminal transmitter release (referred to as CaV channels). These channels are distinguished on the basis of their voltage sensitivity, their location, and the agents which block them. The best known of these channels are the N-type calcium channel blocked by the therapeutic agent ziconotide. Block of this channel will block the release of many afferent terminal transmitters [11].

Spinal Afferent Terminal Transmitters

Sensory afferent uniformly releases excitatory transmitters. In terms of transmitters (Table 1.1), virtually all afferents contain and release the excitatory amino acid glutamate. Small afferent releases not only glutamate but also one or

Table 1.1 Overview of classes of primary afferents characterized by common transmitter and cell markers

Fiber	Spinal termination	Cell marker		Channel/receptor		Transmitter	
		NF200	IB4	TRPV1 channel	Mu opioid receptor	Glutamate	Peptide (sP)
Aβ	III–VI	X				X	
A∂	II, III–V1	X				X	
C	I–II		X	X	X	X	X
C	II					X	

IB4 Isolectin B4, *NF200* Neurofilament 200

more of several peptides, such as substance P or calcitonin gene-related peptide (CGRP) (Fig. 1.2c). These transmitters in turn act postsynaptically upon eponymous receptors present on several of populations of dorsal horn neurons (Fig. 1.2d) [12]:

(i) Glutamate exerts the primary depolarizing effect through the activation of the AMPA receptor which leads to a short lasting increase in sodium conductance yielding a potent and short lasting depolarization of the membrane.

(ii) Substance P acts upon a G protein-coupled receptor that leads to a long slow depolarization of the membrane. Importantly, such receptors lead not only to a depolarization of the membrane, but to an increase in intracellular calcium, the glutamate by activating voltage-sensitive calcium channel and the NK1 by mobilizing intracellular calcium stores.

Laminar Organization of Spinal Dorsal Horn

The spinal dorsal horn is organized transversely in laminae (Rexed laminae), ranging from the most superficial dorsal horn marginal layer (lamina I), the substantia gelatinosa (lamina II), and the deeper nucleus proprius (laminae III–VI) [13].

Primary Afferent Projections

There are several important principles reflecting the pattern of termination of afferent terminals in the dorsal horn (Fig. 1.3) [14]:

(i) Small afferents (A∂/C) terminate superficially in the lamina I (marginal layer) and lamina II. In contrast, the large afferents (Aβ) project deep into the dorsal horn and curve upwards to terminate just deep to lamina III.

(ii) Observing the spinal cord from the dorsal surface, it is noted that the central processes of the afferents collateralize, sending processes rostrally and caudally up to several segments into the dorsal columns (large afferents)

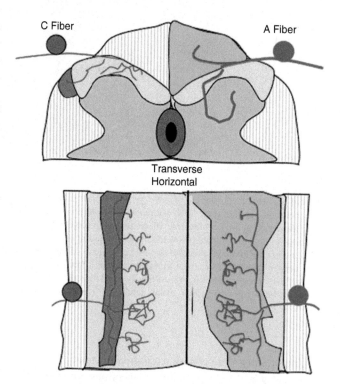

Fig. 1.3 Schematic presenting the spinal cord in transverse section (*top*) and horizontal (*bottom*) and showing: (i) (*left*) the ramification of C fibers in the superficial dorsal horn (laminae I and II) and collateralization into the tract of Lissauer and (ii) (*right*) the ramification of A fibers in the dorsal horn (terminating in the deep dorsal horn) and collateralization rostrocaudally into the dorsal columns and at each segment into the dorsal horn. The densest terminations are within the segment of entry. There are less dense collateralizations into the dorsal horns at the more distal spinal segments. This density of collateralization corresponds to the potency of the excitatory drive into these distal segments. Thus, distal segments may receive input from a given segment, but the input is not sufficiently robust to initiate activation of the neurons in the distal segment under normal circumstances

or in the tract of Lissauer (small C-fiber afferents). Periodically, these collaterals send sprays into the dorsal horn at distal segments. Thus, neurons up to several segments distal to a given root entry zone of any given segment will receive afferent input from a given root (e.g., the L5 root will make synaptic contact with dorsal horn cells as far rostral as spinal segment L1).

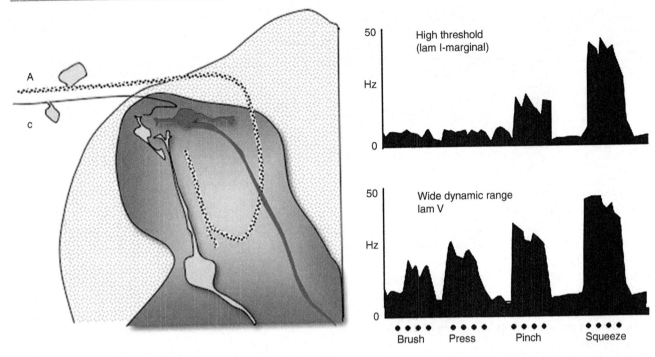

Fig. 1.4 Schematic displays (*left*) two principal classes of second-order neurons. As indicated, small afferents tend to terminate superficially (laminae I and II), while large afferents tend to project deep into the dorsal horn and terminate below lamina II. Accordingly, cells lying in lamina I (marginal layer) receive largely high-threshold input. Cells lying deeper (lamina V) received input from large afferents on their proximal dendrites and can receive excitatory input directly or through excitatory interneurons on their distal dendrites. (*right*) Single-unit recording from spinal dorsal horn, showing firing pattern (impulses/s) of a (*top*) high-threshold (nociceptive-specific marginal) neuron and (*bottom*) a horn wide-dynamic-range neuron, (WDR) located primarily in lamina V in response to graded intensities of mechanical stimulation (brush, pressure, pinch, squeeze) applied to the receptive fields of each cell. Both cells project supraspinally. Note the relationship between firing patterns and the response properties of the afferents with which each cell makes contact

Importantly, the primary excitation occurs at the level of entry where the synaptic connections are strongest. At more distal segments, the degree of excitation from the proximal root is progressively reduced.

Dorsal Horn Neurons

Based on the organization of afferent termination, one can appreciate that superficial lamina I marginal neurons are primarily activated by small, high-threshold afferent input; hence they are "nociceptive specific." In contrast, the deeper lying cells have their cell bodies in lamina V and are hence called lamina V neurons but send their dendrites up into the superficial laminae. Interestingly, they receive input from Aβ (low-threshold) input on their ascending dendrites and C-fiber (high-threshold) input on their distal terminals (Fig. 1.4). Accordingly, these cells with their convergent input show activation at low intensities (mediated by the Aβ input) and increasing activation as the intensity rise (mediated by the C-fiber input). Accordingly, as shown in Fig. 1.2e, the cell shows increasing discharge rates over the range from very

low to very high-threshold stimuli. Accordingly, these cells are referred to as wide-dynamic-range (WDR) neurons [15].

Dorsal Horn Projections

These lamina I and lamina V neurons then project via the ventrolateral tracts to higher centers and thence to cortical levels. Projections may occur ipsilaterally or contralaterally in the ventrolateral tracts. Ipsilaterally projecting axons typically project to terminate in the medial brainstem reticular nuclei. Cells receiving these projections then project to the thalamus. Contralateral axons project into several thalamic nuclei [13, 16].

Supraspinal Organization

The supraspinal projections can be broadly classified in two motifs (Fig. 1.2e) [13]:

(i) Dorsalhorn, ventrobasalthalamiccomplex-somatosensory cortex. This is the classic somatosensory pathway. In these cases, the nervous system undertakes to maintain a specific intensity-, spatial-, and modality-linked encoding of the somatic stimulus, as summarized in Fig. 1.2. This pathway possesses the characteristics that relate to the psychophysical report of pain sensation in humans and the vigor of the escape response in animals. In the absence of tissue injury, removal of the stimulus leads to a rapid abatement of the afferent input and disappearance of the pain sensation. At all levels, the intensity of the message is reflected by the specific populations of axons which are activated and by the frequency of depolarization: the more intense the stimulation, the more frequent is the firing of the afferent; the greater is the dorsal horn transmitter release, the greater is the evoked discharge and the higher is the frequency of firing in the ascending pathway.

(ii) Dorsal horn-medial thalamus-limbic cortex. Here, there appears to be little precise anatomical mapping. Cells in this region project to regions such as the anterior cingulate cortex or inferior insula. The anterior cingulate is part of the older limbic cortex and is believed to be associated with emotional content.

The above subdivision reflects the orthogonal component of the pain experience, notably the "sensory-discriminative" components ("I hurt here on a scale of 1–10, 6") and the "affective-motivational" component of the pain pathway ("I have cancer, I am mortal") as proposed by Ronald Melzack and Kenneth Casey.

Encoding of Nociception After Tissue Injury

As reviewed above, with tissue injury, a distinct pattern of aversive sensations is observed. The psychophysical profile noted with injury or inflammation is composed of (i) an ongoing sensory experience that is described as dull throbbing aching ongoing pain, (ii) enhanced responsiveness to subsequent stimulation (e.g., hyperalgesia/tactile allodynia), and (iii) secondary pain referral (e.g., sensations which are aversive when applied to adjacent uninjured areas).

Peripheral Changes in Afferent Transmission Resulting from Tissue

As described in Fig. 1.1, in the event that a stimulus leads to a local injury, as in a tissue crush (trauma) or an incision, such stimuli may lead to the subsequent local elaboration of active products that directly activate the local terminals of afferents (that are otherwise silent) innervating the injury region and facilitating their discharge in response to otherwise submaximal stimuli. This then leads to an ongoing afferent barrage and enhanced response to any given stimulus (e.g., peripheral sensitization) (Fig. 1.5).

Origin of Ongoing Activity and Enhanced Terminal Responsiveness After Tissue Injury

The source of these active factors may be considered in terms of their source including the following (Fig. 1.5):

(i) Damaged cells which yield increased extracellular contents (potassium).

(ii) Products of plasma extravasation (clotting factors, cellular products such as platelets and erythrocytes which release products including amines (5HT), peptides (bradykinin), and various lipidic acids (prostaglandins)).

(iii) Innate immune cascade wherein given the chemoattractants present in the injury site, there will be a migration of inflammatory cells including neutrophils and macrophages. These contribute products such as myeloperoxidases, cytokines (TNF/IL1β), nerve growth factors (NGF), and serine proteases (trypsin).

(iv) Terminal of primary afferent C fibers activated by the local milieu will lead to a local release of sP and CGRP which respectively cause vasodilation (erythema) and capillary leakiness (e.g., tissue swelling).

Importantly, these products have several effects on terminal function that are dependent upon the presence of the eponymous receptors on those terminals (e.g., trypsin activates proteinase-activated receptors: PARs; TNF) and the concentrations of the ligand (Fig. 1.6) [17].

(i) Activate the sensory terminal, increase intracellular calcium, and initiate a conducted action potential.

(ii) Activate terminal kinases which serve to phosphorylate many membrane channels (e.g., sodium channels) and receptors (TRPV receptors) to increase their excitability. These actions are generally considered to result in spontaneous "afferent discharges" and to an enhanced responsiveness of the terminal to subsequent stimuli manifested by a left shift in the stimulus response curve for the sensory afferent. Overall, these properties are consistent with an ongoing pain stimulus and the ability of a given stimulus applied to that afferent in innervating the injured tissue to show a greater response (Fig. 1.2a).

It should be noted that these events are ubiquitous. This scenario has been demonstrated in numerous body systems, for example, cornea of the eye (sensitivity to light touch after abrasion), joint (pain of modest movement after inflammation of the knee), tooth pulp (sensory experience of cardiac-induced pressure changes in the tooth after inflammation of the pulp), and migraine (activation of the meningeal afferents which, like those in the tooth pulp, are not activated by normal mechanical movement or vascular pulsation). Indeed, think of any disease pathology described by the suffix "-itis" (Fig. 1.6).

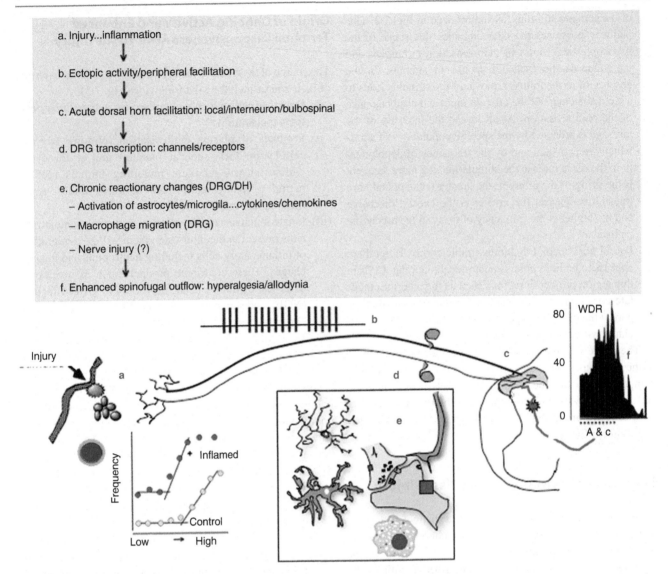

Fig. 1.5 This schematic provides an overview of the organization of events that initiate pain state after a tissue injuring stimulus of the skin. (**a**) Local tissue injury leads to the initiation of an innate immune response that yields the release of a variety of active factors. The factors acting through eponymous receptors on the terminals of C fibers lead to an activation of the C fiber and a state of sensitization. Accordingly, such products initiate an ongoing activity and an enhanced response to an otherwise innocuous stimulus. (**b**) The injury thus leads to an ongoing activity in small afferent. (**c**) The ongoing activity activates dorsal horn neurons and initiates a state of facilitation (windup). (**d**) The ongoing afferent traffic and injury products lead to a change in the tropic functions of the dorsal root ganglion leading to changes in protein synthesis and the expression of various receptors and channels which serve to enhance afferent responsiveness. (**e**) In the dorsal horn, the ongoing afferent drive initiates additional changes related to the activation of microglia and astrocytes as well as the invasion of typically non-neuronal cells including neutrophils and lymphocytes in the extreme. The net effect is to enhance the outflow initiated by any given stimulus, for example, hyperalgesia and allodynia. (**f**) With facilitation, the wide dynamic range neurons (WDR) are activated in response to stimuli that would normally not activate these neurons.[AW1]

Spinal Changes in Afferent Transmission Resulting from Tissue Injury

As reviewed above, acute activation of small afferents by extreme stimuli results in a spinal activation of dorsal horn neurons, the magnitude of which is proportional to the frequency (and identity) of the afferent input (Fig. 1.2e). Factors increasing that input-output relationship will cause a given stimulus to appear more intense (e.g., hyperalgesia). Conversely, factors reducing that function will cause a more intense stimulus to be encoded as less intense (e.g., analgesia). In the preceding section, it was appreciated that inflammation causes an enhanced response at the peripheral level. It is appreciated that there is also an enhanced response mediated in the spinal dorsal horn.

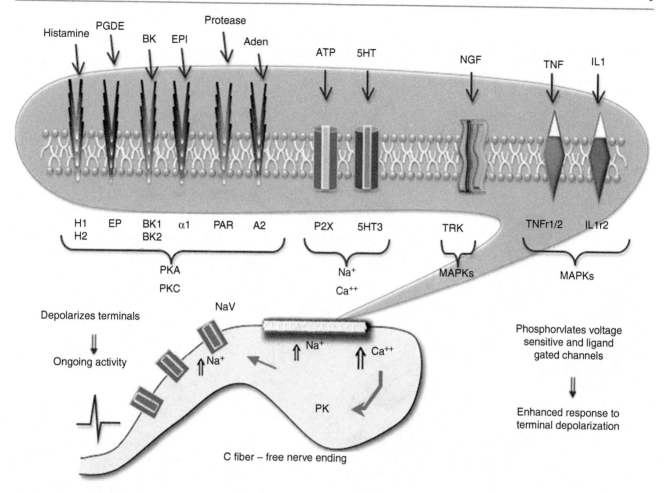

Fig. 1.6 This schematic provides an overview of the organization of events that initiate pain state after an injury to soft tissue. In the face of tissue injury, a variety of active products are released from local tissues, inflammatory cells, and the blood. These products exert a direct effect upon the small afferent terminal, free nerve endings, through specific receptors on the terminal. These receptors are coupled through a variety of second messengers which can lead to a local depolarization because of increased sodium and calcium influx. This leads to the activation of voltage-sensitive sodium channels (*NaV*) that initiate the regenerative action potential. In addition, the kinases and the increased intracellular calcium can initiate phosphorylation (*PK*) of channels and receptors, leading to an enhanced responsiveness of these channels and receptors. The net effect is to initiate an ongoing activity after the injuring stimulus has been removed and an increase in the discharge arising from any given stimulus

Central (Spinal) Facilitation

Animal research has demonstrated that repetitive afferent activation causes dorsal horn wide-dynamic-range (WDR) neurons to show evident signs of facilitation, labeled "windup" by Lorne Mendell and Patrick Wall (Fig. 1.4). This facilitation is characterized by following properties [18]:

(i) High-frequency repetitive stimulation of C (but not A) fibers results in a progressively facilitated discharge of the WDR neurons.

(ii) The receptive field of the WDR neuron showing windup was significantly expanded acutely following the conditioning afferent stimulation, for example, stimulation of an adjacent dermatome which hitherto did not activate that cell, would now lead to activity in that neuron (Fig. 1.7).

Enhanced Response of WDR Neuron

The enhanced responsiveness of the cell was shown by intracellular recording to reflect a progressive and sustained (after termination of the stimulation) excitability of the neuron of the cell, rendering the membrane increasingly susceptible to even weak afferent inputs.

The enlarged receptive field can be explained by the ability of subliminal input coming from afferent input arising from an adjacent non-injured receptive field which was otherwise insufficient to activate a normally excitable cell.

Pharmacology of Central Facilitation

The enhanced excitability of dorsal horn neurons secondary to repetitive small afferent input reflects a series of

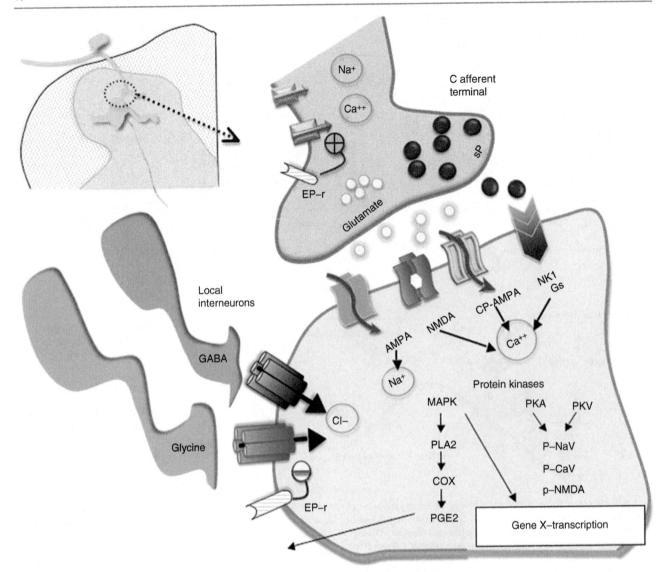

Fig. 1.7 This schematic provides an overview of the organization of the events transpiring at the level of the first-order synapse. (i) As indicated, the presynaptic effects of depolarization lead to opening of voltage-sensitive calcium and sodium channels with increases in intracellular sodium and calcium and mobilization and release of transmitters (*sP* and glutamate). (ii) These act upon eponymous receptors (see text), leading to depolarization and increase in intracellular calcium. (iii) Activation of kinases which phosphorylate a variety of channels and receptors activates intracellular enzyme cascades such as for PLA2 and increasing gene transcription. (iv) Release of products such as prostanoids (*PGE2*) which can act upon the local membrane through their eponymous receptors (*EP-r*) where presynaptically they enhance the opening of voltage-sensitive calcium channels and postsynaptically reduce the activity of glycine receptors. (v). As indicated in addition, the first-order synapse is regulated by inhibitor interneurons such as those release GABA and glycine. These interneurons can be activated by afferent collaterals and by descending pathways to downregulate the excitability of this synapse

complex mechanistic motifs that have a diverse pharmacology which will be briefly reviewed below. These can be broadly considered in terms of those systems which are (i) postsynaptic to the primary afferent and (ii) mediated by local neuronal networks, extraspinal networks, and nonneuronal networks. Examples will be reviewed below (Fig. 1.8).

Primary Afferents

Small afferents release peptides (e.g., sP/CGRP) and excitatory amino acids (glutamate) which evoke excitation in second-order neurons through their eponymous receptors (Table 1.2; Fig. 1.7) [19–22].

(i) AMPA. Activation of the AMPA receptor leads to a short lasting but prominent increase in sodium conductance, yielding a robust, transient depolarization. Direct monosynaptic afferent-evoked excitation is largely mediated by the AMPA receptors, for example, AMPA receptor antagonists will block most acute excitatory input and produce an acute analgesia. A subtype of AMPA receptor is Ca permeable. For example, activation of these receptors leads to large increases in intracellular calcium.

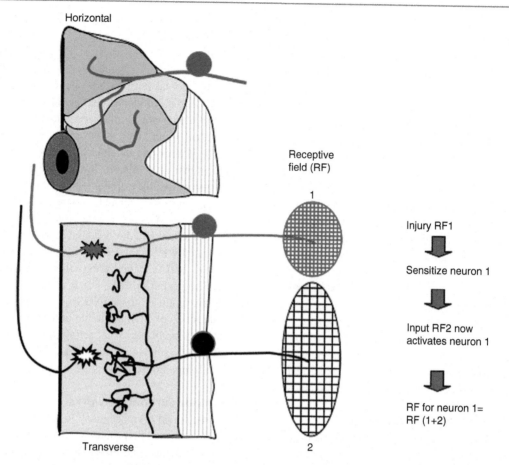

Fig. 1.8 Schematic presents the spinal cord in horizontal section (see Fig. 1.3). Receptive field of dorsal horn neuron depends upon the origin of its segmental input and the input from other segments, which can activate it. Thus, neuron 1 receives strong input from RF1 and very weak (ineffective) input from RF2. After injury in receptive field (*RF*) 1, neuron 1 becomes "sensitized." Collateral input from RF2 normally is unable to initiate sufficient excitatory activity to activate neuron 1, but after sensitization, RF2 input is sufficient. Now, the RF of neuron 1 is effectively RF1 + RF2. Thus, local injury can by a spinal mechanism leads acutely to increased receptive fields such that stimuli applied to a non-injured RF can contribute to the post-tissue injury sensation

Table 1.2 Summary of classes of spinal receptors postsynaptic to primary afferents

Transmitter	Receptor	Receptor type	Ion permeability
Glutamate	AMPA	Ionophore	Na
	AMPA-Ca permeable	Ionophore	Na, Ca
	NMDA	Ionophore	Na, Ca
sP	NK1	G protein cAMP dependent	None (Ca)
CGRP	CGRP1	G protein cAMP dependent	None (Ca)
BDNF	TRK B	Tyrosine kinase	–

sP substance P, *NMDA* N-methyl-D-aspartate, *BDNF* brain-derived neurotrophic factor, *NK1* neurokinin 1, *TRK B* tyrosine-related kinase B, *AMPA* α-amino-3-hydroxy-5-methyl-4-isoxazolepropionic acid

(ii) NMDA. NMDA is a glutamate-activated ionophore that passes sodium and calcium. At normal resting membrane potential, the NMDA receptor is blocked by a magnesium ion. In this condition, occupancy by glutamate will not activate the ionophore. If there is a modest depolarization of the membrane (as produced during repetitive stimulation secondary to the activation of AMPA (glutamate) and neurokinin 1 (NK1) (substance P)

receptors), the Mg block is removed, permitting glutamate to now activate the NMDA receptor. When this happens, the NMDA channel permits the passage of Ca. Accordingly, block of the NMDA receptor has no effect upon acute activation but will prevent windup.

(iii) NK1 and CGRP. For sP and CGRP, excitation is through G protein-coupled receptors, neurokinin 1 (NK1) and CGRP, the effects of which are cAMP dependent and couple through the activation of phospholipase C. Activation of these receptors leads to slow, relatively long-lasting membrane depolarization accompanied by an increase in intracellular calcium. Agents which block the NK1 or CGRP receptor will produce minor effects upon the behavior evoked by acute excitation but will reduce the onset of the facilitated state and behaviorally defined hyperalgesia.

(iv) Growth factors. In addition to classic transmitters, growth factors such as brain-derived nerve growth factor (BDNF) is synthesized by small DRGs and released from spinal terminals, packaged in dense-cored vesicles, and transported within axons into terminals in the dorsal horn of the spinal cord. BDNF has potent sensitizing effect on spinal neurons mediated through TRK receptors.

As noted, with ongoing afferent drive, a progressive increase in excitation is noted. Aside from activation of the NMDA receptors, other components to this facilitatory process can be noted. These can be broadly considered in terms of those systems which are local to the neuronal networks in the dorsal horn, extraspinal networks, and nonneuronal networks. Several examples of each will be reviewed below.

Postsynaptic to the Primary Afferents

Repetitive activation of the primary afferent yields membrane depolarization and a significant increase in intracellular calcium. The increased intracellular calcium activates a series of intracellular cascades. Several examples are given below (Fig. 1.6):

(i) Activation of kinases. Persistent afferent input leads to a marked increase in intracellular Ca^{++} which leads to activation of a wide variety of phosphorylating enzymes, including protein kinase A and C, calcium calmodulin-dependent protein kinases, as well as mitogen-activated kinases (MAPKs) including p38 MAP kinase and ERK. Each of these kinases leads to a variety of downstream events which serve to increase the excitability of the neuron [23, 24].

(ii) Channel phosphorylation. The excitability of many channels is controlled by phosphorylation. Several examples may be cited. (1) PKA- and PKC-mediated phosphorylation of the NMDA ionophore leads to a facilitated removal of the Mg^{++} block and an increase in calcium current. (2) P38 leads MAPK activation to activation of phospholipase A2 (PLA2) which initiates the release of arachidonic acid and provides the substrate for cyclooxygenase (COX) to synthesize prostaglandins. In addition, this MAPK activates transcription factors such as NFKβ, which in turn activates synthesis of a variety of proteins, such as the inducible cyclooxygenase, COX2. Spinal P38 MAPK inhibitors thus reduce acutely initiated hyperalgesia and reduce the upregulation of COX2 otherwise produced by injury [23, 24].

(iii) Lipid cascades. A variety of phospholipases, cyclooxygenases, and lipoxygenases are constitutively expressed in the dorsal horn in both neuronal and nonneuronal cells. Lipid products including prostaglandins and other eicosanoids are synthesized and released after small afferent input. They serve to enhance the opening of voltage-sensitive calcium channels, augmenting afferent transmitter release. In addition, prostaglandins act postsynaptically to *reduce* glycine-mediated inhibition on second-order dorsal horn neurons. Such reduction in glycine or GABA interneuron activity leads to an increase in dorsal horn excitability (to be discussed further below). Spinal delivery of PGE will increase, while PLA2 or COX inhibitors will reduce, injury-induced hyperalgesia [25, 26].

(iv) Nitric oxide synthase (NOS). The neuronal and inducible forms of NOS are found in the spinal cord, and NO plays a facilitatory role, acting presynaptically through cGMP to enhance transmitter release. Spinal NOS inhibitors reduce post-tissue injury hyperalgesia [27].

Local Interneuronal Networks

The spinal dorsal horn has many local interneuronal circuits which are activated by primary afferent input:

(i) These interneurons may contain and release glutamate to act upon AMPA and NMDA receptors and are intrinsically excitatory. This polyneuronal chain can enhance the excitatory drive from a given afferent.

(ii) In addition, there are a wide variety of local interneurons which contain and release inhibitory amino acids such as GABA and glycine which act respectively on GABA A receptors and glycine receptors which are chloride ionophores that serve typically to downregulate the excitability of the membrane. These interneurons may project onto primary afferent terminals (presynaptic) and onto higher-order neurons (postsynaptic inhibition). The net excitatory outflow from the dorsal horn depends upon this local inhibitory regulation. Anything that increases that activity will diminish outflow, while events that inhibit the functionality of these inhibitory circuits will increase excitatory outflow.

As noted above, second-order deep dorsal horn neurons can receive excitatory input from large (Aβ) afferents. In spite of this afferent input onto dorsal horn neurons which are believed to play a role in nociceptive processing, this Aβ input will not typically evoke a pain state. However, after tissue injury such low-threshold mechanical stimuli may initiate a pain state (tactile allodynia). An element of this transition is believed to reflect a loss of local GABA or glycine inhibition. Thus, block of spinal GABA A and glycine receptors yields a markedly enhanced response of these

WDR neurons to Aβ input and a behaviorally defined tactile allodynia. As noted above, repetitive small afferent input leads to a dorsal horn release of PGE2 which in turn reduces glycine-mediated opening of the glycine receptor and leads to a reduction in this local inhibition. The net effect is a corresponding increase in excitation evoked by low-threshold afferents.

Bulbospinal Systems

Serotonergic pathways (arising from the midline raphe nuclei of the medulla) project into the spinal dorsal horn. The effects of this bulbospinal projection are mediated by the presence of a variety of dorsal horn 5HT receptors. Some are inhibitory (5HT1a,b), and some are directly excitatory (5HT 2,3,7). The net effect is complexly defined by the nature of the neurons upon which the receptor is located. Inhibitory receptors on an excitatory neuron will lead to an inhibition of excitation. Conversely, inhibition of an inhibition will lead to an excitation.

The most prominent effect however appears to be a net increase in excitability mediated by 5HT3 bearing dorsal horn neurons. A particularly interesting circuit involves the observation that lamina I (marginal) neurons project into the medullary brainstem to activate these bulbospinal serotonin neurons to activate deep dorsal horn neurons through the 5HT3 receptor. This spino-bulbo-spinal feedback pathway is believed to play an important role in afferent-driven spinal facilitation (Fig. 1.9) [28].

Nonneuronal Cells

Within the spinal parenchyma, there are a variety of nonneuronal cells. These include (i) astrocytes which arise from a multipotent neural stem cells, (ii) monocyte-derived cells (e.g., macrophages) which enter the nervous systems around parturition to become resident microglia, and (iii) circulating cells which enter the nervous systems during the course of peripheral injury and inflammation (neutrophils, lymphocytes, and macrophages). Classically, astrocytes were believed to play a role in trophic systems function. The microglia were considered to be activated by CNS injury, and the circulating cells were part of the response to catastrophic injury and infection.

Current thinking now emphasizes the enormous constitutive contributions of these cells to the excitability of local neuronal circuits. While there are no direct synaptic linkages, neuraxial astrocytes and microglia can be activated by several linkages [29–32]:

(i) High-intensity afferent input leading to synaptic overflow of products such as glutamate, substance P, and BDNF.
(ii) Networks of astrocytes which may communicate over a distance by the spread of excitation through local nonsynaptic contacts ("gap" junctions) and by ATP acting on purine receptors on the glia.

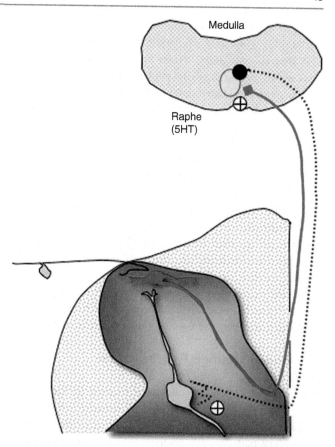

Fig. 1.9 Schematic shows bulbospinal 5HT arising from caudal raphe projects to the dorsal horn to synapse on 5HT3 cells and enhance excitability. This pathway may be activated by projections from lamina I neurons projecting to the raphe resulting in a spino-bulbo-spinal positive feedback loop

(iii) Release of products from neurons. Microglia can be activated by release of chemokines (fractalkine) from the neuronal membrane. In addition to afferent input after tissue injury and inflammation, *circulating* cytokines (such as IL1β/TNF) can activate perivascular astrocytes/microglia.
(iv) Circulating products such as cytokines and lipids can activate these perivascular nonneuronal cells.
(v) Activation of spinal innate immune systems. It is appreciated that glial cells express a variety of toll-like receptors (TLRs). These TLRs are primitive recognition sites (first discovered in fruit flies) that can lead to glial activation. While these recognition sites have classically been considered relevant to recognizing membrane or molecular components of nonself entities such as viruses and bacteria, it is now appreciated that in the course of inflammation there are products that are released that can also activate these TLRs and their intracellular cascades. Activation of these receptors can initiate hyperalgesic states, while their blockade or knockout can minimize post-inflammatory hyperalgesia [33].

When activated, these glial cells can regulate synaptic excitability by (i) releasing excitatory products including ATP, free radicals, nitric oxide, lipid mediators, and cytokines and (ii) regulating extracellular parenchymal glutamate (by transporter-mediated uptake and release).

Preclinical work with spinal inhibitors of microglial activation such as minocycline (a second-generation tetracycline) and pentoxyfiline that have been reported to block indices of an acute or chronic glial activation and diminish hyperalgesic states has supported the role of nonneuronal cells in inflammation and injury-induced pain. These agents, while not clinically useful, suggest important directions in drug therapy development [34].

These events outlined above involving the nonneuronal cells are referred to broadly as "neuroinflammation." The work emphasizes that astrocytes and microglia are *constitutively* active and contributing to acute changes in spinal network excitability and can contribute to the enhanced response of the dorsal horn after peripheral tissue injury and inflammation.

Evolution of a Chronic Pain State After Acute Injury

In the preceding sections, we have focused on the events which occur after tissue injury and inflammation. After such tissue injury and inflammation, for example, as after trauma and surgery, pain typically resolves with a time course that is typically consistent with the resolution of the inflammation, a consequence which parallels the healing process. In a variable but significant fraction of patients, a failure to resolve the pain state in spite of healing may be noted. The persistency may be the result of an occult inflammation (e.g., failure to heal) or perhaps injury to the nerve which leads to events that are evidently unable to heal (see below). Alternatively, there is increasing evidence that in the face of persistent inflammation (as say in arthritis) that there may be fundamental changes in the functionality of the afferent/DRG to yield a state of persistent sensitization. For example, in the face of a persistent (weeks) inflammation in animal models, an allodynic state is noted that continues after the resolution of the inflammation. Importantly, the knockout of the TLR4 receptors has no effects upon the inflammation but prevents the evolution of the persistent tactile allodynia. This is an important area of ongoing research [35, 36].

Summary

Tissue injury and inflammation initiate a behavioral phenotype characterized by ongoing pain and the appearance of states where mildly aversive or innocuous stimuli lead to an enhanced pain state at the site of injury (primary) and adjacent to the site of injury (secondary). The mechanisms underlying these behavioral states reflect release of "active factors" at the injury site initiating afferent traffic and sensitizing the afferent

terminal, yielding an enhanced response to a given stimulus. The ongoing afferent activity leads to a complex series of events in the dorsal horn representing local changes in membrane excitability, activation of local facilitatory circuits, blocking local inhibitory circuits, activation of spino-bulbo-spinal links, and engaging a complex "neuroinflammatory" process involving spinal nonneuronal cells.

Encoding of Nociception After Nerve Injury

The mechanisms underlying the spontaneous pain and the miscoding of low-threshold tactile input are not completely understood. However, the organizing concept is that these events reflect (i) an increase in spontaneous activity the injured afferent and (ii) an exaggerated response of spinal neurons to low-threshold afferent input (Fig. 1.10).

Events Initiated by Nerve Injury

Injury leads to prominent changes at the site of nerve injury and in the DRG of the injured axon [8, 9, 37, 38]:

(i) Injury site: After acute injury of the peripheral afferent axon, there is an initial dying back (retrograde chromatolysis) until the axon begins to sprout, sending growth cones forward. Such axonal growth cone often fails to contact with the original target, and these sprouts show proliferation. Collections of these proliferated sprouts form neuromas.

(ii) DRG: Although the original injury is restricted to the peripheral nerve site, the distal injury has an enormous impact upon the dorsal root ganglion. Several events should be emphasized. (i) Markers of neuronal injury (such as ATF-3, an injury-evoked transcription factor) show a large-scale increase in expression in the DRG of the injured axons. (ii) There is an increased activation of the glial satellite cells (expressing GFAP) present. The DRG neurons are markedly enhanced. (iii) The DRG neurons show prominent increases in the expression of a variety of proteins such as those for sodium channels, calcium channels, and auxiliary calcium channel proteins (such as the alpha 2 delta subunit) and (iv) conversely decreases in the expression of other proteins such as those for certain potassium channels.

Origins of Spontaneous Pain State

As reviewed in the preceding sections, under normal conditions, the normal primary afferent axons show little of any spontaneous activity. After acute injury, the afferent axons display (i) an initial burst of afferent firing secondary to the injury, (ii) silence for intervals of hours to days, and (iii)

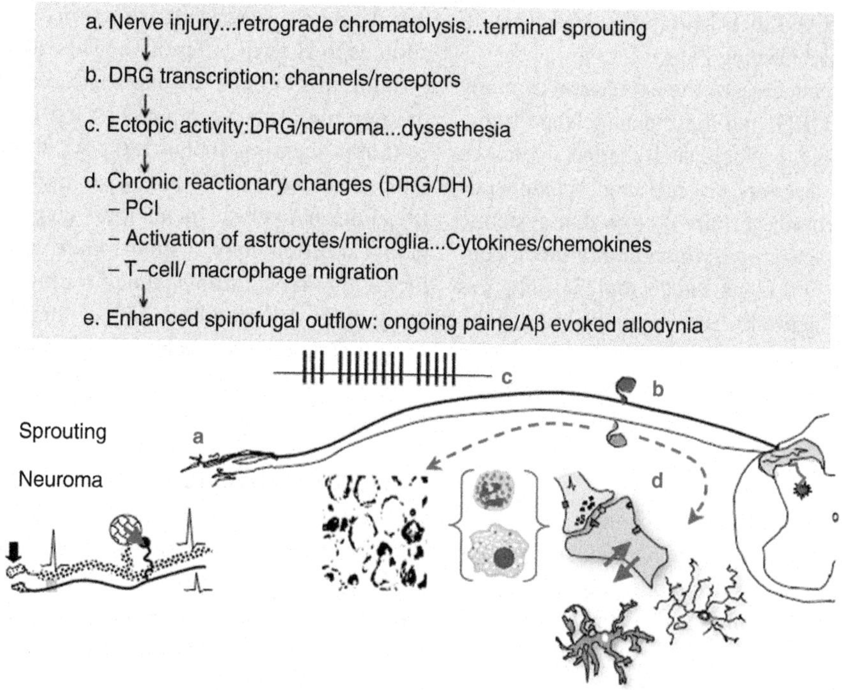

a. Nerve injury...retrograde chromatolysis...terminal sprouting

b. DRG transcription: channels/receptors

c. Ectopic activity:DRG/neuroma...dysesthesia

d. Chronic reactionary changes (DRG/DH)
 – PCI
 – Activation of astrocytes/microglia...Cytokines/chemokines
 – T–cell/ macrophage migration

e. Enhanced spinofugal outflow: ongoing paine/Aβ evoked allodynia

Sprouting

Neuroma

Fig. 1.10 This schematic provides an overview of the organization of events that initiate pain state after a peripheral nerve injury. (**a**) Nerve injury leads to retrograde chromatolysis and then sprouting to form local neuromas. (**b**) In addition to the changes in the terminals, there are trophic changes in the DRG leading to significant changes in the expression of a variety of channel and receptor proteins. (**c**) Over time, there is the appearance of ectopic activity in the injured axon. This activity arises from both the neuroma as well as the dorsal root ganglion. (**d**, **e**) In the dorsal horn, there are a series of reactive changes which lead to a reorganization of nociceptive processing. These changes include changes in the excitability of the second-order neurons, changes in the inhibitory control which normally regulates dorsal horn excitability, and then the activation of nonneuronal cells which contribute to the pro-excitatory nature of the nerve injury

development over time of spontaneous afferent traffic in both myelinated and unmyelinated axons.

Ongoing afferent input origin of ongoing pain. The ongoing afferent input is believed to provide the source of the afferent activity that leads to spontaneous ongoing sensation (Fig. 1.4). Evidence for this assertion that the ectopic afferent activity is in part responsible for the associated pain behavior is based on the observations that (i) parallel onset of pain and ectopic activity in neuroma and DRG, (ii) pain behavior blocked by application of TTX/local anesthetics to neuroma/DRGs, (iii) dorsal rhizotomy transiently reverse the pain behavior, and (iv) irritants applied to DRG initiate activity and importantly, evoke pain behavior [39].

Site of Origin of Spontaneous Afferent Traffic

Recording from the afferent axon has indicated that origin of the spontaneous activity in the injured afferent arises *both* from the neuroma and from the DRG of the injured axon (Fig. 1.4).

Mechanisms of Ongoing Activity

The generation of ongoing activity in the neuroma/DRG of the injured axon results from upregulation of excitable channels/receptors and appearance of excitatory substances in the DRG/neuroma.

Increased Sodium Channel Expression

Cloning shows that there are multiple populations of sodium channels, differing in their current activation properties and structure contributing to the action potential [8, 9].

Multiple sodium channels have been identified based on structure (NaV 1.1–NaV 1.9), whether they are tetrodotoxin sensitive (TTX), and their activation kinetics. Based on these designations, some subtypes are spatially limited in their distribution. Thus, NaV 1.8 and 1.9 are present in small primary afferents.

Importance of sodium channel subtypes in humans has been shown in identified loss- and gain-of-function mutations. The SCN9A gene encodes the voltage-gated sodium channel NaV 1.7, a protein highly expressed in pain-sensing dorsal root ganglion neurons and sympathetic ganglion neurons. Mutations in SCN9A cause three human pain disorders:

(i) Loss of function: Loss-of-function mutations results in insensitivity to pain, no pain perception, and anosmia, but patients are otherwise normal.

(ii) Gain of function: Activating mutations cause severe episodic pain in paroxysmal extreme pain disorders with episodic burning pain in mandibular, ocular, and rectal areas as well as flushing, and primary erythermalgia, a peripheral pain disorder in which blood vessels are episodically blocked then become hyperemic with associated with severe burning pain.

Peripheral nerve injury increases the expression of many sodium channels in the DRG, and these channels are transported to the distal terminals. Increased channel increases ionic conductance and appears to increase spontaneous activity in the sprouting axon terminal. Note that systemic (IV/IP) lidocaine at concentrations which do *not* block conducted action potentials will block the "ectopic" discharges originating in DRG and neuroma. These concentrations are notable in that they will correspondingly block hyperpathia in the nerve jury pain state otherwise observed in humans and in animal models.

Decreased K Channel Expression

Many classes of types of gated $K+$ channels have been described. Opening of $K+$ channels yields membrane hyperpolarization and a reduced excitability. In the face of nerve injury, a reduced expression of such channels has been described, and it is hypothesized that this may contribute to the increased ectopic afferent activity observed after nerve injury [40].

Inflammatory Products

The sprouted terminals of the injured afferent axon display transduction properties that were not possessed by the original axon, including mechanical (e.g., compression) and chemical sensitivity. Thus, neuromas display sensitivity humoral factors, such as prostanoids, catecholamines, and cytokines (TNF). DRGs also respond to these products.

These products are released from local sources such as satellite cells in the DRG and Schwann cells in the periphery. The DRG is of particular interest as it lies outside the blood-brain barrier, for example, it can be influenced by circulating factors. This evolving sensitivity is of particular importance given that following local nerve injury, there is the release of a variety of cytokines, particularly TNF, which can thus directly activate the nerve and neuroma.

Following nerve injury, there is an important sprouting of postganglionic sympathetic efferents that can lead to the local release of catecholamines. This scenario is consistent with the observation that following nerve injury, the postganglionic axons can initiate excitation in the injured axon (see below). These events are believed to contribute to the development of spontaneous afferent traffic after peripheral nerve injury.

Origins of Evoke Hyperpathia

The observation that low-threshold tactile stimulation yields a pain states has been the subject of considerable interest. The psychophysical properties of this state emphasize that the pain results from activation of low-threshold mechanoreceptors (Aβ afferents). This ability of light touch evoking this anomalous pain state is *de facto* evidence that the peripheral nerve injury has led to a reorganization of central processing, that is, it is not a simple case of a peripheral sensitization of otherwise high-threshold afferents. In addition to these behavioral changes, the neuropathic pain condition may display other contrasting anomalies, including on occasion an ameliorating effect of sympathectomy of the afflicted limb and an attenuated responsiveness to spinal analgesics such as opiates. Several underlying mechanisms have been proposed to account for this seemingly anomalous linkage.

Dorsal Root Ganglion Cell Cross Talk

Following nerve injury, evidence suggests that "cross talk" develops between afferents in the DRG and in the neuroma. Here, action potentials in one axon generate depolarizing currents in an adjacent quiescent axon. Thus, activity arising in one axon (a large afferent) would drive activity on a second axon (small C fiber) [41].

Afferent Sprouting

Under normal circumstances, large myelinated (Aβ) afferents project into the spinal Rexed lamina III and deeper (see above). Small afferents (C fibers) tend to project into spinal laminae II and I, a region consisting mostly of nocisponsive neurons. Following peripheral nerve injury, it has been argued that the central terminals of these myelinated afferents (A fibers) sprout into lamina II of the spinal cord. With this synaptic reorganization, stimulation of low-threshold mechanoreceptors (Aβ fibers) could produce excitation of these neurons and be perceived as painful. The degree to which this sprouting occurs is a point of current discussion, and while it appears to occur, it is less prominent than originally reported.

Loss of Intrinsic GABAergic/Glycinergic Inhibitory Control

As reviewed above, GABA/glycinergic interneurons display a potent regulation of large afferent-evoked WDR excitation. The relevance of this intrinsic inhibition to pain processing is evidenced by the observation that spinal delivery of GABA A receptor or glycine receptor antagonists yields a powerful behaviorally defined tactile allodynia [42, 43].

In general, while there are changes in dorsal horn after nerve injury, the predominant evidence does not support a loss of dorsal horn inhibitory amino acids circuitry. Recent observations now suggest an important alternative. After nerve injury, spinal neurons regress to a neonatal phenotype in which GABA A activation becomes excitatory. As noted, the GABA A and glycine channels are chloride ionophores, wherein their activation (increasing Cl permeability) normally leads to a mild hyperpolarization of the postsynaptic membrane as Cl moves inside the cell. After injury, there is a loss of the Cl exporter (so-called KCC2), and there is an accumulation of Cl inside the cell. Now, increasing conductance leads to an extracellular movement of the Cl. This loss of negative charge causes the cell to mildly hypopolarize. This accordingly would turn an inhibitory regulation circuit for larger afferent to a facilitatory circuit for large afferent drive of the WDR neuron [44, 45].

Nonneuronal Cells and Nerve Injury

Nerve section or compression leads to activation of spinal microglia and astrocytes in spinal segments receiving input from injured nerves with a time course that parallels the changes in pain states. While the origin of this activation is not clear, it will lead to an increased spinal expression of COX/NOS/glutamate transporters/proteinases. The effects of such changes in spinal cord afferent processing have been previously reviewed above [46].

Sympathetic Dependency

Following peripheral nerve injury, an increased innervation by postganglionic sympathetic terminals of the neuroma and of the DRG of the injured axons is reliably noted. In the DRG, these postganglionic fibers form baskets of terminals around the ganglion cells. Several properties of this hyperinnervation are noteworthy [47, 48]:

(i) They invest ganglion cells of all sizes, but particularly large ganglion cells (so-called type A).
(ii) Postganglionic innervation occurs largely in the ipsilateral DRG but also occurs to a lesser degree in the contralateral DRG.
(iii) Activation of the preganglionic efferents (traveling in the ventral roots) will activate the sensory axon by an interaction at the site of injury or at the level of the DRG.
(iv) Activation is blocked by intravenous phentolamine, emphasizing an adrenergic effect.

Generalization to Many Nerve Injury Pain States

After nerve injury, there evolves an increase in ongoing dysesthesia and an enhanced response to low-threshold mechanical stimuli (allodynia). These effects are believed to reflect an increase in ectopic activity that arises from the neuromas well as the injured axon. The origin of the ectopic activity is believed to reflect an increased expression of sodium channel, decreased expression of K channels in the neuroma, and DRG leading to enhanced excitability. The allodynia is considered to reflect an alteration in the activation produced by large low-threshold afferents (Aβ). This alteration may result from cross talk between axons and/or a loss of inhibitory regulation.

It should be noted that the above review generically considers the "injured" axon. These changes reviewed above have been observed in animal models following chemotherapy, varicella zoster, extruded intervertebral disks (compressing the nerve root), and osteosarcoma. Accordingly, these changes described in preclinical models are believed to have a great likelihood of being relevant to the human condition.

Conclusions

In the preceding sections, we have provided an overview of the various systems that underlie the three heuristic subdivisions of acute, post-tissue injury and post-nerve injury pain states. An important concept is that in many clinical conditions, it is virtually certain that the clinical state is not one or the other, but rather a combination. Table 1.3 presents a superficial analysis of the types of mechanisms which may be involved in, for example, cancer pain. It is compelling to consider that such a patient may experience a pain state that reflects all three conditions between the events that arise from the tumor itself, the chemotherapy and the surgery (Tables 1.3 and 1.4).

Table 1.3 Summary of primary classes of analgesic therapeutics, mechanisms of action, and pain sites targeted by the agent as defined preclinical models [49–53]

Drug class	Mechanisms	Pain classification		
		Acute	Tissue injury	Nerve injury
Opiate (morphine)	Opiate receptors on high-threshold C fibers	X	X	x
NMDA antagonist (ketamine)	Blocks spinal glutamate-evoked facilitation	O	X	X
NSAID (ibuprofen)	Inhibits cyclooxygenase at injury site and in cord	O	X	O
Local anesthetic (IV lidocaine)	Sodium channel blocker	O	X	X
Anticonvulsant (gabapentin)	Reduces spontaneously active neuronal activity	O	X	X
Tricyclic antidepressant	Increase catecholamine levels	O	X	X
N-type calcium channel blocker (ziconotide)	Blocks spinal N-type calcium channel	O	X	X

Representative preclinical pain models include: Acute nociception: thermal-hot plate/tail flick; Tissue injury: intraplantar carrageenan-hyperalgesia, intraplantar formalin; Nerve injury: nerve ligation, nerve compression yielding tactile allodynia
X significant action, x minimal action, O no activity

Table 1.4 Summary of multiple mechanisms involved in the pain state of a cancer patient

Cancer	Acute Spinal neurons A∂/C	Tissue injury Sensitization (peripheral central)	Nerve injury Ectopic activity Spinal inhibition Sprouting
Tumor erosion (bone/tissue)		X	
Tumor release of factors	X	X	
Immune response (paraneoplastic)			X
Movement (incident pain)	X	X	
Tumor compression			X
Radiation			X
Chemotherapy			X
Surgery		X	X

A∂ lightly myelinated, *C* unmyelinated

The likelihood of multiple mechanisms mediating a particular pain state has an important ramification when it comes to the appropriateness of any particular analgesic therapy. Table 1.3 presents a summary of the basic mechanisms of actions of several classes of analgesic agents. Though not specifically discussed in this chapter (see elsewhere in this text), it is appreciated that they act to alter nociceptive transmission in a variety of ways. Opiates have a potent effect upon spinal transmission initiated by small primary afferents, whereas an NSAID largely has an effect when there is a facilitated state initiated by local inflammation. As reviewed above, there is in addition a central role for NSAIDs because of the constitutive expression of COX in the spinal dorsal horn and the role of prostaglandins in enhancing presynaptic transmitter release and diminish the inhibitory efficacy of the glycine receptor. In the face of multiple pain mechanisms, it can be appreciated that to minimize any pain state may well require addressing multiple therapeutic targets. Hence, it is not surprising that the profile of analgesic management of complex states, such as cancer, often shows 3–4 analgesic agents being employed.

References

1. Dougherty PM. Central sensitization and cutaneous hyperalgesia. Semin Pain Med. 2003;1:121–31.
2. Johanek L, Shim B, Meyer RA. Chapter 4 Primary hyperalgesia and nociceptor sensitization. Handb Clin Neurol. 2006;81:35–47.
3. Mayer EA, Gebhart GF. Basic and clinical aspects of visceral hyperalgesia. Gastroenterology. 1994;107:271–93.
4. Baron R. Neuropathic pain: a clinical perspective. Handb Exp Pharmacol. 2009;194:3–30.
5. Stucky CL, Dubin AE, Jeske NA, Malin SA, McKemy DD, Story GM. Roles of transient receptor potential channels in pain. Brain Res Rev. 2009;60:2–23.
6. Binshtok AM. Mechanisms of nociceptive transduction and transmission: a machinery for pain sensation and tools for selective analgesia. Int Rev Neurobiol. 2011;97:143–77.
7. Cortright DN, Szallasi A. TRP channels and pain. Curr Pharm Des. 2009;15(15):1736–49.
8. Dib-Hajj SD, Black JA, Waxman SG. Voltage-gated sodium channels: therapeutic targets for pain. Pain Med. 2009;10(7):1260–9.
9. Cohen CJ. Targeting voltage-gated sodium channels for treating neuropathic and inflammatory pain. Curr Pharm Biotechnol. 2011; 12:1715–9.
10. Raja SN, Meyer RA, Campbell JN. Peripheral mechanisms of somatic pain. Anesthesiology. 1988;68:571–90.
11. Yaksh TL. Calcium channels as therapeutic targets in neuropathic pain. J Pain. 2006;7(1 Suppl 1):S13–30.
12. Ruscheweyh R, Forsthuber L, Schoffnegger D, Sandkühler J. Modification of classical neurochemical markers in identified primary afferent neurons with abeta-, adelta-, and C-fibers after chronic constriction injury in mice. J Comp Neurol. 2007;502:325–36.
13. Willis Jr WD. The somatosensory system, with emphasis on structures important for pain. Brain Res Rev. 2007;55:297–313.
14. Todd AJ, Spike RC. The localization of classical transmitters and neuropeptides within neurons in laminae I-III of the mammalian spinal dorsal horn. Prog Neurobiol. 1993;41:609–45.
15. Todd AJ. Neuronal circuitry for pain processing in the dorsal horn. Nat Rev Neurosci. 2010;11:823–36.
16. Ralston 3rd HJ. Pain and the primate thalamus. Prog Brain Res. 2005;149:1–10.
17. Reichling DB, Levine JD. Critical role of nociceptor plasticity in chronic pain. Trends Neurosci. 2009;32:611–8.
18. Herrero JF, Laird JM, López-García JA. Wind-up of spinal cord neurones and pain sensation: much ado about something? Prog Neurobiol. 2000;61:169–203.
19. Dickenson AH, Chapman V, Green GM. The pharmacology of excitatory and inhibitory amino acid-mediated events in the transmission and modulation of pain in the spinal cord. Gen Pharmacol. 1997;28:633–8.
20. Bleakman D, Alt A, Nisenbaum ES. Glutamate receptors and pain. Semin Cell Dev Biol. 2006;17:592–604.
21. Luo C, Seeburg PH, Sprengel R, Kuner R. Activity-dependent potentiation of calcium signals in spinal sensory networks in inflammatory pain states. Pain. 2008;140:358–67.
22. Latremoliere A, Woolf CJ. Central sensitization: a generator of pain hypersensitivity by central neural plasticity. J Pain. 2009;10: 895–926.
23. Ji RR, Kawasaki Y, Zhuang ZY, Wen YR, Zhang YQ. Protein kinases as potential targets for the treatment of pathological pain. Handb Exp Pharmacol. 2007;177:359–89.
24. Velázquez KT, Mohammad H, Sweitzer SM. Protein kinase C in pain: involvement of multiple isoforms. Pharmacol Res. 2007;55: 578–89.
25. Svensson CI, Yaksh TL. The spinal phospholipase-cyclooxygenase-prostanoid cascade in nociceptive processing. Annu Rev Pharmacol Toxicol. 2002;42:553–83.

26. Zeilhofer HU. The glycinergic control of spinal pain processing. Cell Mol Life Sci. 2005;62:2027–35.

27. Tang Q, Svensson CI, Fitzsimmons B, Webb M, Yaksh TL, Hua XY. Inhibition of spinal constitutive NOS-2 by 1400 W attenuates tissue injury and inflammation-induced hyperalgesia and spinal p38 activation. Eur J Neurosci. 2007;25:2964–72.

28. Suzuki R, Rygh LJ, Dickenson AH. Bad news from the brain: descending 5-HT pathways that control spinal pain processing. Trends Pharmacol Sci. 2004;25:613–7.

29. Milligan ED, Watkins LR. Pathological and protective roles of glia in chronic pain. Nat Rev Neurosci. 2009;10:23–36.

30. Ren K, Dubner R. Neuron-glia crosstalk gets serious: role in pain hypersensitivity. Curr Opin Anaesthesiol. 2008;21:570–9.

31. Abbadie C, Bhangoo S, De Koninck Y, Malcangio M, Melik-Parsadaniantz S, White FA. Chemokines and pain mechanisms. Brain Res Rev. 2009;60:125–34.

32. Clark AK, Staniland AA, Malcangio M. Fractalkine/CX3CR1 signalling in chronic pain and inflammation. Curr Pharm Biotechnol. 2011;12:1707–14.

33. Grace PM, Rolan PE, Hutchinson MR. Peripheral immune contributions to the maintenance of central glial activation underlying neuropathic pain. Brain Behav Immun. 2011;25:1322–32.

34. Ledeboer A, Sloane EM, Milligan ED, Frank MG, Mahony JH, Maier SF, Watkins LR. Minocycline attenuates mechanical allodynia and proinflammatory cytokine expression in rat models of pain facilitation. Pain. 2005;115:71–83.

35. Kehlet H, Jensen TS, Woolf CJ. Persistent postsurgical pain: risk factors and prevention. Lancet. 2006;367:1618–25.

36. Xu Q, Yaksh TL. A brief comparison of the pathophysiology of inflammatory versus neuropathic pain. Curr Opin Anaesthesiol. 2011;24:400–7.

37. Tuchman M, Barrett JA, Donevan S, Hedberg TG, Taylor CP. Central sensitization and Ca(V) α2δ ligands in chronic pain syndromes: pathologic processes and pharmacologic effect. J Pain. 2010;12:1241–9.

38. Bráz JM, Ackerman L, Basbaum AI. Sciatic nerve transection triggers release and intercellular transfer of a genetically expressed macromolecular tracer in dorsal root ganglia. J Comp Neurol. 2011;519:2648–57.

39. Zimmermann M. Pathobiology of neuropathic pain. Eur J Pharmacol. 2001;429:23–37.

40. Takeda M, Tsuboi Y, Kitagawa J, Nakagawa K, Iwata K, Matsumoto S. Potassium channels as a potential therapeutic target for trigeminal neuropathic and inflammatory pain. Mol Pain. 2011;7:5.

41. Devor M, Wall PD. Cross-excitation in dorsal root ganglia of nerve-injured and intact rats. J Neurophysiol. 1990;64(6):1733–46.

42. Yaksh TL. Behavioral and autonomic correlates of the tactile evoked allodynia produced by spinal glycine inhibition: effects of modulatory receptor systems and excitatory amino acid antagonists. Pain. 1989;37:111–23.

43. Sivilotti L, Woolf CJ. The contribution of GABAA and glycine receptors to central sensitization: disinhibition and touch-evoked allodynia in the spinal cord. J Neurophysiol. 1994;72:169–79.

44. Polgár E, Hughes DI, Riddell JS, Maxwell DJ, Puskár Z, Todd AJ. Selective loss of spinal GABAergic or glycinergic neurons is not necessary for development of thermal hyperalgesia in the chronic constriction injury model of neuropathic pain. Pain. 2003;104:229–39.

45. Price TJ, Cervero F, de Koninck Y. Role of cation-chloride-cotransporters (CCC) in pain and hyperalgesia. Curr Top Med Chem. 2005;5(6):547–55.

46. Cao H, Zhang YQ. Spinal glial activation contributes to pathological pain states. Neurosci Biobehav Rev. 2008;32(5):972–83.

47. McLachlan EM, Jänig W, Devor M, Michaelis M. Peripheral nerve injury triggers noradrenergic sprouting within dorsal-root ganglia. Nature. 1993;363:543–6.

48. Drummond PD. Involvement of the sympathetic nervous system in complex regional pain syndrome. Int J Low Extrem Wounds. 2004;3:35–42.

49. Borsook D, Becerra L. CNS animal fMRI in pain and analgesia. Neurosci Biobehav Rev. 2011;35:1125–43.

50. D'Souza WN, Ng GY, Youngblood BD, Tsuji W, Lehto SG. A review of current animal models of osteoarthritis pain. Curr Pharm Biotechnol. 2011;12:1596–612.

51. Mogil JS. Animal models of pain: progress and challenges. Nat Rev Neurosci. 2009;10:283–94.

52. Waszkielewicz AM, Gunia A, Słoczyńska K, Marona H. Evaluation of anticonvulsants for possible use in neuropathic pain. Curr Med Chem. 2011;18:4344–58.

53. Xu J, Brennan TJ. The pathophysiology of acute pain: animal models. Curr Opin Anaesthesiol. 2011;24:508–14.

Pharmacogenomics of Pain Management

Piotr K. Janicki

Key Points

- Individual pain variability and differences in the efficacy of analgesic drugs are genetically controlled.
- Drug-metabolizing enzymes represent a major target of current effort to identify associations between individuals' analgesic drug response and genetic profile.
- Genetic variants in other candidate genes influencing drug effector sites, such as those encoding receptors, transporters, and other molecules important for pain transmission represent another, less well-defined target.
- The pharmacogenomics-based approach to pain management represents a potential tool to improve the effectiveness and the side effect profile of therapy; however, well-designed prospective studies are needed to demonstrate superiority to conventional dosing regimes.

Introduction

Medicine has been continuously challenged, as well as stimulated, by the extraordinary variability in patient response to pharmacotherapy. The new age of identification of risk factors associated with pharmacotherapy using the methods of molecular medicine focuses on generating predictions regarding clinical outcome on the basis of each individual's unique DNA sequence. This new field has been coined *pharmacogenomics*. The goal of pharmacogenomics is to use information provided by advances in human genetics to identify patients at risk for significantly altered response during pharmacotherapy. The field of pharmacogenomics represents the major drive behind the introduction of the concept of *personalized medicine* in which the medical treatment is customized according to the individual patient genomic signature [1].

Background

Association of genome variability with increased or decreased pain, or modified effects of analgesics, has demonstrated that pain therapy is subject to pharmacogenomics [2–6].

There are two major components of pain management and pharmacogenomics (see Fig. 2.1). The use of genetic information from basic science and clinical studies to examine the impact of genetic variability on factors modulating the risk of developing pain, its clinical course, and intensity is called *functional pain genomics*. Functional pain genomics aims to discover the biologic function of particular genes and to uncover how a set of genes and their products work together in regulating the response to pain.

The second, more traditional, and better established component of pain related genomics is called *pharmacogenomics of pain management* and aims to characterize how genetic variations contribute to an individual's sensitivity and response to a variety of drugs important to pain management practice. Pharmacogenomics is traditionally divided into two parts describing genetic variants influencing pharmacokinetics and pharmacodynamics.

The molecular basis for the observed variability in patient response is defined by different forms of the detected genetic variants. These variants, consisting of the interindividual differences in the DNA sequences, produce the individual *phenotypes* of the human being. There are many different types of genetic variants (see Fig. 2.2). The most common (more than ten million types known so far) are single *nucleotide polymorphisms (or SNP)*, which represent a point mutation (change of one base) in the DNA fragments.

P.K. Janicki, M.D., Ph.D., DSci, DABA (✉)
Department of Anesthesiology, Pennsylvania State Milton S. Hershey Medical Center, 500 University Drive, Mailcode H187, Hershey, PA 17033, USA

Laboratory of Perioperative Genomics, Pennsylvania State University College of Medicine, Hershey, PA, USA
e-mail: pjanicki@hmc.psu.edu

T.R. Deer et al. (eds.), *Treatment of Chronic Pain by Medical Approaches: the AMERICAN ACADEMY of PAIN MEDICINE Textbook on Patient Management*, DOI 10.1007/978-1-4939-1818-8_2,
© American Academy of Pain Medicine 2015

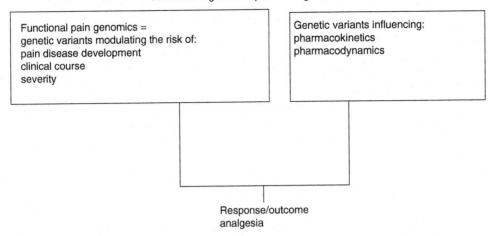

Fig. 2.1 Framework of genetic background influencing the response to analgesic drugs

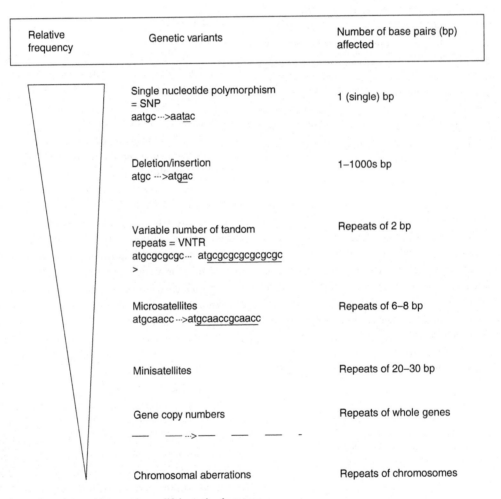

Fig. 2.2 Types of genetic variants taking part in modifying pain phenotype

Other allelic mutations include insertion or deletion of a single base (*indels*), multiple, continuous repeats of 2–4 bases (*variable number of tandem repeats or VNTR*); repeats of longer DNA fragments (*micro- and mini-satellites*); *copy number variants* (CNV, deletion or multiplication of large, >1,000 bases fragments of chromosomes); and finally *chromosomal aberrations*. The genetic variants may produce alterations in the protein's function through either changes in the protein expression or its structure.

Functional Genomics of Pain

Pain as a complex trait is expected to have a polygenic nature shaped by the environmental pressures. Identification of specific genetic elements of pain perception promises to be one of the key elements for creating novel and individualized pain treatments. It was demonstrated previously that both rare deleterious genetic variants and common genetic polymorphisms are mediators of human pain perception and clinical pain phenotypes [7, 8]. A higher or lower intensity of pain is very likely to require higher or lower doses of analgesics for efficient pain management. The genetic control of human pain perception and processing is therefore likely to modulate analgesic therapy.

The complete inability to sense pain in an otherwise healthy individual is a very rare phenotype. At present, five types of congenital insensitivity to pain (or HSAN = hereditary sensory and autonomic neuropathy) were identified which are caused by mutations in five different genes [9].

Recently, several new genomic mutations were identified which are described as "channelopathy-associated insensitivity to pain" [10] which are characterized by complete and selective inability to perceive any form of pain. It includes mutations in the alpha-subunit of sodium channel $Na_v1.7$ (SCN9A), causing the loss of function in this specific form of sodium channel [10, 11]. By contrast, mutations in SCN9A that leads to excessive channel activity trigger activation of pain signaling in humans and produce primary erythermalgia (more frequently used term is erythromelalgia), which is characterized by burning pain in response to exposure to mild warmth [12, 13]. Mutations in this gene also produce a rare condition referred to as "paroxysmal extreme pain disorder," which is characterized by rectal, ocular, and submandibular pain [14].

These syndromes probably have no importance in the everyday clinical pain management as they are very rare, and the affected people probably do not require pain therapy (with exception of erythromelalgia which causes severe pain that is considered a true pain-related emergency). However, defining the molecular causes for hereditary insensitivity to pain may serve as an important source of information to find new targets for analgesic drugs. This assumption was con-

firmed in the recently published study, in which the authors after investigating 27 common polymorphisms in the SCN9A gene found out that the minor A allele of the SNP rs6746030 was associated with an altered pain threshold and the effect was mediated through C-fiber activation [15]. They concluded that individuals experience differing amounts of pain, per nociceptive stimulus, on the basis of their SCN9A rs6746030 genotype.

Pain in the average population is controlled by fairly frequent genetic variants (allelic frequency > 10 %). Each of them, however, modifies the pain phenotype to only modest degree, and in the majority of cases, the evidence for their involvement in the efficacy of analgesics is either lacking or remains controversial [7, 8]. The involvement of common variants of the opioid receptors, kappa and mu, are discussed below in the part describing pharmacodynamic modifications of activity of opioid analgesics. A variant of third type of opioid receptor, delta, has been associated with lower thermal pain intensity with no association, so far, with the efficacy of opioid analgesics [16].

GTP cyclohydrolase (GCH1), recently implicated in shaping pain responses in humans, regulates production of tetrahydrobiopterin (BH4), an essential factor for the synthesis of dopamine, serotonin, and nitric acid. Tegeder et al. discovered a haplotype associated with reduction of experimental pain in normal volunteers and a favorable outcome with regard to long-term pain reduction that underwent pain (did you mean "a painful surgery"?) surgery [17]. In another study, Tegeder et al. showed that carriers of the particular GCH1 haplotype had higher pain threshold to mechanical and thermal pain following capsaicin sensitization [18]. However, Kim and Dionn and Lazarev et al. failed to replicate significant associations between the same GCH1 genomic variants and pain responses, both in assessment of experimental pain and postoperative pain after dental surgery, as well chronic pancreatic pain [19, 20]. Conversely, the most recent study confirmed again that the five previously identified GCH1 SNPs were profoundly affecting the ratings of pain induced by capsaicin in healthy human volunteers [21]. It was also suggested that the carriers of this particular GCH1 haplotype (which may be responsible for the decreased function of GCH1) display delayed need for pain therapy [2, 22].

Pharmacogenomics of Pain Therapy and Its Usefulness in Clinical Practice

Pharmacogenomics of pain management represents the most familiar area of practical pain genomics. It includes several examples of genomic variations, dramatically changing response to analgesic drugs through either change in their metabolism or receptor targets.

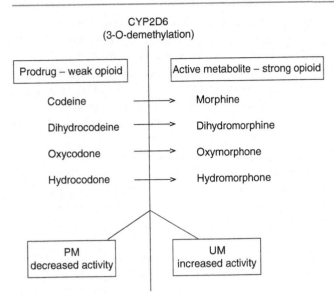

CYP2D6
(3-O-demethylation)

Prodrug – weak opioid   Active metabolite – strong opioid

Codeine   ———→   Morphine

Dihydrocodeine   ———→   Dihydromorphine

Oxycodone   ———→   Oxymorphone

Hydrocodone   ———→   Hydromorphone

PM
decreased activity

UM
increased activity

Fig. 2.3 Opioid analgesics influenced by polymorphic CYP2D6 metabolism (3-O-demethylation)

The current list of genetic polymorphisms which may affect the action of analgesic drugs is quite long and appears to be growing rapidly. The best known mechanisms involved in the altered effects of analgesics involve polymorphic changes in its metabolism. In this respect, three major mechanisms have been identified, involving genetic variations in the metabolic activation of the analgesics administered as an inactive or less active prodrug, variations in the metabolic degradation of the active components, and variations in its transmembrane transport.

Genetic Variations in the Prodrug Activation

The better known example involves polymorphisms in genes of the liver isoforms of the cytochrome P450 system (CYP) [23]. In particular, the most well-characterized *CYP2D6* polymorphism is responsible for the considerable variation in the metabolism (and clinical responses) of drugs from many therapeutic areas, including several analgesics (Fig. 2.3) [24–26]. More than 100 CYP2D6 alleles have been identified, ranging from nonsynonymous mutations to SNPs that either alter RNA splicing or produce deletions of the entire gene [27]. Of these, *3, *4, and *8 are nonfunctional, *9, *10, and *41 have reduced function, and *1,*2, *35, and *41 can be duplicated, resulting in greatly increased expression of functional CYP2D6. There are also interethnic differences in the frequencies of these variant alleles. Allele combinations determine phenotype: two nonfunctional = poor metabolizer (PM); at least one reduced functional = intermediate metabolizer (IM); at least one functional = extensive

metabolizers (EM); and multiple copies of a functional and/or allele with promoter mutation = ultrarapid metabolizer (UM). The most recent update of CYP2D6 nomenclature and terminology could be found on home Web page of the Human Cytochrome P450 (CYP) Allele Nomenclature *at* http://www.cypalleles.ki.se/.

Codeine and other weak opioids are extensively metabolized by polymorphic CYP2D6 which regulates its O-demethylation to more potent metabolites (e.g., after a single oral dose of 30 mg codeine, 6 % is eventually transformed to morphine). The clinical analgesic effect of codeine is mainly attributed to its conversion to morphine, which has a 200 times higher affinity and 50 times higher intrinsic activity at MOR than codeine itself [28]. Since CYP2D6 is genetically highly polymorphic, the effects of codeine are under pharmacogenetic control.

Genetically, altered effects of codeine may occur in subjects with either decreased, absent, or highly increased CYP2D6 activity when compared with the population average [29, 30]. Decreased or absent CYP2D6 activity in PMs causes production of only very low or absent amount of morphine after codeine administration. The ultrafast metabolizers (UM) produce on the other hand excessive amount of morphine after typical dose of codeine. Roughly, one out of seven Caucasians is at risk of either failure or toxicity of codeine therapy due to extremely low or high morphine formation, respectively. Recent case reports of codeine fatalities highlighted that the use of this weak opioid, particularly in young children, is associated with a substantial risk in those subjects displaying UM genotype [31–37]. The polymorphic variants in the CYP2D6 system are responsible for some but not all variability observed after codeine administration. The other causes for the observed high variability in codeine efficacy include both polymorphisms in other genes involved in opioid expression or trafficking, as well as nongenetic factors. In addition to differences in codeine metabolism between EM and PM, the differences between EM of various ethnicities have also been highlighted. The Chinese EM reported having a lower rate of codeine O-demethylation when compared with the Caucasian EM, because of the much higher frequency (50 %) of the *10 (reduced function) allele in the Chinese [27].

Other popular analgesic drug which depends on activation by the CYP2D6 includes *tramadol*. Tramadol is a mu-opioid receptor (MOR) agonist but has a lower affinity at MORs than its active metabolite O-desmethyltramadol. Tramadol itself has weak analgesic activity which becomes evident when CYP2D6 is blocked and also acts through nonopioid-dependent mechanisms which involve serotonin- and noradrenaline-mediated pain inhibition originating in brain stem. The analgesic activity of tramadol is strongly modulated by CYP2D6 activity. The analgesic activity on experimental pain is reduced in CYP2D6 PMs, a finding later confirmed in pain patients [38–42]. It is interesting to note that the pharmacokinetics of tramadol (which is administered as racemic substance containing equal amount of (−) and (+) optical isomers producing analgesia by a synergistic action of its two enantiomers and their metabolites) is enantioselective in CYP2D6 poor and extensive metabolizers, meaning that the production of either optical isomer differs depending on the metabolic status [41, 43, 44]. The clinical significance of this finding for pain management remains to be further explored.

As far as other CYP2D6 substrates with active analgesic metabolites are concerned (see Fig. 2.3), the evidence for variation in its analgesic with altered CYP2D6 function is less evident when compared with codeine or tramadol. These examples are either negative, such as for dihydrocodeine [45, 46], or explained at a nongenetic level, such as for oxycodone. In other cases, the evidence is based only on animal studies, such as hydrocodone, or restricted to single case reports for inadequate activity of oxycodone [3].

Tilidine (an opioid analgesic) is activated to active metabolite nortilidine, and *parecoxib* (an NSAID) is activated into valdecoxib by CYP3A system. This enzyme is phenotypically highly variable, but only a minor part of this variability can be attributed to genetics [2]. Individuals with at least one CYP3A5*1 allele copy produce fully active active copy of CYP3A5 enzyme; however, the majority of Caucasians have no active CYP3A5 due to a premature stop codon.

Genetic Variations in the Elimination of Analgesic Drugs

Many of the opioids contain hydroxyl group at position 6, and the potent opioids have a hydroxyl at position 3 of the 4,5-methoxymorphinan structure. The glucuronidation of morphine, codeine, buprenorphine, dihydrocodeine, dihydromorphine, hydromorphone, dihydromorphine, oxymorphone, as well as opioid receptor antagonists (naloxone and naltrexone) is mainly mediated by the uridine diphosphate (UDP) glucuronyltransferase (UGT)2B7 [3]. Similar to CYP genes, the UGT2B7 gene is also polymorphic, although less than 20 allelic variants have been identified. The main proportion of morphine is metabolized to morphine-6-glucuronide, M6G (approximately 70 %), and to lesser degree to morphine-3-glucuronide (M3G). Both metabolites are active, with effects opposite to each other, consisting in excitation and anti-analgesia for M3G and in typical opioid agonist effects for M6G. Despite the role of UGT2B7 in the formation of M6G and M3G, the clinical effect of the UGT2B7*2 (268Y) variant has only produced conflicting results so far. Different variants in the 5′ untranslated region of UGT2B7 are associated with reduced M6G/morphine ratios in patients. In addition, it was reported that UGT2B7

*2/*2 genotypes and CYP2D6 UM phenotypes were associated with severe neonatal toxicity after breast-feeding and oral ingestion of opioids. The above preliminary data indicate that the consequences of UGT variants were so far restricted to alterations of plasma concentrations, while none of the UGT variants alone have been associated with the altered efficacy of opioid analgesics [3, 4].

The increased enzyme activity associated with the CYP3A5*1 allele may cause accelerated elimination of CYP3A substrates, such as alfentanil, fentanyl, or sufentanil. However, positive associations of CYP3A polymorphisms with analgesic actions have not been reported so far. The CYP3A5 genotype did not affect the systemic or apparent oral clearance as well as the pharmacodynamics of alfentanil and levomethadone [47, 48].

In addition to CYP2D6 and CYP2A5, there is also clinical evidence about the involvement of other CYP systems in the metabolism of frequently used nonsteroid anti-inflammatory drugs (NSAIDs). Human CYP2C9 metabolizes numerous drugs (e.g., warfarin, oral sulfonylurea hypoglycemics, antiepileptics, and others) [49]. In addition, CYP2C9 polymorphism might play a significant role in the analgesic efficacy and toxicity of traditional NSAIDs, for example, diclofenac, ibuprofen, naproxen, tenoxicam, and piroxicam, as well as selective COX-2 inhibitors such as celecoxib and valdecoxib [50]. More than 33 variants and a series of subvariants have been identified for CYP2C9 to date. The two missense mutations, CYP2C9*2 (rs1799853) and CYPC9*3 (rs1057910), yield enzymes with decreased activity [51]. These alleles are mainly present in Caucasians, while their frequency is lower in African and Asian subjects. More than twofold reduced clearance after oral intake of celecoxib was observed in homozygous carriers of CYP2C9*3 compared with carriers of the wild-type genotype CYP2C9*1/*1 [52]. Similarly, ibuprofen-mediated inhibition of COX-1 and COX-2 is significantly decreased (by 50 %) in carriers of two CYP2C9*3 alleles [53]. Further investigations demonstrating the relevance of the CYP2C9*3 allele for naproxen, tenoxicam, piroxicam, and lornoxicam pharmacokinetics have been also published [4, 54]. Although CYP2C9 is the major determinant of clearance, it is necessary to also consider CYP2C8 genotype, as it contributes to some smaller extent in NSAIDs metabolism. In the study performed in healthy volunteers, it was demonstrated that metabolism of diclofenac was significantly slower in individuals carrying CYP2C8*3 (rs10509681) or CYP2C8*4 (rs1058930) allele than in those homozygous for the wild-type allele [55].

Whereas numerous clinical trials have demonstrated the impact of CYP2C9*3 on therapy with Coumadin, less information is available on the CYP2C9 genotype-related efficacy of NSAIDs in the pain management. Some publications focus, however, on the incidence and severity of adverse effects (e.g., gastrointestinal (GI) bleeding, effects on coagulation). It was that the combined presence of CYP2C8*3 and CYP2C9*2 was a relevant determinant in the risk of developing GI bleeding in patients receiving NSAIDs metabolized by CYP2C8/9 [56]. Similar results were also presented by Agundez et al. [57]. However, to date, the study results from other authors are conflicting, with several other trials reporting no association [58, 59]. More studies are clearly necessary to confirm the relevance of CYP2C8/9 genotype with increased incidence of GI bleeding.

Another typical adverse effect is the influence of classical NSAIDs on coagulation. The risk of altered coagulation was substantially increased in patients with either CYP2C9*3 and CYP2C9*3 (mentioned twice) genotypes taking Coumadin together with NSAIDs which are known CYP2C9 substrates [60].

Genetic Variations in the Transmembrane Transport of Analgesics

P-glycoprotein (P-gp) coded by the ATP-binding cassette subfamily (ABCB1)/multidrug resistance (MDR1) gene is mainly located in organs with excretory functions (e.g., liver, kidneys). It is also expressed at the blood-brain barrier where it forms an outward transporter. Therefore, functional impairment of P-gp-mediated drug transport may be expected to result in increased bioavailability of orally administered drugs, reduced renal clearance, or an increased brain concentration of its substrates. Some opioids are P-gp substrates. The ABCB1 3435 C > T variant (rs1045642) is associated with decreased dosage requirements in opioids that are P-gp substrates, as assessed in outpatients. Moreover, a diplotype consisting of three polymorphic positions in the ABCB1 gene (1236TT-rs1128503, 2677TT-rs2032582, and 3435TT) is associated with increased susceptibility to respiratory depression caused by fentanyl in Korean patients [61]. The results suggest that analysis of ABCB1 polymorphisms may have clinical relevance in the prevention of respiratory suppression by intravenous fentanyl or to anticipate its clinical effects. With the OPRM1 118 A > G variant (see below), the ABCB1 3435 C > T predicted the response to morphine in cancer patients with a sensitivity close to 100 % and a specificity of more than 70 % [62]. Trials in patients suffering from chronic and cancer pain had shown decreased opioid consumption in carriers of the 3435T allele [63, 64]. Finally, methadone analgesia may be subject to P-gp pharmacogenetic modulation. The pupillary effects of orally administered methadone are increased following the pharmacological blockade of P-gp by quinidine, and the methadone dosing for heroin substitution can be decreased in carriers of ABCB1 variants associated with decreased transporter expression, for example, ABCB1 2435 C > T and others [65, 66].

Pharmacodynamics of Pain Therapy

The alterations in effects of analgesics may also result from pharmacodynamic interferences, consisting of altered receptor binding, activation or signaling mechanisms, or of altered expression of the drug's target, such as opioid receptors or cyclooxygenases. Genetic factors have been found to act via any of these mechanisms.

Opioid Receptors

The mu-opioid receptor (MOR) is part of the family of several types of opioid receptors which are 7-transmembrane domain, G-protein-coupled receptors (GPCR), and inhibit cellular activity. MOR is clinically most relevant target of opioid analgesics. The OPRM1 gene coding for MOR in humans is highly polymorphic, with excess of 1,800 SNPs listed in the current edition (2010) of the NCBI SNP database (http://www.ncbi.nlm.nih.gov/snp). Coding mutations affecting the third intracellular loop of MOR (e.g., 779 G > A, 794 G > A, 802 T > C) result in reduced G-protein coupling, receptor signaling, and desensitization, leading to an expectation that opioids should be almost ineffective in patients carrying those polymorphisms. However, these polymorphisms are extremely rare (<0.1 % population) and are therefore restricted to very rare single cases.

Evidence for a function of OPRM1 variants with allelic frequencies >5 % is sparse, except for the 118 A > G polymorphism (rs1799971). This SNP causes an amino acid exchange of the aspartate with an asparagine at position 40 of extracellular part of MOR, deleting one of a putative glycosylation sites. This change can cause altered expression of MOR or its signaling [67–69]. The OPRM1 118 A > G polymorphism has an allele frequency of 8–17 % in Caucasians and considerably higher in Asians, with a frequency of 47 % reported from Japan. It is also worth noting that the frequency of homozygotes for the GG allele is by much higher in Asian population with only very rare (<1 %) occurrence in Caucasian population [70]. The data obtained so far with the OPRM1 118 A > G polymorphism have been controversial [71]. The molecular changes associated with SNP 118 A > G translate to a variety of clinical effects (predominantly decrease) of many opioids in experimental settings and clinical studies [72–81]. The consequences of the SNP 118 A > G have consistently been related to a decrease in opioid potency for pupil constriction (e.g., for morphine, M6G, methadone). For analgesia, the SNP decreases the concentration-dependent effects of alfentanil on experimental pain. Specifically, the variant decreases the effect of opioids on pain-related activation mainly in those regions of the brain that are processing the sensory dimension of pain including the primary and secondary somatosensory cortex and posterior insular cortex [82]. In clinical settings, greater postoperative requirements of alfentanil and morphine have been reported for carriers of the variant, and higher concentrations of alfentanil of M6G were needed to produce analgesia in experimental pain models [2, 48, 83–87]. It should be noted that other studies described only moderate to no significant effects of the OPRM1 118 A > G polymorphism on opioid requirements or pain relief. Several studies did not demonstrate any association between OPRM1 variant and analgesic needs [88–92]. Contradictory results were reported by Landau et al. who investigated the influence of OPRM1 118 A > G polymorphism on the analgesic effectiveness of fentanyl in females after its intrathecal administration during labor and delivery. The analgesic requirements in this study were increased in homozygous carriers of AA allele, the opposite effect compared with most other studies [93]. In the chronic pain patients, it was reported that in the high-quartile opioid utilization group, the homozygous carriers of the minor allele required significantly higher opioid doses than the carriers of the minor allele [91]. In another studies, GG homozygote patients were characterized by higher morphine consumption than carriers of the major AA allele [76, 94]. In summary, an influence of OPRM1 genetic variants on opioid requirements and degree of pain relief under opioid medication has been demonstrated in some studies; however, this could not be replicated in all subsequent investigations. Patients stratification; a low number of patients with the GG genotype (in particular in studies performed in Caucasian populations); presence of multiple, uncontrolled co-variables influencing the phenotype; and a clinically questionable reduction in opioid consumption are some major concerns. The requirements of high opioid doses may in part reflect an addiction component or a higher/faster rate of tolerance development in certain pain patients. It was reported that OPRM1 A118G polymorphism is a major determinant of striatal dopamine responses to alcohol. Social drinkers recruited based on OPRM1 genotype were challenged in separate sessions with alcohol and placebo under pharmacokinetically controlled conditions and examined for striatal dopamine release using positron emission tomography and [(11)C]-raclopride displacement. A striatal dopamine response to alcohol was restricted to carriers of the minor 118G allele. Based on the results of this study, it was concluded that OPRM1 A118G variation is a genetic determinant of dopamine responses to alcohol, a mechanism by which it likely modulates alcohol reward [95].

In addition, the most recent study seems to suggest that some of the effect of SNP A > G could be explained by the linkage disequilibrium with other functional SNPs located in the OPRM1 region [96]. For example, SNP rs563649 is located within a structurally conserved internal ribosome entry site in the 5′-UTR of a novel exon 13-containing OPRM1 isoforms (MOR-1K) and affects both mRNA levels and translation efficiency of these variants. Furthermore, rs563649 exhibits very strong linkage disequilibrium throughout the entire OPRM1 gene locus and thus affects the functional contribution of the corresponding haplotype that includes other functional OPRM1 SNPs. These results might provide evidence for an essential role for MOR-1K isoforms in nociceptive signaling and suggest that genetic variations in alternative OPRM1 isoforms may contribute to individual differences in opiate responses.

Catechol-O-Methyltransferase (COMT)

CMOT degrades catecholamine neurotransmitters such as norepinephrine, epinephrine, and dopamine. Increased dopamine concentrations suppress the production of endogenous opioid peptides. Opioid receptor expression is in turn upregulated, which has been observed with the Val158Met variant of COMT, coded by the COMT 772 G > A (rs4680) SNP in human postmortem brain tissue and in vivo by assessing radiolabeled 11C-carfentanil MOR binding [97, 98]. This variant leads to a low-function COMT enzyme that fails to degrade dopamine, which may cause a depletion of enkephalin. Patients with cancer carrying the Val158Met variant needed less morphine for pain relief than patients not carrying this variant. Finally, the variants exerts its opioid enforcing effects also in cross relation with the OPRM1 118 A > G variant [94, 97–101]. During the past decade, several new polymorphisms were identified in the COMT gene which contains at least five functional polymorphisms that impact its biological activity and associated phenotypes (including pain). The potentially complex interactions of functional variations in COMT imply that the overall functional state of the gene might not be easily deduced from genotype information alone, which presumably explains the inconsistency in the results from association studies that focus on the V158Met polymorphism [102, 103].

Melanocortin 1 Receptor (MC1R)

Nonfunctional variants of the MC1R which produces bright red hair and fair skin phenotype were associated with an increased analgesic response to kappa opioid receptors (KOR)-mediated opioid analgesia. Red-headed women required less of the KOR agonist drug – pentazocine – to reach a specific level of analgesia compared with all other groups [104, 105]. This study presented the first strong evidence for a gene-by-sex interaction in the area of pain genetics, because the authors also showed that red-headed men did not experience enhanced KOR analgesia.

Cyclooxygenases (COX)

Polymorphisms in the prostaglandin endoperoxidase synthase 2 gene (PTGS2) coding for COX-2 may modulate the development of inflammation and its response to treatment with inhibitors of COXs, especially those specific for COX-2 [106]. This has been proposed for the PTGS2-765 G > C SNP (rs20417), which was reported to be associated with more than a twofold decrease in COX-2 expression [107]. By altering a putative Sp1 binding site in the promoter region of PTGS2, this gene variant was found to decrease the promoter activity by 30 % [108]. However, the controversial results were reported so far in clinical studies with this polymorphisms and different COX-2 inhibitors. The inhibitory effect of celecoxib on COX-2 was not associated with the presence of this variant in volunteers [109]; conversely, significantly decreased analgesic effects of rofecoxib were observed in the homozygous carriers of this variant [110].

Future Direction of Pharmacogenomics in Pain Treatment

The influence of different genetic variants on analgesic requirements and degree of pain relief has been demonstrated in some studies; however, there is relatively less information available about the interactions between these variants. Each of the genetic variants investigated up to now seems to contribute in a modest way to the modulation of analgesic response [111]. However, a global approach investigating multiple possible variables within one trial has not been performed. After more than a decade of identifying genetic associations, the current challenge is to intensify compilation of this information for precisely defined clinical settings for which improved pain treatment is possible.

The current knowledge about the impact of genetics in the pain management is based on the association studies. In contrast to traditional family or pedigree-based studies (linkage analysis), in this type of studies, two cohorts of unrelated patients (with and without the observed phenotype, i.e., changes in the efficacy of analgesics) are compared in respect to the frequency of different genetic variants (adjusted for other known risk factors and for environmental differences). Candidate-gene association studies are focused on selected genes which are thought to be relevant for a specific observed outcome.

The alternative to targeted association studies are genomewide association studies (GWAS). In this type of studies, there is no a priori hypothesis about the gene candidates. Instead, the microarray-based genomic scans are performed throughout the whole genome in order to find all SNPs possibly associated with observed phenotypic changes in the cohorts of patients with investigated traits (and controls). The modern microarray platforms allow for the cost-effective, parallel analysis of approximately one million genomic variants in one sample (or pooled samples) and, using sophisticated computer strategy, enable finding the most relevant statistical associations between control and

affected patients. The main advantage of GWAS is that it is an unbiased hypothesis-free approach. In contrast to other areas of medicine, the GWAS approach lags behind in pain genomics, but the next few years should bring about the results of several studies currently being performed in the area of pain medicine. One of the first pain pharmacogenomic studies using GWAS technology was recently published by Kim et al. and demonstrated association of minor allele variant in a zinc finger protein (ZNF429) gene with delayed onset of action of ketorolac in the oral surgery patients [112].

Summary

In summary, genetics continues to make rapid progress in terms of technology and understanding, but there are still, as yet, no large randomized, multicenter controlled trials to support the use of widespread genetic screening to predict an individual's response to pain medication (Table 2.1) [113]. Despite intensive research, genetics-based personalized pain therapy has yet to emerge. Monogenetic heredity of pain conditions seems to be restricted to very rare and extreme phenotypes, whereas common phenotypes are very complex and multigenetic. Many common variants, of which only a fraction have been identified so far, produce only minor effects that are sometimes partly canceled out. For most clinical settings and analgesic drug effects, common genetic variants cannot yet be used to provide a relevant prediction of individual pain and analgesic responses. However, genetics has

Table 2.1 List of the most common analgesic drugs and polymorphic genes for which some evidence exists that the pharmacokinetics and/or pharmacodynamics of these analgesic drugs are modulated by functional genetic variants

Analgesic drug	Genes
Opioid analgesics	
Codeine	CYP2D6, UGT2B7, ABCB1, OPRM1
Pentazocine	MC1R
Tramadol	CYP2D6
Morphine	UGT2B7, ABCB1, COMT, OPRM1, CGH1
Methadone	CYP2D6, UGT2B7, ABCB1, OPRM1
Tilidine	CYP3A
Dihydrocodeine, hydrocodone, oxycodone	CYP2D6, ABCB1, COMT, OPRM1
NSAIDs	
Ibuprofen	CYP2C9
Diclofenac	CYP2C9
Naproxen	CYP2C9
Valdecoxib	CYP2C9, PTGS2
Celecoxib	CYP2C9, PTGS2
Parecoxib	CYP3A, CYP2C9, PTGS2

some potential practical uses: CYP2D6, MC1R, and potentially PTGS2 could provide guidance on the right choice of analgesics. We still have a way to go before genetic screening becomes a routine practice and much further still before the contribution of gene-environment interactions is fully realized. However, continued identification of genotypes which are predictive of efficacy of pain management may not only further our understanding of the pain mechanisms but also potentially help discover new potential molecular targets for pain therapy.

References

1. Eichelbaum M, Ingelman-Sundberg M, Evans WE. Pharmacogenomics and individualized drug therapy. Annu Rev Med. 2006;57:119–37.
2. Lotsch J, Geisslinger G, Tegeder I. Genetic modulation of the pharmacological treatment of pain. Pharmacol Ther. 2009;124:168–84.
3. Somogyi AA, Barratt DT, Coller JK. Pharmacogenetics of opioids. Clin Pharmacol Ther. 2007;81:429–44.
4. Stamer UM, Zhang L, Stuber F. Personalized therapy in pain management: where do we stand? Pharmacogenomics. 2010;11:843–64.
5. Lacroix-Fralish ML, Mogil JS. Progress in genetic studies of pain and analgesia. Annu Rev Pharmacol Toxicol. 2009;49:97–121.
6. Landau R. One size does not fit all: genetic variability of mu-opioid receptor and postoperative morphine consumption. Anesthesiology. 2006;105:235–7.
7. Diatchenko L, Nackley AG, Tchivileva IE, Shabalina SA, Maixner W. Genetic architecture of human pain perception. Trends Genet. 2007;23:605–13.
8. Fillingim RB, Wallace MR, Herbstman DM, Ribeiro-Dasilva M, Staud R. Genetic contributions to pain: a review of findings in humans. Oral Dis. 2008;14:673–82.
9. Nagasako EM, Oaklander AL, Dworkin RH. Congenital insensitivity to pain: an update. Pain. 2003;101:213–9.
10. Cox JJ, Reimann F, Nicholas AK, et al. An SCN9A channelopathy causes congenital inability to experience pain. Nature. 2006;444:894–8.
11. Goldberg YP, MacFarlane J, MacDonald ML, et al. Loss-of-function mutations in the Nav1.7 gene underlie congenital indifference to pain in multiple human populations. Clin Genet. 2007;71:311–9.
12. Waxman SG. Neurobiology: a channel sets the gain on pain. Nature. 2006;444:831–2.
13. Waxman SG, Dib-Hajj SD. Erythromelalgia: a hereditary pain syndrome enters the molecular era. Ann Neurol. 2005;57:785–8.
14. Fertleman CR, Baker MD, Parker KA, et al. SCN9A mutations in paroxysmal extreme pain disorder: allelic variants underlie distinct channel defects and phenotypes. Neuron. 2006;52:767–74.
15. Reimann F, Cox JJ, Belfer I, et al. Pain perception is altered by a nucleotide polymorphism in SCN9A. Proc Natl Acad Sci USA. 2010;107:5148–53.
16. Kim H, Mittal DP, Iadarola MJ, Dionne RA. Genetic predictors for acute experimental cold and heat pain sensitivity in humans. J Med Genet. 2006;43:e40.
17. Tegeder I, Costigan M, Griffin RS, et al. GTP cyclohydrolase and tetrahydrobiopterin regulate pain sensitivity and persistence. Nat Med. 2006;12:1269–77.
18. Tegeder I, Adolph J, Schmidt H, Woolf CJ, Geisslinger G, Lotsch J. Reduced hyperalgesia in homozygous carriers of a GTP cyclohydrolase 1 haplotype. Eur J Pain. 2008;12:1069–77.
19. Kim H, Dionne RA. Lack of influence of GTP cyclohydrolase gene (GCH1) variations on pain sensitivity in humans. Mol Pain. 2007;3:6.
20. Lazarev M, Lamb J, Barmada MM, et al. Does the pain-protective GTP cyclohydrolase haplotype significantly alter the pattern or severity of pain in humans with chronic pancreatitis? Mol Pain. 2008;4:58.
21. Campbell CM, Edwards RR, Carmona C, et al. Polymorphisms in the GTP cyclohydrolase gene (GCH1) are associated with ratings of capsaicin pain. Pain. 2009;141:114–8.
22. Lotsch J, Klepstad P, Doehring A, Dale O. A GTP cyclohydrolase 1 genetic variant delays cancer pain. Pain. 2010;148:103–6.
23. Ingelman-Sundberg M, Sim SC, Gomez A, Rodriguez-Antona C. Influence of cytochrome P450 polymorphisms on drug therapies: pharmacogenetic, pharmacoepigenetic and clinical aspects. Pharmacol Ther. 2007;116:496–526.
24. Wang B, Yang LP, Zhang XZ, Huang SQ, Bartlam M, Zhou SF. New insights into the structural characteristics and functional relevance of the human cytochrome P450 2D6 enzyme. Drug Metab Rev. 2009;41:573–643.
25. Zhou SF. Polymorphism of human cytochrome P450 2D6 and its clinical significance: Part I. Clin Pharmacokinet. 2009;48:689–723.
26. Zhou SF, Liu JP, Lai XS. Substrate specificity, inhibitors and regulation of human cytochrome P450 2D6 and implications in drug development. Curr Med Chem. 2009;16:2661–805.
27. Zanger UM, Raimundo S, Eichelbaum M. Cytochrome P450 2D6: overview and update on pharmacology, genetics, biochemistry. Naunyn Schmiedebergs Arch Pharmacol. 2004;369:23–37.
28. Mignat C, Wille U, Ziegler A. Affinity profiles of morphine, codeine, dihydrocodeine and their glucuronides at opioid receptor subtypes. Life Sci. 1995;56:793–9.
29. Thorn CF, Klein TE, Altman RB. Codeine and morphine pathway. Pharmacogenet Genomics. 2009;19:556–8.
30. Zhou SF. Polymorphism of human cytochrome P450 2D6 and its clinical significance: part II. Clin Pharmacokinet. 2009;48:761–804.
31. Ciszkowski C, Madadi P, Phillips MS, Lauwers AE, Koren G. Codeine, ultrarapid-metabolism genotype, and postoperative death. N Engl J Med. 2009;361:827–8.
32. Gasche Y, Daali Y, Fathi M, et al. Codeine intoxication associated with ultrarapid CYP2D6 metabolism. N Engl J Med. 2004;351:2827–31.
33. Koren G, Cairns J, Chitayat D, Gaedigk A, Leeder SJ. Pharmacogenetics of morphine poisoning in a breastfed neonate of a codeine-prescribed mother. Lancet. 2006;368:704.
34. Madadi P, Koren G. Pharmacogenetic insights into codeine analgesia: implications to pediatric codeine use. Pharmacogenomics. 2008;9:1267–84.
35. Madadi P, Koren G, Cairns J, et al. Safety of codeine during breastfeeding: fatal morphine poisoning in the breastfed neonate of a mother prescribed codeine. Can Fam Physician. 2007;53:33–5.
36. Madadi P, Ross CJ, Hayden MR, et al. Pharmacogenetics of neonatal opioid toxicity following maternal use of codeine during breastfeeding: a case-control study. Clin Pharmacol Ther. 2009;85:31–5.
37. Voronov P, Przybylo HJ, Jagannathan N. Apnea in a child after oral codeine: a genetic variant – an ultra-rapid metabolizer. Paediatr Anaesth. 2007;17:684–7.
38. Enggaard TP, Poulsen L, Arendt-Nielsen L, Brosen K, Ossig J, Sindrup SH. The analgesic effect of tramadol after intravenous injection in healthy volunteers in relation to CYP2D6. Anesth Analg. 2006;102:146–50.
39. Poulsen L, Arendt-Nielsen L, Brosen K, Sindrup SH. The hypoalgesic effect of tramadol in relation to CYP2D6. Clin Pharmacol Ther. 1996;60:636–44.
40. Stamer UM, Lehnen K, Hothker F, et al. Impact of CYP2D6 genotype on postoperative tramadol analgesia. Pain. 2003;105:231–8.

41. Stamer UM, Musshoff F, Kobilay M, Madea B, Hoeft A, Stuber F. Concentrations of tramadol and O-desmethyltramadol enantiomers in different CYP2D6 genotypes. Clin Pharmacol Ther. 2007;82:41–7.

42. Stamer UM, Stuber F, Muders T, Musshoff F. Respiratory depression with tramadol in a patient with renal impairment and CYP2D6 gene duplication. Anesth Analg. 2008;107:926–9.

43. Musshoff F, Madea B, Stuber F, Stamer UM. Enantiomeric determination of tramadol and O-desmethyltramadol by liquid chromatography- mass spectrometry and application to postoperative patients receiving tramadol. J Anal Toxicol. 2006;30:463–7.

44. Pedersen RS, Damkier P, Brosen K. Enantioselective pharmacokinetics of tramadol in CYP2D6 extensive and poor metabolizers. Eur J Clin Pharmacol. 2006;62:513–21.

45. Hufschmid E, Theurillat R, Wilder-Smith CH, Thormann W. Characterization of the genetic polymorphism of dihydrocodeine O-demethylation in man via analysis of urinary dihydrocodeine and dihydromorphine by micellar electrokinetic capillary chromatography. J Chromatogr B Biomed Appl. 1996;678:43–51.

46. Wilder-Smith CH, Hufschmid E, Thormann W. The visceral and somatic antinociceptive effects of dihydrocodeine and its metabolite, dihydromorphine. A cross-over study with extensive and quinidine-induced poor metabolizers. Br J Clin Pharmacol. 1998;45:575–81.

47. Kharasch ED, Walker A, Isoherranen N, et al. Influence of CYP3A5 genotype on the pharmacokinetics and pharmacodynamics of the cytochrome P4503A probes alfentanil and midazolam. Clin Pharmacol Ther. 2007;82:410–26.

48. Lotsch J, Skarke C, Wieting J, et al. Modulation of the central nervous effects of levomethadone by genetic polymorphisms potentially affecting its metabolism, distribution, and drug action. Clin Pharmacol Ther. 2006;79:72–89.

49. Zhou SF, Zhou ZW, Huang M. Polymorphisms of human cytochrome P450 2C9 and the functional relevance. Toxicology. 2010;278:165–88. Epub 2009 Aug 26.

50. Rodrigues AD. Impact of CYP2C9 genotype on pharmacokinetics: are all cyclooxygenase inhibitors the same? Drug Metab Dispos. 2005;33:1567–75.

51. Kirchheiner J, Brockmoller J. Clinical consequences of cytochrome P450 2C9 polymorphisms. Clin Pharmacol Ther. 2005;77:1–16.

52. Kirchheiner J, Stormer E, Meisel C, Steinbach N, Roots I, Brockmoller J. Influence of CYP2C9 genetic polymorphisms on pharmacokinetics of celecoxib and its metabolites. Pharmacogenetics. 2003;13:473–80.

53. Kirchheiner J, Meineke I, Freytag G, Meisel C, Roots I, Brockmoller J. Enantiospecific effects of cytochrome P450 2C9 amino acid variants on ibuprofen pharmacokinetics and on the inhibition of cyclooxygenases 1 and 2. Clin Pharmacol Ther. 2002;72:62–75.

54. Bae JW, Kim JH, Choi CI, et al. Effect of CYP2C9*3 allele on the pharmacokinetics of naproxen in Korean subjects. Arch Pharm Res. 2009;32:269–73.

55. Dorado P, Cavaco I, Caceres MC, Piedade R, Ribeiro V, Llerena A. Relationship between CYP2C8 genotypes and diclofenac 5-hydroxylation in healthy Spanish volunteers. Eur J Clin Pharmacol. 2008;64:967–70.

56. Blanco G, Martinez C, Ladero JM, et al. Interaction of CYP2C8 and CYP2C9 genotypes modifies the risk for nonsteroidal anti-inflammatory drugs-related acute gastrointestinal bleeding. Pharmacogenet Genomics. 2008;18:37–43.

57. Agundez JA, Garcia-Martin E, Martinez C. Genetically based impairment in CYP2C8- and CYP2C9-dependent NSAID metabolism as a risk factor for gastrointestinal bleeding: is a combination of pharmacogenomics and metabolomics required to improve personalized medicine? Expert Opin Drug Metab Toxicol. 2009;5:607–20.

58. Ma J, Yang XY, Qiao L, Liang LQ, Chen MH. CYP2C9 polymorphism in non-steroidal anti-inflammatory drugs-induced gastropathy. J Dig Dis. 2008;9:79–83.

59. Vonkeman HE, van de Laar MA, van der Palen J, Brouwers JR, Vermes I. Allele variants of the cytochrome P450 2C9 genotype in white subjects from The Netherlands with serious gastroduodenal ulcers attributable to the use of NSAIDs. Clin Ther. 2006;28:1670–6.

60. Visser LE, van Schaik RH, van Vliet M, et al. Allelic variants of cytochrome P450 2C9 modify the interaction between nonsteroidal anti-inflammatory drugs and coumarin anticoagulants. Clin Pharmacol Ther. 2005;77:479–85.

61. Park HJ, Shinn HK, Ryu SH, Lee HS, Park CS, Kang JH. Genetic polymorphisms in the ABCB1 gene and the effects of fentanyl in Koreans. Clin Pharmacol Ther. 2007;81:539–46.

62. Zwisler ST, Enggaard TP, Noehr-Jensen L, et al. The antinociceptive effect and adverse drug reactions of oxycodone in human experimental pain in relation to genetic variations in the OPRM1 and ABCB1 genes. Fundam Clin Pharmacol. 2010;24:517–24. Epub 2009 Oct 21.

63. Campa D, Gioia A, Tomei A, Poli P, Barale R. Association of ABCB1/MDR1 and OPRM1 gene polymorphisms with morphine pain relief. Clin Pharmacol Ther. 2008;83:559–66.

64. Lotsch J, von Hentig N, Freynhagen R, et al. Cross-sectional analysis of the influence of currently known pharmacogenetic modulators on opioid therapy in outpatient pain centers. Pharmacogenet Genomics. 2009;19:429–36.

65. Coller JK, Barratt DT, Dahlen K, Loennechen MH, Somogyi AA. ABCB1 genetic variability and methadone dosage requirements in opioid-dependent individuals. Clin Pharmacol Ther. 2006;80:682–90.

66. Levran O, O'Hara K, Peles E, et al. ABCB1 (MDR1) genetic variants are associated with methadone doses required for effective treatment of heroin dependence. Hum Mol Genet. 2008;17:2219–27.

67. Beyer A, Koch T, Schroder H, Schulz S, Hollt V. Effect of the A118G polymorphism on binding affinity, potency and agonist-mediated endocytosis, desensitization, and resensitization of the human mu-opioid receptor. J Neurochem. 2004;89:553–60.

68. Margas W, Zubkoff I, Schuler HG, Janicki PK, Ruiz-Velasco V. Modulation of Ca^{2+} channels by heterologously expressed wild-type and mutant human micro-opioid receptors (hMORs) containing the A118G single-nucleotide polymorphism. J Neurophysiol. 2007;97:1058–67.

69. Kroslak T, Laforge KS, Gianotti RJ, Ho A, Nielsen DA, Kreek MJ. The single nucleotide polymorphism A118G alters functional properties of the human mu opioid receptor. J Neurochem. 2007;103:77–87.

70. Tan EC, Lim EC, Teo YY, Lim Y, Law HY, Sia AT. Ethnicity and OPRM variant independently predict pain perception and patient-controlled analgesia usage for post-operative pain. Mol Pain. 2009;5:32.

71. Walter C, Lotsch J. Meta-analysis of the relevance of the OPRM1 118A > G genetic variant for pain treatment. Pain. 2009;146:270–5.

72. Bruehl S, Chung OY, Donahue BS, Burns JW. Anger regulation style, postoperative pain, and relationship to the A118G mu opioid receptor gene polymorphism: a preliminary study. J Behav Med. 2006;29:161–9.

73. Chou WY, Wang CH, Liu PH, Liu CC, Tseng CC, Jawan B. Human opioid receptor A118G polymorphism affects intravenous patient-controlled analgesia morphine consumption after total abdominal hysterectomy. Anesthesiology. 2006;105:334–7.

74. Chou WY, Yang LC, Lu HF, et al. Association of mu-opioid receptor gene polymorphism (A118G) with variations in morphine consumption for analgesia after total knee arthroplasty. Acta Anaesthesiol Scand. 2006;50:787–92.

75. Fillingim RB, Kaplan L, Staud R, et al. The A118G single nucleotide polymorphism of the mu-opioid receptor gene (OPRM1) is associated with pressure pain sensitivity in humans. J Pain. 2005;6:159–67.

76. Klepstad P, Rakvag TT, Kaasa S, et al. The 118 A > G polymorphism in the human micro-opioid receptor gene may increase

morphine requirements in patients with pain caused by malignant disease. Acta Anaesthesiol Scand. 2004;48:1232–9.

77. Oertel BG, Schmidt R, Schneider A, Geisslinger G, Lotsch J. The mu-opioid receptor gene polymorphism 118A > G depletes alfentanil-induced analgesia and protects against respiratory depression in homozygous carriers. Pharmacogenet Genomics. 2006;16:625–36.

78. Sia AT, Lim Y, Lim EC, et al. A118G single nucleotide polymorphism of human mu-opioid receptor gene influences pain perception and patient-controlled intravenous morphine consumption after intrathecal morphine for postcesarean analgesia. Anesthesiology. 2008;109:520–6.

79. Wand GS, McCaul M, Yang X, et al. The mu-opioid receptor gene polymorphism (A118G) alters HPA axis activation induced by opioid receptor blockade. Neuropsychopharmacology. 2002;26:106–14.

80. Ginosar Y, Davidson EM, Meroz Y, Blotnick S, Shacham M, Caraco Y. Mu-opioid receptor (A118G) single-nucleotide polymorphism affects alfentanil requirements for extracorporeal shock wave lithotripsy: a pharmacokinetic-pharmacodynamic study. Br J Anaesth. 2009;103:420–7.

81. Wu WD, Wang Y, Fang YM, Zhou HY. Polymorphism of the micro-opioid receptor gene (OPRM1 118A > G) affects fentanyl-induced analgesia during anesthesia and recovery. Mol Diagn Ther. 2009;13:331–7.

82. Lotsch J, Stuck B, Hummel T. The human mu-opioid receptor gene polymorphism 118A > G decreases cortical activation in response to specific nociceptive stimulation. Behav Neurosci. 2006;120:1218–24.

83. Lotsch J, Freynhagen R, Geisslinger G. Are polymorphisms in the mu-opioid receptor important for opioid therapy? Schmerz. 2005;19:378–82. 384–95.

84. Lotsch J, Geisslinger G. Relevance of frequent mu-opioid receptor polymorphisms for opioid activity in healthy volunteers. Pharmacogenomics J. 2006;6:200–10.

85. Lotsch J, Geisslinger G. Current evidence for a genetic modulation of the response to analgesics. Pain. 2006;121:1–5.

86. Lotsch J, Skarke C, Grosch S, Darimont J, Schmidt H, Geisslinger G. The polymorphism A118G of the human mu-opioid receptor gene decreases the pupil constrictory effect of morphine-6-glucuronide but not that of morphine. Pharmacogenetics. 2002;12:3–9.

87. Lotsch J, Zimmermann M, Darimont J, et al. Does the A118G polymorphism at the mu-opioid receptor gene protect against morphine-6-glucuronide toxicity? Anesthesiology. 2002;97:814–9.

88. Coulbault L, Beaussier M, Verstuyft C, et al. Environmental and genetic factors associated with morphine response in the postoperative period. Clin Pharmacol Ther. 2006;79:316–24.

89. Fukuda K, Hayashida M, Ide S, et al. Association between OPRM1 gene polymorphisms and fentanyl sensitivity in patients undergoing painful cosmetic surgery. Pain. 2009;147:194–201.

90. Huehne K, Leis S, Muenster T, et al. High post surgical opioid requirements in Crohn's disease are not due to a general change in pain sensitivity. Eur J Pain. 2009;13:1036–42.

91. Janicki PK, Schuler G, Francis D, et al. A genetic association study of the functional A118G polymorphism of the human mu-opioid receptor gene in patients with acute and chronic pain. Anesth Analg. 2006;103:1011–7.

92. Hayashida M, Nagashima M, Satoh Y, et al. Analgesic requirements after major abdominal surgery are associated with OPRM1 gene polymorphism genotype and haplotype. Pharmacogenomics. 2008;9:1605–16.

93. Landau R, Kern C, Columb MO, Smiley RM, Blouin JL. Genetic variability of the mu-opioid receptor influences intrathecal fentanyl analgesia requirements in laboring women. Pain. 2008;139:5–14.

94. Reyes-Gibby CC, Shete S, Rakvag T, et al. Exploring joint effects of genes and the clinical efficacy of morphine for cancer pain: OPRM1 and COMT gene. Pain. 2007;130:25–30.

95. Ramchandani VA, Umhau J, Pavon FJ, et al. A genetic determinant of the striatal dopamine response to alcohol in men. Mol Psychiatry. 2011;16:809–17. Epub 2010 May 18.

96. Shabalina SA, Zaykin DV, Gris P, et al. Expansion of the human mu-opioid receptor gene architecture: novel functional variants. Hum Mol Genet. 2009;18:1037–51.

97. Berthele A, Platzer S, Jochim B, et al. COMT Val108/158Met genotype affects the mu-opioid receptor system in the human brain: evidence from ligand-binding, G-protein activation and preproenkephalin mRNA expression. Neuroimage. 2005; 28:185–93.

98. Zubieta JK, Heitzeg MM, Smith YR, et al. COMT val158met genotype affects mu-opioid neurotransmitter responses to a pain stressor. Science. 2003;299:1240–3.

99. Rakvag TT, Klepstad P, Baar C, et al. The Val158Met polymorphism of the human catechol-O-methyltransferase (COMT) gene may influence morphine requirements in cancer pain patients. Pain. 2005;116:73–8.

100. Rakvag TT, Ross JR, Sato H, Skorpen F, Kaasa S, Klepstad P. Genetic variation in the catechol-O-methyltransferase (COMT) gene and morphine requirements in cancer patients with pain. Mol Pain. 2008;4:64.

101. Ross JR, Riley J, Taegetmeyer AB, et al. Genetic variation and response to morphine in cancer patients: catechol-O-methyltransferase and multidrug resistance-1 gene polymorphisms are associated with central side effects. Cancer. 2008;112:1390–403.

102. Nackley AG, Shabalina SA, Lambert JE, et al. Low enzymatic activity haplotypes of the human catechol-O-methyltransferase gene: enrichment for marker SNPs. PLoS One. 2009;4:e5237.

103. Nackley AG, Shabalina SA, Tchivileva IE, et al. Human catechol-O-methyltransferase haplotypes modulate protein expression by altering mRNA secondary structure. Science. 2006;314:1930–3.

104. Mogil JS, Ritchie J, Smith SB, et al. Melanocortin-1 receptor gene variants affect pain and mu-opioid analgesia in mice and humans. J Med Genet. 2005;42:583–7.

105. Mogil JS, Wilson SG, Chesler EJ, et al. The melanocortin-1 receptor gene mediates female-specific mechanisms of analgesia in mice and humans. Proc Natl Acad Sci USA. 2003;100:4867–72.

106. Esser R, Berry C, Du Z, et al. Preclinical pharmacology of lumiracoxib: a novel selective inhibitor of cyclooxygenase-2. Br J Pharmacol. 2005;144:538–50.

107. Cipollone F, Patrono C. Cyclooxygenase-2 polymorphism: putting a brake on the inflammatory response to vascular injury? Arterioscler Thromb Vasc Biol. 2002;22:1516–8.

108. Papafili A, Hill MR, Brull DJ, et al. Common promoter variant in cyclooxygenase-2 represses gene expression: evidence of role in acute-phase inflammatory response. Arterioscler Thromb Vasc Biol. 2002;22:1631–6.

109. Skarke C, Reus M, Schmidt R, et al. The cyclooxygenase 2 genetic variant -765 G > C does not modulate the effects of celecoxib on prostaglandin E2 production. Clin Pharmacol Ther. 2006;80: 621–32.

110. Lee YS, Kim H, Wu TX, Wang XM, Dionne RA. Genetically mediated interindividual variation in analgesic responses to cyclooxygenase inhibitory drugs. Clin Pharmacol Ther. 2006;79: 407–18.

111. Lotsch J, Fluhr K, Neddermayer T, Doehring A, Geisslinger G. The consequence of concomitantly present functional genetic variants for the identification of functional genotype-phenotype associations in pain. Clin Pharmacol Ther. 2009;85:25–30.

112. Kim H, Ramsay E, Lee H, Wahl S, Dionne RA. Genome-wide association study of acute post-surgical pain in humans. Pharmacogenomics. 2009;10:171–9.

113. Lotsch J, Geisslinger G. A critical appraisal of human genotyping for pain therapy. Trends Pharmacol Sci. 2010;31:312–7.

Nonsteroidal Anti-inflammatory Drugs

3

Asokumar Buvanendran

Key Points

- NSAIDs are analgesic compounds with anti-inflammatory activity determined by their ability to decrease prostaglandin formation through inhibition of COX following tissue injury.
- There are two major isoforms of COX. COX-1 is largely constitutive and is responsible for the production of prostaglandins involved in homeostatic processes in the gastric protection, kidney, and platelet aggregation. COX-2 is an inducible form created in the presence of inflammation and is largely responsible for the production of prostaglandins involved in pain and inflammation. Selective COX-2 inhibitors are capable of producing the same analgesic effect of the nonselective NSAIDs but without affecting platelet function and gastropathy.
- Initiation of NSAIDs should occur with the patient education of side effects and should be prescribed with the lowest effective dose and for the shortest duration.
- Combination medications (opioid/NSAID) should occur with patient education of the contents of the combination medication.
- The NSAIDs are extremely effective as part of a multimodal perioperative analgesic regimen. Selective COX-2 inhibitors provide an additional advantage in the perioperative period of not affecting platelet coagulation profile.

Introduction

Nonsteroidal anti-inflammatory drugs (NSAIDs) are the most widely used analgesic medications in the world because of their ability to reduce pain and inflammation [1–3].

A. Buvanendran, M.D. (✉)
Department of Anesthesiology, Rush Medical College, Chicago, IL, USA

Orthopedic Anesthesia, Rush University Medical Center, Chicago, IL, USA
e-mail: asokumar@aol.com

The NSAIDs are structurally diverse, but all have antipyretic, anti-inflammatory, and analgesic properties. The salicylates (aspirin-like medications) have been used to treat pain conditions for thousands of years [4]. Greater than 100 million prescriptions for NSAIDS are written by clinicians in the United States each year, and more than 30 million Americans use prescription or over-the-counter (OTC) NSAIDs regularly [5, 6]. This class of medications contains compounds that are often chemically diverse which are grouped together based on their therapeutic actions. Many of these NSAIDs used today are available as OTC products with greater than 14 million patients use NSAIDs for relief of symptoms associated with arthritis alone [7]. NSAIDs are the most widely prescribed drugs in the world with sales in the United States alone of nearly five billion dollars [3]. They have even demonstrated clear clinical utility in such severe pain states as osteoarthritis, rheumatoid arthritis, and metastatic spread of cancer to bone, usually supplementing rather than replacing the role of opioids [8, 9].

Often labeled as a NSAID, acetaminophen and NSAIDs have important differences such as acetaminophen's weak anti-inflammatory effects and its generally poor ability to inhibit COX in the presence of high concentrations of peroxides, as are found at sites of inflammation [10, 11] nor does it have an adverse effect on platelet function [12] or the gastric mucosa [11].

Mechanism of Action

The mechanism of action of the NSAIDs is inhibition of prostaglandin production from arachidonic acid by either reversible or irreversible acetylation of the cyclooxygenase (Fig. 3.1). Cyclooxygenase (COX) is present in at least two isoforms (COX-1 and COX-2) and is dispersed throughout the body. The COX-1 isoform is constitutive, causing hemostasis, platelet aggregation, and the production of prostacyclin, which is gastric mucosal protective. The inhibition of

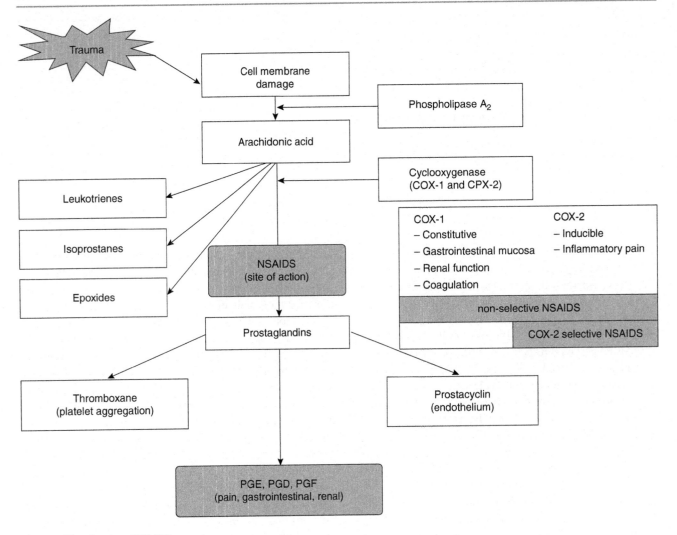

Fig. 3.1 Site of action of NSAIDs

COX-1 isoform may be responsible for the adverse effects related to the nonselective NSAIDs [13]. It is the COX-2 isoform that is induced by pro-inflammatory stimuli and cytokines causing fever, inflammation, and pain and thus the target for antipyresis, anti-inflammation, and analgesia by NSAIDs [4]. COX-1, as the constitutive isoform, is necessary for normal functions and is found in most cell types. COX-1 mediates the production of prostaglandins that are essential in the homeostatic processes in the stomach (gastric protection), kidney, and platelet aggregation. The COX-2 is generally considered to be an inducible enzyme, induced pathologic processes such as fever, pain, and inflammation. COX-2, despite being the inducible isoform, is expressed under normal conditions in a number of tissues, which probably include brain, testis, and kidney. In inflammatory states, COX-2 becomes expressed in macrophages and other cells propagating the inflammatory process [14]. The pain associated with inflammation and prostaglandin production results from the production of prostanoids in the inflamed body tissues that sensitize nerve ending and leads to the sensation of pain [15].

Originally thought of as possessing solely peripheral inhibition of prostaglandin production, more recent research indicates that NSAIDs have peripheral and central mechanisms of action [2, 16, 17]. Peripherally, prostaglandins contribute to hyperalgesia by sensitizing nociceptive sensory nerve endings to other mediators (such as histamine and bradykinin) and by sensitizing nociceptors to respond to non-nociceptive stimuli (e.g., touch) [16, 18]. Peripheral inflammation induces a substantial increase in COX-2 [19] and prostaglandin synthase expression in the central nervous system. Centrally, prostaglandins are recognized to have direct actions at the level of the spinal cord enhancing nociception, notably the terminals of sensory neurons in the dorsal horn [20]. Both COX-1 and COX-2 are expressed constitutively in dorsal root ganglia and spinal dorsal and ventral gray matter, but inhibition of COX-2 and not COX-1 reduces hyperalgesia [21]. Additionally, the pro-inflammatory cytokine interleukin-1beta (IL-1β) plays a major role in inducing COX-2 in local inflammatory cells by activating the transcription factor NF-κB. In the central nervous system (CNS), IL-1β causes increased production of COX-2 and PGE$_2$, producing hyperalgesia, but this is not the result of neural activity arising from the sensory fibers innervating the inflamed tissue or of systemic IL-1β in the plasma [22]. Peripheral inflammation possibly produces other signal molecules that enter the circulation, crossing the blood-brain barrier, and act to elevate IL-1β, leading to COX-2 expression in neurons and nonneuronal cells in many different areas of the spinal cord [22, 23]. At present, evidence suggests that interleukin-6 (IL-6) triggers the formation of IL-1β in the CNS, which in turn causes increased production of COX-2 and PGE$_2$ [22].

There appear to be two forms of input from peripheral-inflamed tissue to the CNS. The first is mediated by electrical activity in sensitized nerve fibers innervating the inflamed area, which signals the location of the inflamed tissue as well as the onset, duration, and nature of any stimuli applied to this tissue [21]. This input is sensitive to peripherally acting COX-2 inhibitors and to neural blockade with local anesthetics [24]. The second is a humoral signal originating from the inflamed tissue, which acts to produce a widespread induction of COX-2 in the CNS.

Pharmacokinetics

NSAIDs are most often administered enterally, but intravenous, intramuscular, rectal, and topical preparations are available. NSAIDs are highly bound to plasma proteins, specifically to albumin (>90 %), and therefore, only a small portion of the circulating drug in plasma exists in the unbound (pharmacologically active) form. The volume of distribution of NSAIDs is low, ranging from 0.1 to 0.3 L/kg, suggesting minimal tissue binding [25]. Most NSAIDs are weak acids with pK_as < 6, and since weak acids will be 99 % ionized two pH units above their pK_a, these anti-inflammatory medications are present in the body mostly in the ionized form. In contrast, the coxibs are nonacidic which may play a role in the favorable tolerability profile.

Absorption

NSAID's pH profile facilitates absorption via the stomach, and the large surface area of the small intestine produces a major absorptive site for orally administered NSAIDs. Most of the NSAIDs are rapidly and completely absorbed from the gastrointestinal tract, with peak concentrations occurring within 1–4 h. The presence of food tends to delay absorption without affecting peak concentration [10]. Ketorolac is one of the few NSAIDs approved for parenteral administration, but most NSAIDs are not available in parenteral forms in the United States. Recently, injectable ibuprofen has been approved as an injectable formulation for pain and fever. Parenteral administration may have the advantage of decreased direct local toxicity in the gastrointestinal tract, but parenteral ketorolac tromethamine does not decrease the risk of adverse events associated with COX-1 inhibition. Topical NSAIDs possess the advantage of providing local action without systemic adverse effects. These medications, such as diclofenac epolamine transdermal patch (Flector®) and diclofenac sodium gel (Voltaren®) are formulated to traverse the skin to reach the adjacent joints and muscles and exert therapeutic activity.

Distribution

The majority of NSAIDs are weakly acidic, highly bound to plasma proteins (albumin), and lipophilic. The relatively low pH of most NSAIDs, in part, determines the distribution too because they are ionized at physiologic pHs. In areas with acidic extracellular pH values, NSAIDs may accumulate (inflamed tissue, gastrointestinal tract, kidneys) [24]. Additionally, the unbound drug is generally considered responsible for pharmacological effects, and the apparent volume of distribution (Vd/F), determined after oral administration, is usually 0.1–0.3 L/kg, which approximates plasma volume [25]. This high-protein binding places only a small portion in the active, unbound form. However, some NSAIDs (i.e., ibuprofen, naproxen, salicylate) have activity that is concentration-dependent because their plasma concentration approaches that of plasma albumin and the Vd/F increases with dose [24]. The high-protein binding (>90 %) of the NSAIDs has particular relevance in the state of hypoalbuminemia or decrease albumin concentrations (e.g., elderly, malnourished). A greater fraction of unbound NSAIDs are present in the plasma which may enhance efficacy, but also increase toxicity.

Elimination

The major metabolic pathway for elimination of NSAIDs is hepatic oxidation or conjugation. The half-lives of NSAIDs vary as active metabolites may be present or the metabolite is the active form when liberated from the prodrug. Also, the elimination of the NSAIDs may determine the dosing frequency as NSAID plasma elimination half-lives vary widely from 0.25 to 70 h [24]. Renal excretion of unmetabolized drug is a minor elimination pathway for most NSAIDs accounting for less than 10 % of the administered dose.

Specific Medications

Salicylates

Aspirin

Acetylsalicylic acid (ASA) is the most widely used analgesic, antipyretic, and anti-inflammatory agent in the world and remains the standard for which all other NSAIDs are compared. Aspirin inhibits the biosynthesis of prostaglandins by means of an irreversible acetylation and consequent inactivation of COX; thus, aspirin inactivates COX permanently. This is an important distinction among the NSAIDs because aspirin's duration action is related to the turnover rate of cyclooxygenases in different target tissues. The duration of action of other NSAIDs, which competitively inhibit the active sites of the COX enzymes, relates more directly to the time course of drug disposition [26]. Platelets are devoid of the ability to produce additional cyclooxygenase; thus, thromboxane synthesis is arrested.

Propionic Acid

Naproxen

Naproxen is a nonprescription NSAID, but a newly formulated controlled-release tablet is available (Naprelan®). It is fully absorbed after enteral administration and has a half-life of 14 h. Peak concentrations in plasma occur within 4–6 h. Naproxen has a volume of distribution of 0.16 L/kg. At therapeutic levels, naproxen is greater than 99 % albumin-bound. Naproxen is extensively metabolized to 6-0-desmethyl naproxen, and both parent and metabolites do not induce metabolizing enzymes. Most of the drug is excreted in the urine, primarily as unchanged naproxen. Naproxen has been used for the treatment of arthritis and other inflammatory diseases. Metabolites of naproxen are excreted almost entirely in the urine. About 30 % of the drug undergoes 6-demethylation, and most of this metabolite, as well as naproxen itself, is excreted as the glucuronide or other conjugates.

Ibuprofen

Ibuprofen is one of the most widely used NSAIDs after ASA, and N-acetyl-p-aminophenol (APAP) in OTC is used for the relief of symptoms of acute pain, fever, and inflammation. Ibuprofen is rapidly absorbed from the upper GI tract, with peak plasma levels achieved about 1–2 h after administration. Ibuprofen is highly bound to plasma proteins and has an estimated volume of distribution of 0.14 L/kg. Ibuprofen is primarily hepatically metabolized (90 %) with less than 10 % excreted unchanged in the urine and bile. and mild-to-moderate pain conditions [27]. Ibuprofen at a dose of 1,200–2,400 mg/day has a predominately analgesic effect for mild-to-moderate pain conditions, with dose of 3,200 mg/day only recommended under continued care of clinical professionals. Even at anti-inflammatory doses of more than 1,600 mg/day, renal side effects are almost exclusively encountered in patients with low intravascular volume and low cardiac output, particularly in the elderly [28]. The effectiveness of ibuprofen has been demonstrated in the treatment of headache and migraine, menstrual pain, and acute postoperative pain [29–31]. The recent injectable formulation will gain increased use for acute pain and fever.

Ketoprofen

The pharmacological properties of ketoprofen are similar to other propionic acid derivative, although the different formulations differ in their release characteristic. Not available in the United States, the optically pure (S) enantiomer (dexketoprofen) is available which is rapidly reabsorbed from the gastrointestinal tract, having a rapid onset of effects. Additionally, capsules release drug in the stomach, whereas the capsule pellets (extended release) are designed to resist dissolution in the low pH of gastric fluid but release drug at a controlled rate in the higher pH environment of the small intestine. Peak plasma levels achieved about 1–2 h after oral administration for the capsules and 6–7 h after administration of the capsule pellets. Ketoprofen has high plasma protein binding (98–99 %) and an estimated volume of distribution of 0.11 L/kg. Ketoprofen is conjugated with glucuronic acid in the liver, and the conjugate is excreted in the urine. The glucuronic acid moiety can be converted back to the parent compound. Thus, the metabolite serves as a potential reservoir for parent drug, and this may be important in persons with renal insufficiency. The extended release ketoprofen is not recommended for the treatment of acute pain because of the release characteristics. Individual patients may show a better response to 300 mg daily as compared to 200 mg, although in well-controlled clinical trials patients on 300 mg did not show greater mean effectiveness. The usual starting dose of ketoprofen is 50 or 75 mg with immediate release capsules every 6–8 h or 200 mg with extended release capsules once daily. The maximum dose is 300 mg daily of immediate release capsules or 200 mg daily of extended release capsules. Ketoprofen has shown statistical superiority over acetaminophen on the time-effect curves for pain relief and pain intensity difference in the treatment of moderate or severe postoperative pain and acute low back pain [32–34].

Oxaprozin

In contrast to the other propionic acid derivatives, oxaprozin peak plasma levels are not achieved until 3–6 h after an oral dose and its half-life of 40–60 h allows for once-daily administration [35]. Oxaprozin is highly bound to plasma proteins and has an estimated volume of distribution of 0.15 L/kg. Oxaprozin is primarily metabolized by the liver, and 65 % of the dose is excreted into the urine and 35 % in the feces as metabolites. Oxaprozin diffuses readily into inflamed synovial tissues after oral administration and is capable of inhibiting both anandamide hydrolase in neurons and NF-kappaB activation in inflammatory cells, which are crucial for synthesis of pro-inflammatory and histotoxic mediators in inflamed joints [36–38].

Acetic Acid

Diclofenac

Diclofenac has COX-2 selectivity, and the selective inhibitor of COX-2 lumiracoxib is an analog of diclofenac. Its potency against COX-2 is substantially greater than that of indomethacin, naproxen, or several other NSAIDs and is similar to celecoxib [10]. Diclofenac is rapidly absorbed after oral administration, but substantial first-pass metabolism of only about 50 % of diclofenac is available systemically. After oral administration, peak serum concentrations are attained within 2–3 h. Diclofenac is highly bound to plasma proteins and has an estimated volume of distribution of 0.12 L/kg. Diclofenac is excreted primarily in the urine (65 %) and 35 % as bile conjugates. Diclofenac is available in two enteral formulations, diclofenac sodium and diclofenac potassium. Diclofenac potassium is formulated to be released and absorbed in the stomach. Diclofenac sodium, usually distributed in enteric-coated tablets, resists dissolution in low-pH gastric environments, releasing instead in the duodenum [39]. Hepatotoxicity, elevated transaminases, may occur, and measurements of transaminases should be measured during therapy with diclofenac. Other formulations of diclofenac include topical gels (Voltaren® Gel) and transdermal patches (Flector® Patch). Additionally, diclofenac is available in a parenteral formulation for infusion (Voltarol® Ampoules), and more recently, a formulation for intravenous bolus has been developed (diclofenac sodium injection [DIC075V; Dyloject®]). Uniquely, diclofenac accumulates in synovial fluid after oral administration [40], which may explain why its duration of therapeutic effect is considerably longer than the plasma half-life of 1–2 h. Oral preparations have been shown to provide significant analgesia in the postoperative period for adults experiencing moderate or severe pain following a surgical procedure [41].

The transdermal application of diclofenac has also shown efficacy in the treatment of musculoskeletal disorders including ankle sprains, epicondylitis, and knee osteoarthritis [42, 43]. The advantage of the transdermal formulation is the lack of appreciable systemic absorption and accumulation of the medication at the site of application, thereby providing local pain relief. In comparison to enteral delivery, topical application of diclofenac provides analgesia by peripheral activity and not central mediation.

Etodolac

Etodolac has some degree of COX-2 selectivity conferring less gastric irritation compared with other NSAIDs [44]. The analgesic effect of full doses of etodolac is longer than that of aspirin, lasting up to 8 h. After oral administration, peak serum concentrations of 16 and 25 mg/L are attained within 2 h of administering 200 and 400 mg, respectively. Etodolac is highly bound to plasma proteins and has an estimated volume of distribution of 0.4 L/kg. Etodolac is excreted primarily in the urine, and 60 % of a dose is recovered within 24 h. Greater than 60 % of the metabolites are hydroxylated with glucuronic conjugation. The half-life of etodolac is approximately 7 h in healthy subjects. When compared with other NSAIDs, etodolac 300 and 400 mg daily has tended to be more effective than aspirin 3–4 g daily and was similar in efficacy to sulindac 400 mg daily [10]. Clinical doses of 200–300 mg twice a day for the relief of low back or shoulder pain have been equated to analgesia with naproxen 500 mg twice a day [45]. In postsurgical pain, etodolac 100–200 mg was approximately equivalent to aspirin 650 mg in providing pain relief, although etodolac had a longer duration of action [46].

Indomethacin

It is a nonselective COX inhibitor introduced in 1963, but has fallen out of favor with the advent of safer alternatives. Indomethacin is a more potent inhibitor of the cyclooxygenases than is aspirin, but patient intolerance generally limits its use to short-term dosing. Oral indomethacin has excellent bioavailability. Peak concentrations occur 1–2 h after dosing. Indomethacin is 90 % bound to plasma proteins and tissues. The concentration of the drug in the CSF is low, but its concentration in synovial fluid is equal to that in plasma within 5 h of administration [10]. Complaints associated with gastrointestinal irritation are common, including diarrhea, and ulcerative lesions are a contraindication to indomethacin use. Indomethacin has FDA approval for closure of persistent patent ductus arteriosus, but side effect profile limits other uses.

Ketorolac

Ketorolac Tromethamine is a NSAID with activity at COX-1 and COX-2 enzymes thus blocking prostaglandin production. After oral administration, peak serum concentrations are attained within 1–2 h. Ketorolac is highly bound to plasma proteins and has an estimated volume of distribution of 0.28 L/kg. Ketorolac is excreted primarily in the urine and has a half-life of approximately 5–6 h in healthy subjects.

Administration of ketorolac is available for enteral, ophthalmic, and parenteral delivery and is the only parenteral NSAID currently available in the United States. Ketorolac has been utilized to treat mild-to-severe pain following major surgical procedures including general abdominal surgery, gynecologic surgery, orthopedic surgery, and dentistry. Multiple studies have investigated the analgesic potency of ketorolac, and in animal models, the analgesic potency has be estimated to be between 180 and 800 times that of aspirin [47, 48]. When compared to morphine, ketorolac 30 mg intramuscular (IM) has been shown to be equivalent to 12 mg morphine IM and 100 mg meperidine IM [49]. It was observed that the mean values for total body clearance of ketorolac were decreased by about 50 % and that the half-life was approximately doubled in patients with renal impairment compared with healthy control subjects [50], and it may precipitate or exacerbate renal failure in hypovolemic, elderly, or especially those with underlying renal dysfunction. Therefore, ketorolac is recommended for limited use (3–5 days). Recently, intranasal route of administration of ketorolac (Sprix™) has been approved by the FDA for acute pain. The CSF penetration of this compound via the nasal route should be superior.

Nabumetone

Nabumetone is a prodrug, which undergoes hepatic biotransformation to the active component, 6-methoxy-2-naphthylacetic acid (6MNA), that has some degree of COX-2 selectivity conferring less gastric irritation compared with other NSAIDs [51]. Nabumetone is highly bound to plasma proteins and has an estimated volume of distribution of 0.68 L/kg. Nabumetone is excreted primarily in the urine and has a half-life of approximately 20–24 h in healthy subjects enabling single-daily dosing. When compared with other NSAIDs, nabumetone has tended to show efficacy [52] and tolerability in the treatment of arthritis [53, 54].

Anthranilic Acid

Mefenamic Acid

Peak serum concentrations are attained within 2–4 h and a half-life of 3–4 h. Mefenamic acid has been associated with severe pancytopenia and many other side effects. Hence, therapy is not to be for more than 1 week [55].

Meloxicam

The enolic acid derivative shows nonselectivity, except for meloxicam which shows relative COX-2 selectivity. For example, meloxicam shows dose-dependent COX selectivity, where 7.5 mg is more selective for COX-2 while at 15 mg meloxicam becomes less selective [56]. After oral administration, peak serum concentrations are attained within 5–10 h after administration. Meloxicam is highly bound to plasma proteins and has an estimated half-life of approximately 15–20 h in healthy subjects.

COX-2 Inhibitors

COX-2 inhibitors (celecoxib, rofecoxib, and valdecoxib) were approved for use in the United States and Europe, but both rofecoxib and valdecoxib have now been withdrawn from the market due to their adverse event profile. Recently, parecoxib and etoricoxib have been approved in Europe. The newest drug in the class, lumiracoxib, is under consideration for approval in Europe. Upon administration, most of the coxibs are distributed widely throughout the body with celecoxib possessing an increased lipophilicity enabling transport into the CNS. Despite these subtle differences, all of the coxibs achieve sufficient brain concentrations to have a central analgesic effect [57] and all reduce prostaglandin formation in inflamed joints. The estimated half-lives of these medications vary (2–6 h for lumiracoxib, 6–12 h for celecoxib and valdecoxib, and 20–26 h for etoricoxib). Likewise, the relative degree of selectivity for COX-2 inhibition is lumiracoxib = etoricoxib > valdecoxib = rofecoxib >> celecoxib [10].

Celecoxib

Currently, celecoxib is the only selective COX-2 inhibitor available in the United States. After oral administration, peak serum concentrations of celecoxib are attained 2–3 h after administration. Celecoxib is highly bound to plasma proteins, is excreted primarily by hepatic metabolism, and has a half-life of approximately 11 h in healthy subjects. Celecoxib does not interfere with platelet aggregation; thus, perioperative administration can be conducted as part of a multimodal analgesic regimen without increased risk of bleeding. Additionally, NSAID-induced GI complications are one of the most common drug-related serious adverse events, but celecoxib preferentially inhibits the inducible COX-2 isoform and not the constitutive COX-1 isoform thus conferring some gastroprotective effect.

The efficacy and tolerability of celecoxib has been studied in multiple studies. Celecoxib has demonstrated effectiveness in both placebo and active-control (or comparator) clinical trials in patients with osteoarthritis, rheumatoid arthritis, and postoperative pain relief [58–60].

Etoricoxib

Etoricoxib is a second-generation, highly selective cyclooxygenase 2 (COX-2) inhibitor with anti-inflammatory and analgesic properties [61]. It shows dose-dependent inhibition of COX-2 across the therapeutic dose range, without inhibition of COX-1, does not inhibit gastric prostaglandin synthesis and has no effect on platelet function [62]. Etoricoxib shows 106-fold selectivity for COX-2 over COX-1 [63], compared with 7.6-fold selectivity observed with celecoxib [62, 63].

Acetaminophen

Acetaminophen (paracetamol – APAP) is an analgesic and antipyretic medication that produces its analgesic effect by inhibiting central prostaglandin synthesis with minimal inhibition of peripheral prostaglandin synthesis [10, 11]. After oral administration, peak serum concentrations are attained within 0.5–3 h. A small portion of acetaminophen is bound to plasma proteins (10–50 %) and has an estimated volume of distribution of 0.95 L/kg. Acetaminophen is eliminated from the body primarily by formation of glucuronide and sulfate conjugates in a dose-dependent manner. The half-life of acetaminophen is approximately 2–3 h in healthy subjects. As previously stated, acetaminophen and NSAIDs have important differences such as acetaminophen's weak anti-inflammatory effects and its generally poor ability to inhibit COX in the presence of high concentrations of peroxides, as are found at sites of inflammation [10, 11] nor does it have an adverse effect on platelet function [12] or the gastric mucosa [11]. It is absorbed rapidly, with peak plasma levels seen within 30 min to 1 h, and is metabolized in the liver by conjugation and hydroxylation to inactive metabolites and has duration of action of 4–6 h [64, 65]. Paracetamol is perhaps the safest and most cost-effective non-opioid analgesic when it is administered in analgesic doses [66]. Paracetamol is available in parenteral form as propacetamol, and 1 g of propacetamol provides 0.5 g paracetamol after hydrolysis [67]. Propacetamol is widely used in many countries other than the United States and has shown to reduce opioid consumption by about 35–45 % [68] in postoperative pain studies [68, 69] including after cardiac surgery [70].

Safety, Toxicity, and Adverse Effects

Although NSAIDs are the most widely used OTC medications, with a long history of use, research, and medication advancements, NSAIDs remain as a source of adverse effects. NSAIDs not only share therapeutic actions but also similar adverse effects that include GI ulceration and bleeding, disturbance of platelet function, sodium and water retention, nephrotoxicity, and hypersensitivity reactions [71]. The adverse effects range from minor (e.g., nausea, gastric irritation, dizziness) to major (e.g., allergic reaction, gastrointestinal, renal and coagulation derangements, and delay in bone healing) in acute use. Chronic use of these medications may increase minor or major adverse effects. The three most common adverse drug reactions to NSAIDs are gastrointestinal,

dermatological, and neuropsychiatric, the last one oddly not being age related [55, 72].

Gastrointestinal

Gastrointestinal bleeding is one of the most frequently reported significant complications of NSAID use. The effects of NSAIDs on gastric mucosa have been estimated to occur in 30–40 % of users [73]. NSAIDs affect the GI tract with symptoms of gastric distress alone and through actual damage with ulceration. Dyspepsia has been shown to have an annual prevalence with NSAID use of about 15 % [55]. One review estimated 7,000 deaths and 70,000 hospitalizations per year in the USA among NSAID users. Among rheumatoid arthritis patients, an estimated 20,000 hospitalizations and 2,600 deaths per year are related to NSAID GI toxicity [55, 74]. Evidence of the association between NSAIDs and gastropathy accrued in the 1970s with the increased use of endoscopy and the introduction of several new NSAIDs [55, 75].

The risk of developing GI complications with the continued and long-term use of NSAIDs is now well recognized. Likewise, risk factors have been identified for the development of NSAID-induced gastropathy. Risk factors include history of GI complications, high-dose or multiple NSAIDs, advanced age, concomitant corticosteroid use, and alcohol use [76]. Administration of GI protective agents (H_2-receptor antagonist and proton pump inhibitors), may attenuate the complications associated with long-term NSAID use. Other strategies include the use of selective COX-2 inhibitors, such as celecoxib, which are less ulcerogenic compared with nonselective NSAIDs.

Renal

NSAIDs can decrease renal function and cause renal failure. Renal impairment has been reported to occur in as many as 18 % of patients using ibuprofen, whereas acute renal failure has been shown to occur in about 6 % of patients using NSAIDs in another study [55, 77, 78]. The proposed mechanism is reduction in prostaglandin production leading to reduced renal blood flow with subsequent medullary ischemia that may result from NSAID use in susceptible individuals [79]. Acute renal failure may occur with any COX-2-selective or nonselective NSAID [80]. The risk factors for NSAID-induced renal toxicity include chronic NSAID use, high-dose or multiple NSAIDs, volume depletion, congestive heart failure, vascular disease, hyperreninemia, shock, sepsis, systemic lupus erythematosus, hepatic disease, sodium depletion, nephrotic syndrome, diuresis, concomitant drug therapy (diuretics, ACE inhibitors, beta blockers, potassium supplements), and advanced age [81].

Hepatic

Hepatotoxicity seems to be a rare complication of most NSAIDs [82]. Hepatic-related side effects of NSAIDs have been reported to occur in 3 % of patients receiving the drugs [83]. In contrast, paracetamol has a recognized potential for hepatotoxicity and is thought to be responsible for at least 42 % of acute liver failure cases observed and has become the most common cause of acute liver failure in the United States [27]. Most of these cases were due to intentional or unintentional overdose with 79 % reported taking the analgesic specifically for pain and 38 % were taking two different preparations of the drug simultaneously [27]. Acetaminophen is almost entirely metabolized in the liver, and the minor metabolites are responsible for the hepatotoxicity seen in overdoses [84]. Mechanisms of acetaminophen hepatotoxicity include depletion of hepatocyte glutathione, accumulation of the toxic metabolite NAPQI, mitochondrial dysfunction, and alteration of innate immunity [85]. Risk factors include concomitant depression, chronic pain, alcohol or narcotic use, and/or take several preparations simultaneously [27]. The lowest dose of acetaminophen to cause hepatotoxicity is believed to be between 125 and 150 mg/kg [86, 87]. The threshold dose to cause hepatotoxicity is 10–15 g of acetaminophen for adults and 150 mg/kg for children [86, 88]. The most recognized dosing limit is 4 g/24 h in healthy adult patients. Clinicians should continually inquire medication usage as many patients are not aware that prescription narcotic–acetaminophen combinations contain acetaminophen and unintentionally combine these medications with OTC acetaminophen.

Cardiovascular

The inhibition of cyclooxygenase reduces the production of thromboxane and prostacyclin. Thromboxane functions as a vasoconstrictor and facilitates platelet aggregation. Thromboxane A_2 (TXA$_2$), produced by activated platelets, has prothrombotic properties, stimulating activation of new platelets as well as increasing platelet aggregation. Endothelium-derived prostacyclin (PGI$_2$) functions in concert with thromboxane, primarily inhibiting platelet activation, thus, preventing the formation of a hemostatic plug. Nonselective NSAIDs inhibit both the COX-1 and COX-2 thus reducing the production of thromboxane and prostacyclin. The nucleated endothelial cells are able to regenerate prostacyclin, but the anucleated platelets are incapable of regenerating this enzyme. The imbalance of thromboxane and prostacyclin may lead a thrombogenic situation. Low-dose aspirin (81 mg/day) has been advocated as a platelet aggregation inhibitor, thus reducing thrombotic events related to platelet aggregation. Aspirin at larger doses 1.5–2 g/day has been described to result in a paradoxical thrombogenic effect [2, 89]. The analgesic effects of aspirin are usually at higher doses, possibly negating the antithrombotic effects of aspirin. Celecoxib is an anti-inflammatory agent that primarily inhibits COX-2, an inducible enzyme not expressed in platelets and thus does not interfere with platelet aggregation. A systematic review and meta-analysis assessing the risks of serious cardiovascular events with selective COX-2 inhibitors and nonselective NSAIDs indicates that rofecoxib was associated with a significant dose-related risk (relative risk, 2.19 [>25 mg daily]) of serious cardiovascular events during the first month of treatment although celecoxib was not associated with an elevated risk. Among the nonselective NSAIDs, diclofenac had the highest risk (relative risk, 1.40), ibuprofen (relative risk, 1.07) and piroxicam (relative risk, 1.06), and naproxen (relative risk, 0.97) [90].

Summary

NSAIDs are useful analgesics for many pain states, especially those involving inflammation. Acetaminophen provides comparable analgesic effects but lacks clinically useful anti-inflammatory activity. The COX-2 selective inhibitors are continuing its development to attenuate the GI and hematological side effects of traditional NSAIDs. Overall, NSAIDs have similar pharmacokinetic characteristics: they are rapidly and extensively absorbed after oral administration, tissue distribution is very limited, they are metabolized extensively in the liver with little dependence on renal elimination, and therefore, the choice of NSAID may be determined by the efficacy and side-effect profile. This chapter has provided an overview of the NSAIDs and acetaminophen, but there remains research to be conducted in newer and more efficacious NSAIDs, adverse effect preventative strategies.

References

1. De Ledinghen V, Heresbach D, Fourdan O, et al. Anti-inflammatory drugs and variceal bleeding: a case-control study. Gut. 999;44(2):270–3.
2. Godal HC, Eika C, Dybdahl JH, et al. Aspirin and bleeding-time. Lancet. 1979;1(8128):1236.
3. Laine L. Approaches to nonsteroidal anti-inflammatory drug use in the high-risk patient. Gastroenterology. 2001;120(3):594–606.
4. Vane JR, Botting RM. Mechanism of action of nonsteroidal anti-inflammatory drugs. Am J Med. 1998;104(3A):2S–8. discussion 21S–22S.
5. Singh G. Gastrointestinal complications of prescription and over-the-counter nonsteroidal anti-inflammatory drugs: a view from the ARAMIS database. Arthritis, rheumatism, and aging medical information system. Am J Ther. 2000;7(2):115–21.
6. Jouzeau JY, Terlain B, Abid A, et al. Cyclo-oxygenase isoenzymes. How recent findings affect thinking about nonsteroidal anti-inflammatory drugs. Drugs. 1997;53(4):563–82.

7. Talley NJ, Evans JM, Fleming KC, et al. Nonsteroidal antiinflammatory drugs and dyspepsia in the elderly. Dig Dis Sci. 1995;40(6):1345–50.

8. Tannenbaum H, Bombardier C, Davis P, et al. An evidence-based approach to prescribing nonsteroidal antiinflammatory drugs. Third Canadian Consensus Conference. J Rheumatol. 2006;33(1):140–57.

9. Eisenberg E, Berkey CS, Carr DB, et al. Efficacy and safety of nonsteroidal antiinflammatory drugs for cancer pain: a meta-analysis. J Clin Oncol. 1994;12(12):2756–65.

10. Burke Anne SE, FitzGerald Garret A. Chapter 26: Analgesic-antipyretic and antiinflammatory agents; pharmacotherapy of gout. In: Goodman & Gilman's the pharmacological basis of therapeutics. 2011. [11th: http://www.accessmedicine.com/content.aspx?aID=942390]. Accessed 11 Feb 2010.

11. Graham GG, Scott KF. Mechanism of action of paracetamol. Am J Ther. 2005;12(1):46–55.

12. Munsterhjelm E, Munsterhjelm NM, Niemi TT, et al. Dose-dependent inhibition of platelet function by acetaminophen in healthy volunteers. Anesthesiology. 2005;103(4):712–17.

13. Lanza FL. A review of gastric ulcer and gastroduodenal injury in normal volunteers receiving aspirin and other non-steroidal anti-inflammatory drugs. Scand J Gastroenterol Suppl. 1989;163:24–31.

14. Seibert K, Zhang Y, Leahy K, et al. Pharmacological and biochemical demonstration of the role of cyclooxygenase 2 in inflammation and pain. Proc Natl Acad Sci USA. 1994;91(25):12013–17.

15. Gordon SM, Brahim JS, Rowan J, et al. Peripheral prostanoid levels and nonsteroidal anti-inflammatory drug analgesia: replicate clinical trials in a tissue injury model. Clin Pharmacol Ther. 2002;72(2):175–83.

16. McCormack K. The spinal actions of nonsteroidal anti-inflammatory drugs and the dissociation between their anti-inflammatory and analgesic effects. Drugs. 1994;47 Suppl 5:28–45; discussion 46–47.

17. Cashman JN. The mechanisms of action of NSAIDs in analgesia. Drugs. 1996;52 Suppl 5:13–23.

18. Bjorkman R. Central antinociceptive effects of non-steroidal anti-inflammatory drugs and paracetamol. Experimental studies in the rat. Acta Anaesthesiol Scand Suppl. 1995;103:1–44.

19. Kroin JS, Buvanendran A, McCarthy RJ, et al. Cyclooxygenase-2 inhibition potentiates morphine antinociception at the spinal level in a postoperative pain model. Reg Anesth Pain Med. 2002;27(5):451–5.

20. Vasko MR. Prostaglandin-induced neuropeptide release from spinal cord. Prog Brain Res. 1995;104:367–80.

21. Svensson CI, Yaksh TL. The spinal phospholipase-cyclooxygenase-prostanoid cascade in nociceptive processing. Annu Rev Pharmacol Toxicol. 2002;42:553–83.

22. Samad TA, Moore KA, Sapirstein A, et al. Interleukin-1beta-mediated induction of Cox-2 in the CNS contributes to inflammatory pain hypersensitivity. Nature. 2001;410(6827):471–5.

23. Samad TA, Sapirstein A, Woolf CJ. Prostanoids and pain: unraveling mechanisms and revealing therapeutic targets. Trends Mol Med. 2002;8(8):390–6.

24. Brune K, Glatt M, Graf P. Mechanisms of action of anti-inflammatory drugs. Gen Pharmacol. 1976;7(1):27–33.

25. Davies NM, Skjodt NM. Choosing the right nonsteroidal anti-inflammatory drug for the right patient: a pharmacokinetic approach. Clin Pharmacokinet. 2000;38(5):377–92.

26. Munir MA, Enany N, Zhang JM. Nonopioid analgesics. Med Clin North Am. 2007;91(1):97–111.

27. Larson AM, Polson J, Fontana RJ, et al. Acetaminophen-induced acute liver failure: results of a United States multicenter, prospective study. Hepatology. 2005;42(6):1364–72.

28. Mann JF, Goerig M, Brune K, et al. Ibuprofen as an over-the-counter drug: is there a risk for renal injury? Clin Nephrol. 1993;39(1):1–6.

29. Silver S, Gano D, Gerretsen P. Acute treatment of paediatric migraine: a meta-analysis of efficacy. J Paediatr Child Health. 2008;44(1–2):3–9.

30. Derry C, Derry S, Moore RA, et al. Single dose oral ibuprofen for acute postoperative pain in adults. Cochrane Database Syst Rev. 2009;3:CD001548.

31. Grimes DA, Hubacher D, Lopez LM, et al. Non-steroidal anti-inflammatory drugs for heavy bleeding or pain associated with intra-uterine-device use. Cochrane Database Syst Rev. 2006;4:CD006034.

32. Olson NZ, Otero AM, Marrero I, et al. Onset of analgesia for liqui-gel ibuprofen 400 mg, acetaminophen 1000 mg, ketoprofen 25 mg, and placebo in the treatment of postoperative dental pain. J Clin Pharmacol. 2001;41(11):1238–47.

33. Barden J, Derry S, McQuay HJ, et al. Single dose oral ketoprofen and dexketoprofen for acute postoperative pain in adults. Cochrane Database Syst Rev. 2009;4:CD007355.

34. Moore RA, Barden J. Systematic review of dexketoprofen in acute and chronic pain. BMC Clin Pharmacol. 2008;8:11.

35. Davies NM. Clinical pharmacokinetics of oxaprozin. Clin Pharmacokinet. 1998;35(6):425–36.

36. Kean WF. Oxaprozin: kinetic and dynamic profile in the treatment of pain. Curr Med Res Opin. 2004;20(8):1275–7.

37. Kurowski M, Thabe H. The transsynovial distribution of oxaprozin. Agents Actions. 1989;27(3–4):458–60.

38. Dallegri F, Bertolotto M, Ottonello L. A review of the emerging profile of the anti-inflammatory drug oxaprozin. Expert Opin Pharmacother. 2005;6(5):777–85.

39. Olson NZ, Sunshine A, Zighelboim I, et al. Onset and duration of analgesia of diclofenac potassium in the treatment of postepisiotomy pain. Am J Ther. 1997;4(7–8):239–46.

40. Davies NM, Anderson KE. Clinical pharmacokinetics of diclofenac. Therapeutic insights and pitfalls. Clin Pharmacokinet. 1997;33(3):184–213.

41. Derry P, Derry S, Moore RA, et al. Single dose oral diclofenac for acute postoperative pain in adults. Cochrane Database Syst Rev. 2009;2:CD004768.

42. Bruhlmann P, de Vathaire F, Dreiser RL, et al. Short-term treatment with topical diclofenac epolamine plaster in patients with symptomatic knee osteoarthritis: pooled analysis of two randomised clinical studies. Curr Med Res Opin. 2006;22(12):2429–38.

43. Petersen B, Rovati S. Diclofenac epolamine (Flector) patch: evidence for topical activity. Clin Drug Investig. 2009;29(1):1–9.

44. Warner TD, Giuliano F, Vojnovic I, et al. Nonsteroid drug selectivities for cyclo-oxygenase-1 rather than cyclo-oxygenase-2 are associated with human gastrointestinal toxicity: a full in vitro analysis. Proc Natl Acad Sci USA. 1999;96(13):7563–8.

45. Pena M. Etodolac: analgesic effects in musculoskeletal and postoperative pain. Rheumatol Int. 1990;10(Suppl):9–16.

46. Lynch S, Brogden RN. Etodolac. A preliminary review of its pharmacodynamic activity and therapeutic use. Drugs. 1986;31(4):288–300.

47. Gillis JC, Brogden RN. Ketorolac. A reappraisal of its pharmacodynamic and pharmacokinetic properties and therapeutic use in pain management. Drugs. 1997;53(1):139–88.

48. Buckley MM, Brogden RN. Ketorolac. A review of its pharmacodynamic and pharmacokinetic properties, and therapeutic potential. Drugs. 1990;39(1):86–109.

49. Morley-Forster P, Newton PT, Cook MJ. Ketorolac and indomethacin are equally efficacious for the relief of minor postoperative pain. Can J Anaesth. 1993;40(12):1126–30.

50. Resman-Targoff BH. Ketorolac: a parenteral nonsteroidal antiinflammatory drug. DICP. 1990;24(11):1098–104.

51. Laneuville O, Breuer DK, Dewitt DL, et al. Differential inhibition of human prostaglandin endoperoxide H synthases-1 and -2 by nonsteroidal anti-inflammatory drugs. J Pharmacol Exp Ther. 1994;271(2):927–34.

52. Lanier BG, Turner Jr RA, Collins RL, et al. Evaluation of nabumetone in the treatment of active adult rheumatoid arthritis. Am J Med. 1987;83(4B):40–3.

53. Appelrouth DJ, Baim S, Chang RW, et al. Comparison of the safety and efficacy of nabumetone and aspirin in the treatment of osteoarthritis in adults. Am J Med. 1987;83(4B):78–81.

54. Krug H, Broadwell LK, Berry M, et al. Tolerability and efficacy of nabumetone and naproxen in the treatment of rheumatoid arthritis. Clin Ther. 2000;22(1):40–52.

55. Katz JA. NSAIDs and COX-2-selective inhibitors. In: Benzon HT, Raja SN, Molloy RE, Liu SS, Fishman SM, editors. Essentials of pain medicine and regional anesthesia. 2nd ed. Philadelphia: Elsevier Churchill Livingstone; 2005. p. 141–58.

56. Patoia L, Santucci L, Furno P, et al. A 4-week, double-blind, parallel-group study to compare the gastrointestinal effects of meloxicam 7.5 mg, meloxicam 15 mg, piroxicam 20 mg and placebo by means of faecal blood loss, endoscopy and symptom evaluation in healthy volunteers. Br J Rheumatol. 1996;35 Suppl 1:61–7.

57. Buvanendran A, Kroin JS, Tuman KJ, et al. Cerebrospinal fluid and plasma pharmacokinetics of the cyclooxygenase 2 inhibitor rofecoxib in humans: single and multiple oral drug administration. Anesth Analg. 2005;100(5):1320–4, table of contents.

58. Derry S, Barden J, McQuay HJ, et al. Single dose oral celecoxib for acute postoperative pain in adults. Cochrane Database Syst Rev. 2008;4:CD004233.

59. Singh G, Fort JG, Goldstein JL, et al. Celecoxib versus naproxen and diclofenac in osteoarthritis patients: SUCCESS-I study. Am J Med. 2006;119(3):255–66.

60. Towheed TE, Maxwell L, Judd MG, et al. Acetaminophen for osteoarthritis. Cochrane Database Syst Rev. 2006;1:CD004257.

61. Takemoto JK, Reynolds JK, Remsberg CM, et al. Clinical pharmacokinetic and pharmacodynamic profile of etoricoxib. Clin Pharmacokinet. 2008;47(11):703–20.

62. Croom KF, Siddiqui MA. Etoricoxib: a review of its use in the symptomatic treatment of osteoarthritis, rheumatoid arthritis, ankylosing spondylitis and acute gouty arthritis. Drugs. 2009;69(11):1513–32.

63. Riendeau D, Percival MD, Brideau C, et al. Etoricoxib (MK-0663): preclinical profile and comparison with other agents that selectively inhibit cyclooxygenase-2. J Pharmacol Exp Ther. 2001;296(2):558–66.

64. Strassels SA, McNicol E, Suleman R. Postoperative pain management: a practical review, part 1. Am J Health Syst Pharm. 2005;62(18):1904–16.

65. Burke Anne SE, FitzGerald Garret A. Analgesic-antipyretic and antiinflammatory agents; pharmacotherapy of gout. 11th ed. New York: The McGraw-Hill Companies, Inc.; 2006.

66. White PF. The changing role of non-opioid analgesic techniques in the management of postoperative pain. Anesth Analg. 2005;101(5 Suppl):S5–22.

67. Flouvat B, Leneveu A, Fitoussi S, et al. Bioequivalence study comparing a new paracetamol solution for injection and propacetamol after single intravenous infusion in healthy subjects. Int J Clin Pharmacol Ther. 2004;42(1):50–7.

68. Delbos A, Boccard E. The morphine-sparing effect of propacetamol in orthopedic postoperative pain. J Pain Symptom Manage. 1995;10(4):279–86.

69. Sinatra RS, Jahr JS, Reynolds LW, et al. Efficacy and safety of single and repeated administration of 1 gram intravenous acetaminophen injection (paracetamol) for pain management after major orthopedic surgery. Anesthesiology. 2005;102(4):822–31.

70. Cattabriga I, Pacini D, Lamazza G, et al. Intravenous paracetamol as adjunctive treatment for postoperative pain after cardiac surgery: a double blind randomized controlled trial. Eur J Cardiothorac Surg. 2007;32(3):527–31.

71. Laffi G, La Villa G, Pinzani M, et al. Arachidonic acid derivatives and renal function in liver cirrhosis. Semin Nephrol. 1997;17(6):530–48.

72. Clark DW, Ghose K. Neuropsychiatric reactions to nonsteroidal anti-inflammatory drugs (NSAIDs). The New Zealand experience. Drug Saf. 1992;7(6):460–5.

73. Garcia Rodriguez LA. Nonsteroidal antiinflammatory drugs, ulcers and risk: a collaborative meta-analysis. Semin Arthritis Rheum. 1997;26(6 Suppl 1):16–20.

74. Fries JF. NSAID gastropathy: the second most deadly rheumatic disease? Epidemiology and risk appraisal. J Rheumatol Suppl. 1991;28:6–10.

75. Wallace JL. Nonsteroidal anti-inflammatory drugs and gastroenteropathy: the second hundred years. Gastroenterology. 1997;112(3):1000–16.

76. Fries JF, Williams CA, Bloch DA, et al. Nonsteroidal anti-inflammatory drug-associated gastropathy: incidence and risk factor models. Am J Med. 1991;91(3):213–22.

77. Murray MD, Brater DC. Adverse effects of nonsteroidal anti-inflammatory drugs on renal function. Ann Intern Med. 1990;112(8):559–60.

78. Corwin HL, Bonventre JV. Renal insufficiency associated with nonsteroidal anti-inflammatory agents. Am J Kidney Dis. 1984;4(2):147–52.

79. Nies AS. Renal effects of nonsteroidal anti-inflammatory drugs. Agents Actions Suppl. 1988;24:95–106.

80. Vonkeman HE, van de Laar MA. Nonsteroidal anti-inflammatory drugs: adverse effects and their prevention. Semin Arthritis Rheum. 2010;39(4):294–312.

81. Taber SS, Mueller BA. Drug-associated renal dysfunction. Crit Care Clin. 2006;22(2):357–74, viii.

82. Garcia Rodriguez LA, Perez Gutthann S, Walker AM, et al. The role of non-steroidal anti-inflammatory drugs in acute liver injury. BMJ. 1992;305(6858):865–8.

83. Rabinovitz M, Van Thiel DH. Hepatotoxicity of nonsteroidal anti-inflammatory drugs. Am J Gastroenterol. 1992;87(12):1696–704.

84. Stewart DM, Dillman RO, Kim HS, et al. Acetaminophen overdose: a growing health care hazard. Clin Toxicol. 1979;14(5):507–13.

85. Chun LJ, Tong MJ, Busuttil RW, et al. Acetaminophen hepatotoxicity and acute liver failure. J Clin Gastroenterol. 2009;43(4):342–9.

86. Makin AJ, Williams R. Acetaminophen-induced hepatotoxicity: predisposing factors and treatments. Adv Intern Med. 1997;42:453–83.

87. Dargan PI, Jones AL. Acetaminophen poisoning: an update for the intensivist. Crit Care. 2002;6(2):108–10.

88. Larson AM. Acetaminophen hepatotoxicity. Clin Liver Dis. 2007;11(3):525–48, vi.

89. Amezcua JL, O'Grady J, Salmon JA, et al. Prolonged paradoxical effect of aspirin on platelet behaviour and bleeding time in man. Thromb Res. 1979;16(1–2):69–79.

90. McGettigan P, Henry D. Cardiovascular risk and inhibition of cyclooxygenase: a systematic review of the observational studies of selective and nonselective inhibitors of cyclooxygenase 2. JAMA. 2006;296(13):1633–44.

The Role of Antidepressants in the Treatment of Chronic Pain

Beth B. Murinson

Key Points

- Selected antidepressants are effective against pain, and these include the tricyclic antidepressants: amitriptyline, desipramine, and imipramine as well as specific selective serotonin and noradrenergic reuptake inhibitors: duloxetine, venlafaxine, and milnacipran.
- Most antidepressants carry a black box warning regarding increased risk of suicidality. This is generally more common in young people including teens and young adults. It is important to remain vigilant for symptoms of suicidal ideation and to provide appropriate guidance and warnings.
- Tricyclic antidepressants are contraindicated in the immediate period following a myocardial infarction and should be used with caution in patients with known heart disease; they are however generally safe and well tolerated over sustained periods of treatment.
- Newer pain-active antidepressants, e.g., duloxetine, have relatively mild side effects and can be quite effective, but clinical trials have indicated that these agents have a lower "number needed to treat" (NNT), meaning that for an individual patient, the chance of experiencing a therapeutic response may be one in four or lower.
- Pain-active antidepressants are an important component of treating chronic pain. They are not "habit forming" and should be used where appropriate in the treatment for persistent pain-producing conditions reducing the requirements for long-term opioids.

B.B. Murinson, M.S., M.D., Ph.D. (✉)
Department of Neurology, Johns Hopkins University School of Medicine, Baltimore, MD, USA

Department of Neurology, Clinical, Technion Faculty of Medicine, Haifa, Israel
e-mail: bethmurinson@hotmail.com

Introduction

A number of antidepressants are essential for the treatment of chronic pain; these are referred to as the "pain-active" antidepressants. As a group, these agents manifest noradrenergic modulation. They have a number of advantages in this context: well-documented efficacy, mechanism or mechanisms of action that are complimentary to other agents used for persistent pain, distinctive and unique side effect profiles, excellent long-term tolerability, and a spectrum of cost-range options. Because the onset of action for the pain-active antidepressants can take days to weeks, these drugs are generally not appropriate for acute pain treatment with notable exceptions [1]. It is because of their numerous advantages including efficacy and tolerability for long-term usage that antidepressants have become a staple of medical management of chronic pain (Table 4.1).

Some antidepressants have not consistently demonstrated clinical efficacy against pain [2]. These include the most commonly prescribed antidepressants: fluoxetine (Prozac) and escitalopram (Lexapro) [3]. Paroxetine (Paxil) has been suggested as an agent that may modulate important pain-signaling events in the dorsal root ganglion; however, clinical trials have been inconsistent in demonstrating efficacy against pain.

As a group, pain-active antidepressants can serve as alternative single-agent therapy or complement the actions of agents in other classes. However, antidepressants used for the treatment of chronic pain have specific advantages. Giannopoulos et al. [4] reported that compliance and mood were higher in those chronic pain patients treated with antidepressants compared to those treated with GBP (gabapentin); however the effect size was small. Overall, both treatments demonstrated efficacy against neuropathic pain in about half of those treated as measured by patient satisfaction (Table 4.1).

T.R. Deer et al. (eds.), *Treatment of Chronic Pain by Medical Approaches: the AMERICAN ACADEMY of PAIN MEDICINE Textbook on Patient Management*, DOI 10.1007/978-1-4939-1818-8_4,
© American Academy of Pain Medicine 2015

Table 4.1 Pain-active antidepressants

Drug (trade name) (trade name)	Class	Available dosages	FDA-approved indication	Side effects, warnings[a,b]	Notes
Imipramine	TCA	75, 100, 125, or 150 mg	Depression	Dry mouth, constipation, tremor black, box warning[a]	Potentially alerting
Desipramine	TCA	10, 25, 50, 75, 100, or 150 mg	Depression	Tachycardia, avoid in those with history of dysrhythmias, black box warning[a]	Metabolite of imipramine Nonsedating
Amitriptyline (Elatrol) (Elavil?)	TCA	10, 25, 50, 75, 100, or 150 mg	Depression	Dental caries with prolonged use, hypersomnia, black box warning[a]	Heavily sedating
Nortriptyline (Pamelor)	TCA	10, 25, 50, and 75 mg	Depression	Constipation, urinary retention, black box warning[a]	Mildly sedating
Venlafaxine (Effexor)	SNRI	25, 37.5, 50, 75, or 100 mg; 37.5, 75, or 150 mg XR	Depression	Nausea, elevated blood pressure, nervousness, insomnia, black box warning[a]	Primarily serotonergic at low-dose Half-life: 4 h short half-life means extended release dosing necessary
Duloxetine (Cymbalta)	SNRI	20, 30, or 60 mg	Depression, GAD[c], diabetic peripheral neuropathic pain, fibromyalgia, chronic musculoskeletal pain	Hepatotoxicity, black box warning[a]	Higher affinity for 5HT than for NE Half-life: 12 h
Milnacipran (Savella)	SNRI	12.5, 25, 50, or 100 mg	Fibromyalgia	Nausea (10 %), headache (<10 %), black box warning[a]	Balanced NE/5HT Half-life: 8 h

[a]Black box warning for suicidality applies to all agents discussed here
[b]MAO inhibitors should not be prescribed with any of these agents
[c]GAD generalized anxiety disorder

In this chapter, seven "pain-active antidepressants" are discussed. The chapter begins with the most recent entry to the field and then takes a step back in time to examine aspects of selected tricyclic antidepressants and finishes with the two newer pain-active antidepressants.

Imipramine

Imipramine is a tricyclic antidepressant, the first to be synthesized and to undergo clinical testing. It was widely marketed as "Tofranil." Imipramine is available in tablets of the following dosages: 75, 100, 125, or 150 mg.

Imipramine carries the same black box warning as amitriptyline and nortriptyline [Imipramine]. It requires special monitoring for clinical worsening, suicidality, and behavior changes that are unusual. The proposed mechanism of action against depression is through the blockage of norepinephrine reuptake. The FDA has approved imipramine for the treatment of the symptoms of depression. It is noted that treatment effects may not be apparent for 1–3 weeks.

The absolute contraindications, as for the other tricyclics, include acute myocardial ischemia and recovery from such, current or recent use of MAO inhibitors, and hypersensitivity to the medication.

The package insert for imipramine notes the necessity for EKG screening prior to administering *larger than usual* doses of the medication. Although it has been recommended that a screening EKG be obtained prior to TCA treatment for all patients over age 40 [5], a recent study suggests that patients without known cardiovascular history in fact have a lower risk for MI during treatment with tricyclic antidepressants [6]. Clinical judgment is clearly appropriate. Abrupt cessation of the medication should be avoided as headache, nausea, and malaise may ensue.

Imipramine is less potent than the other tricyclic antidepressants, and the recommended starting dose is 75 mg daily, with lower starting doses recommended for older adults and those younger. The medication is not recommended for use in children [Imipramine].

Imipramine was among the earliest antidepressants to demonstrate efficacy against neuropathic pain [7]. It has been shown in repeated clinical studies to have good efficacy against the symptoms of diabetic neuropathy; however, side effects may interfere with successful management [8, 9]. A recent Cochrane Database Review indicates that imipramine is efficacious against neuropathic pain with a NNT of 2.2 [10]. Among the earliest references to imipramine in the treatment of pain is the efficacy of amitriptyline and imipramine in the treatment of tension headache [11]. Amitriptyline was superior to all other therapies attempted in this early study.

Desipramine

Desipramine is a tricyclic antidepressant and a metabolite of imipramine. It is available in tablets of 10, 25, 50, 75, 100, or 150 mg dosage. Widely marketed as "Norpramin," it should not be confused with nortriptyline.

Relative to amitriptyline, desipramine is a more potent as a relative inhibitor of norepinephrine reuptake, compared with inhibition of serotonin reuptake. Relative to imipramine, it is noted that the onset of treatment effects with desipramine is more rapid and benefits may be observed as soon as 2–5 days following the initiation of treatment [Desipramine]. An additional potential benefit of desipramine is that it is relatively nonsedating and is well tolerated when taken twice daily. Thus, in those patients for whom pain is a more constant feature of their daily routine, desipramine may be an excellent choice. There are those patients who are very busy with work demands and for whom the residual sedating effects of amitriptyline, which may persist even with nighttime administration, preclude successful dose titration for pain relief. In these patients also, desipramine may represent a useful alternative. It was shown in one high-quality study to have efficacy against PHN, and it is observed to work well with gabapentin in clinical practice.

Desipramine is metabolized in the liver but largely excreted in the urine. There is a wide range in serum levels among individuals receiving the same dose. Serum levels are generally higher with fixed doses in the elderly, consistent with decreased renal function. Cimetidine impedes metabolism and raises serum levels, whereas tobacco, barbiturates, and alcohol resulted in induced metabolic losses. It is recommended that caution be exercised in considering coadministration of SSRIs with desipramine as metabolic interactions will result in increased concentrations of desipramine.

TCAs have idiosyncratic metabolism, and serum levels can vary widely potentially accounting for variations in clinical responses. Metabolism is markedly decreased in a small but significant percentage of patients. Partially due to a polymorphism in CYP2D6 metabolizing protein transcripts, variants result in higher than anticipated serum drug levels [12].

The contraindications for desipramine are similar to those for other tricyclics that are discussed here and include MAO inhibitor administration, recent myocardial ischemia, and allergy to the medication.

The black box warning for the tricyclic antidepressants pertains also to desipramine. Patients should be monitored during therapy, and caregivers should receive appropriate instructions regarding behavioral changes and the need to contact health providers with concerns.

"Extreme caution" is urged in considering use of this medication in those with cardiovascular disease, a family history of sudden death, difficulty with urination, glaucoma, thyroid disease, or seizure disorder. It is established that desipramine can lower the seizure threshold.

The usual adult dosage is noted as 100–200 mg daily with recommendations not to exceed 300 mg daily. The starting dose should be lower than the usual dosage. Dosage adjustment for adolescents and geriatric patients includes recommendations for doses of 25–100 mg daily.

Although desipramine does not carry FDA approval for the treatment of any pain condition, it has been investigated for such in clinical trials and may be used at the discretion of the prescribing physician. In 1990, desipramine was described as effective against pain in patients with postherpetic neuralgia. In this randomized, double-blind crossover trial, the average desipramine dose was 167 mg daily. Compared with placebo, desipramine provided significant pain relief beginning at week 3 of the active treatment [13]. A study of desipramine for the treatment of painful diabetic neuropathy found that somewhat higher doses were prescribed following titration (201 mg daily) and that significant pain relief was demonstrable following week 5 of the treatment period [14]. Comparison with amitriptyline and fluoxetine demonstrated that amitriptyline and desipramine were both efficacious in relieving the pain of diabetic neuropathy while fluoxetine was not significantly different from placebo. The mean titrated dose of desipramine was 111 mg daily which compared to 105 for amitriptyline [15]. Recent Cochrane Database Review indicates that desipramine is efficacious against neuropathic pain with a NNT of 2.6 [10]. The use of TCAs for acute pain management is not common practice; however, in a trial of preemptive analgesia for pain following dental surgery, desipramine was effective in reducing opioid requirements [1]. Other applications for acute or subacute pain have not been extensively studied.

Amitriptyline

Amitriptyline was approved by the FDA for the relief of symptoms of depression in 1961 and widely prescribed as "Elavil." It is metabolized to nortriptyline, another "pain-active" antidepressant described below. Although amitriptyline is not FDA approved for indications other than depression, it is used for a variety of conditions including diabetic neuropathy, fibromyalgia, migraine prophylaxis, neuropathic pain, postherpetic neuralgia, and tension headache [11].

Amitriptyline has multiple mechanisms of action that may be important for notable activity against neuropathic pain. These include both central (noradrenergic) and peripheral (sodium channel blocking) mechanisms.

Nortriptyline

Nortriptyline is a tricyclic antidepressant, widely prescribed as "Pamelor." It is a metabolite of amitriptyline but is relatively less sedating. Nortriptyline is FDA approved for the relief of symptoms of depression [Nortriptyline]. It has multiple potential mechanisms of action but clearly "interferes with the transport, release, and storage of catecholamines" [Nortriptyline]. According to the package insert, preclinical trials of nortriptyline indicated that it has both "stimulant and depressant properties."

Nortriptyline carries the same black box warning as amitriptyline and imipramine. It requires special monitoring for clinical worsening, suicidality, and behavior changes that are unusual. The absolute contraindications, as for the other tricyclics, include acute myocardial ischemia and recovery from such, current or recent use of MAO inhibitors, and hypersensitivity to the medication. It has been written that nortriptyline carries significant cardiovascular dangers [5], but the study that supports this compared nortriptyline to a SSRI that was not pain-active, in patients who were post-MI and who were depressed. Relative to the SSRI used for the treatment of depression, nortriptyline did produce an increase in average heart rate (eight beats per minute) and did result in more patients discontinuing therapy for cardiac-related side effects (sinus tachycardia and ventricular ectopy) [16]. In follow-up studies of this effect, it was shown that these effects of nortriptyline relate to the vagolytic activity of nortriptyline relative to paroxetine [17], an aspect of this medication that may have a significant relationship to its mechanism of action against pain. There is little evidence to support the notion that nortriptyline is more pronounced in this effect than other pain-active antidepressants. One point of interest is that in recent preclinical studies screening a large compound library for efficacy against hypoxic injury, nortriptyline has in fact shown a neuroprotective effect in models of *cerebral* ischemia [18].

Caveats aside, nortriptyline is an important medication option in the management of persistent pain. For many pain specialists, it is the tricyclic of choice. In a clinical trial of postherpetic neuralgia, nortriptyline and desipramine showed similar efficacy to morphine [19]. In diabetic and postherpetic neuralgia, nortriptyline has been shown to be at least as effective as gabapentin in the treatment of these disorders [20]. It is accompanied by dry mouth in the majority of patients, but nortriptyline in combination with gabapentin provided additional incremental pain relief [20].

Contraindications for Imipramine, Desipramine, Amitriptyline, and Nortriptyline

Amitriptyline and other tricyclic antidepressants (nortriptyline, desipramine) are contraindicated for concomitant prescription with MAO inhibitors. MAO inhibitors block the metabolism of catecholamines, and in concert with agents which block the reuptake of amines from the synaptic cleft can produce a life-threatening syndrome of elevated temperature and seizures. It is recommended that tricyclics should not be started sooner than 14 days after discontinuation of MAO inhibitors [Amitriptyline]. Amitriptyline and the tricyclic antidepressants are also contraindicated during the acute recovery phase following myocardial ischemia. One of the important side effects of tricyclic antidepressants and a serious problem in the setting of medication overdose is the prolongation of the Q-T interval. TCAs should be avoided in patients with conduction defects such as AV block [5]. Patients with hypersensitivity to amitriptyline or other tricyclic antidepressants should not receive this drug [Amitriptyline].

Although there is a strong contraindication for using tricyclic antidepressants in the acute period following MI, an important recent study indicates no hazard in using antidepressants for those who do not have an established history of cardiovascular disease [6]. The findings of this study suggest that those patients who complete at least 12 weeks of treatment with antidepressant medications have a reduced risk for MI and lower all causes of mortality.

Black Box Warnings for Imipramine, Desipramine, Amitriptyline, and Nortriptyline

Amitriptyline and all tricyclic antidepressants carry a black box warning indicating that patients receiving these medications may be at increased risk for suicide. The warning indicates that providers prescribing these medications should monitor patients for clinical worsening and suicidality. They are further instructed to advise caregivers and family members about the need for close observation and specifically to watch for signs of irritability, agitation, and worsening of depression.

Coadministration of tricyclic antidepressants with SSRIs may produce a metabolic interaction such that the resulting plasma levels are markedly and variably elevated. Caution, clinical experience, and clear-cut therapeutic rationale should dictate the use of these agents in combination.

Amitriptyline was noted from the earliest studies of pharmacological treatment of chronic pain to be highly effective against persistent pain and provide the added benefit of improved sleep [11]. Although early dosing regimens involved three-times daily dosing, daytime sedation is a frequent concomitant of this approach. Switching patients to single-dose administration at bedtime resolves many of the concerns with hypersomnia and has the added benefit of mitigating the effects of amitriptyline in producing orthostatic hypotension. The sedation of amitriptyline may ameliorate with time; however, the sedation when present can be profound so that patients should be instructed not to drive following the evening medication dose. Dry mouth is a prominent side effect of amitriptyline. This phenomenon goes beyond being a minor annoyance and can have a devastating effect by accelerating dental caries. Diligent attention to professional dental care and enhanced attention to daily dental hygiene should be urged for patients receiving amitriptyline long-term.

The sedating effects of amitriptyline can be used to great advantage in patients with increased pain severity at night or in the evening. It is typical that patients with painful small fiber neuropathy will describe pain that is markedly worse once they get into bed for the evening or even once they put their feet up to rest. Patients with neuropathy will also describe difficulty tolerating sheets on the feet at night, a phenomenon that may represent mechanical allodynia, or may represent aberrant sensory processing that occurs with mild warming of the feet. In either case, a burning, occasionally searing pain is provoked by resting the feet under covers. The ordinary comfort that comes from climbing under warm blankets is completely replaced by spontaneous dysesthesias for these patients with early neuropathy. The elicitation of a night pain history is quickly accomplished with the question "At what time of day is your pain the worst?" The patient with night pain or with sleep disruption due to neuropathic pain may find that amitriptyline provides excellent therapeutic relief.

Amitriptyline is available in a wide range of doses including 10, 25, 50, 75, 100, or 150 mg tablets. The half-life is relatively short, but the therapeutic benefit can be obtained with once daily dosing over the longer treatment intervals. Amitriptyline is not appropriate for the treatment of acute pain.

Amitriptyline has not been shown to provide significant pain relief in the treatment of HIV-associated sensory neuropathy [21].

Amitriptyline at low dose (25 mg daily) has been found in meta-analysis to provide relief from symptoms of fibromyalgia including pain relief, sleep, and fatigue at the 6-week time point [22].

Amitriptyline has shown consistent efficacy against neuropathic pain as assessed by recent meta-analysis; the number needed to treat (NNT) is in the range of 3.1 [10].

Venlafaxine

Venlafaxine (marketed as Effexor) is an SNRI that has FDA approval for the treatment of depression [Venlafaxine]. It is available in tablets of 2, 37.5, 50, 75, or 100 mg and extended release capsules of 37.5, 75, or 150 mg XR. Among the major potential side effects are nausea, persistently elevated blood pressure, nervousness, and insomnia. Like all of the antidepressants, it carries a black box warning indicating that patients should be monitored for increased suicidality and unusual behavior changes that might herald suicide attempts or worsening depression. The drug has activity against serotonin and norepinephrine reuptake pumps but is primarily serotonergic at low dose. Venlafaxine has a short half-life of about 4 h. The short half-life means extended release dosing is generally necessary for efficacy.

Venlafaxine has been demonstrated in randomized controlled trials to be efficacious in the treatment of painful neuropathy [23]. In comparison to imipramine, it is indistinguishably effective; however, the NNT for venlafaxine, around 4.5, is higher than that of the TCAs [8, 9]. Although generally used in the context of treating established chronic pain, a recent randomized study has shown that venlafaxine provides pain relief in the first 10 days after mastectomy, superior even to gabapentin [24]. Venlafaxine, although having an NNT higher than the TCAs, is valuable medication in the armamentarium against neuropathic pain as it has a more targeted mechanism of action, and for many patients, the side effects are more tolerable.

Duloxetine

Duloxetine, trade name Cymbalta, is an SNRI that is FDA approved for the treatment of depression as well as diabetic peripheral neuropathic pain, fibromyalgia, and chronic musculoskeletal pain [Duloxetine]. In this respect, the medication has a significant advantage over the other pain-active antidepressants as it clearly has a stamp of approval from the FDA for a wide range of pain-associated conditions. One limitation of duloxetine that may frustrate its use in clinical practice is the observation that the NNT is estimated at 5.7. This could be expected to mean that a number of patients will try the treatment and not obtain clinically significant relief. The NNT for duloxetine compares with more favorable NNTs, less than 3, for the tricyclic antidepressants. Duloxetine is available in delayed release capsules of the following dosages: 20, 30, or 60 mg.

Like the other pain-active antidepressants, duloxetine carries a black box warning for the worsening of depression and the risk for increased suicidality. Patients should be monitored for suicidality. In some cases, patients with no prior experience of suicidal ideation will find the emergence of suicidal ideation to be deeply troubling. Immediate discontinuation is appropriate for patients who develop these intrusive and emotionally disturbing thoughts. Caregivers should also receive appropriate guidance to observe patients for irritability, aggression, and unusual behavior changes.

Contraindications for duloxetine include the prohibition against co-prescribing with MAO inhibitors due to the severe serotonin syndrome effects that result. There is also a contraindication for prescribing this medication to patients with untreated narrow-angle glaucoma.

Elevation of liver transaminases and fatal liver failure has been observed in patients taking duloxetine. These patients present with jaundice, abdominal pain, or elevated transaminases. Elevated transaminases resulted in the discontinuation of duloxetine in 0.3 % of patients in clinical trials, and in placebo-controlled trials, significant elevations of ALT occurred in an excess of 0.8 % of treated patients relative to placebo. For these reasons, duloxetine should not be prescribed to patients with "substantial alcohol use or evidence of chronic liver disease." Other potential side effects include nausea, somnolence, orthostatic hypotension, hyponatremia, and worsening of glycemic control in diabetes.

Duloxetine is metabolized by both CYP1A2 and CYP2D6, and drug interactions reflect this. Concomitant administration with desipramine resulted in increased desipramine concentrations. Drug interactions should be reviewed as appropriate for this medication.

Duloxetine is significantly more potent in blocking serotonin reuptake than norepinephrine. For this reason, at lower doses, serotonergic effects may dominate.

Duloxetine has been found to provide pain relief comparable to gabapentin and pregabalin in patients with diabetic peripheral neuropathy (meta-analysis) [25].

A recent Cochrane Database Review of duloxetine indicated efficacy for the treatment of both diabetic peripheral neuropathy and fibromyalgia at doses of 60 and 120 mg daily. The NNT to treat for these conditions was quite high however at 6 and 8, respectively. Despite the potential for side effects and adverse events, these events are relatively uncommon compared with side effect profiles of other pain-active antidepressants. In those patients who do respond to the pain-relieving effects, duloxetine is usually a well-tolerated medication that dramatically improves quality of life. For these reasons, duloxetine has become a valued treatment option for patients with neuropathic pain [26].

Milnacipran

Milnacipran is one of the newer SNRIs approved for the treatment of chronic pain conditions, specifically fibromyalgia. Distinctive from the other two SNRIs discussed here,

it has nearly balanced efficacy against serotonin and norepinephrine reuptake [27]. Although milnacipran is Food and Drug Administration (FDA) approved for fibromyalgia and not for depression, it is used internationally for depression and there is literature to suggest that milnacipran has efficacy against depression that is comparable to imipramine [28]. It is generally well tolerated with most side effects being comparable to placebo. Exceptions to this are infrequent, occurring in fewer than 5 % of the patients studied in meta-analysis, but include dysuria, palpitations, hot flushes, anxiety, sweating, and vertigo.

Milnacipran is available as tablets of 12.5, 25, 50, or 100 mg. Rapidly absorbed, milnacipran has high bioavailability (85 %). The half-life of milnacipran is around 8 h which suggests that twice daily dosing may provide better efficacy. The prescribing information for milnacipran indicates that titration is recommended when starting this medication with an initial dose of 12.5 mg tapered upward over the course of a week to 50 mg twice daily. There is no significant inhibition or induction of metabolic enzymes, and for this reason, milnacipran has relatively few drug-drug interactions. It is excreted largely unmetabolized.

There are important absolute contraindications to prescribing this medication: concurrent irreversible MAO inhibitors such as selegiline may result in serotonergic crisis. Recent (within 14 days) use of MAO inhibitors is also contraindicated. Milnacipran is contraindicated in patients with untreated narrow-angle glaucoma. The medication is also not to be used concurrently with digitalis glycosides or with 5HT-1D agonists (triptans) as myocardial ischemia may result. Hepatotoxicity has been observed, and mild elevations in blood pressure and heart rate have been reported.

As with all of the antidepressants discussed in this chapter, Milnacipran carries a black box warning for increased risk of suicidality especially in children, adolescents, and young adults. Patients of all ages who are starting this medication are required to have appropriate monitoring and should be "observed closely for clinical worsening, suicidality or unusual changes in behavior."

Summary

Antidepressants are widely used in the treatment of neuropathic pain. Though the number of agents that are FDA approved for use in chronic pain states are very limited at this time, there is now good evidence from a wide range of clinical trials and meta-analysis studies that specific antidepressants are very effective in particular circumstances. Pain-associated conditions that may respond well to treatment with antidepressants include diabetic peripheral neuropathy, postherpetic neuralgia, fibromyalgia, tension headache, migraine prophylaxis, chronic musculoskeletal pain, and fibromyalgia. It is important to understand the particulars of each agent and its demonstrated efficacy from clinical trials to appropriately select therapies. Although the pain-active antidepressants offer significant advantages in terms of complementary mechanisms of action and long-term tolerability, it is important to prescribe these agents only when appropriate and with the recognition that increased suicidality, concomitant use of MAO inhibitors, cardiac disease, and allergies remain important impediments to broader, freer use of these agents. On a positive note, it is a monumental advance in the treatment of pain that so many diverse and generally effective agents are available today [29].

Electronic Sources for Prescribing Information

Duloxetine. Eli Lilly and Company. http://dailymed.nlm.nih.gov/dailymed/lookup.cfm?setid=2f7d4d67-10c1-4bf4-a7f2-c185fbad64ba. Accessed October 2, 2011.

Venlafaxine. Wyeth Pharmaceuticals Company. http://dailymed.nlm.nih.gov/dailymed/lookup.cfm?setid=53c3e7ac-1852-4d70-d2b6-4fca819acf26. Accessed September 28, 2011.

Milnacipran. Forrest Laboratories. http://dailymed.nlm.nih.gov/dailymed/lookup.cfm?setid=16a4a314-f97e-4e91-95e9-576a3773d284. Accessed October 2, 2011.

Amitriptyline. Sandoz Inc. http://dailymed.nlm.nih.gov/dailymed/lookup.cfm?setid=705a2bae-031d-4218-82fe-4346542c0baa. Accessed September 27, 2011.

Nortriptyline. Mallinckrodt Inc. http://dailymed.nlm.nih.gov/dailymed/lookup.cfm?setid=e17dc299-f52d-414d-ab6e-e809bd6f8acb. Accessed September 27, 2011.

Desipramine. Sanofi-Aventis Inc. http://dailymed.nlm.nih.gov/dailymed/lookup.cfm?setid=3e593725-3fc9-458e-907d-19d51d5a7f9c. Accessed October 2, 2011.

Imipramine. Sandoz Inc. http://dailymed.nlm.nih.gov/dailymed/lookup.cfm?setid=7d52c40c-bbcb-4698-9879-d40136301d31. Accessed October 2, 2011.

References

1. Levine JD, Gordon NC, Smith R, McBryde R. Desipramine enhances opiate postoperative analgesia. Pain. 1986;27(1):45–9.
2. Watson CP, Gilron I, Sawynok J, Lynch ME. Nontricyclic antidepressant analgesics and pain: are serotonin norepinephrine reuptake inhibitors (SNRIs) any better? Pain. 2011;152(10):2206–10.
3. Dharmshaktu P, Tayal V, Kalra BS. Efficacy of antidepressants as analgesics: a review. J Clin Pharmacol. 2011. doi:10.1177/0091270010394852.
4. Giannopoulos S, Kosmidou M, Sarmas I, Markoula S, Pelidou SH, Lagos G, Kyritsis AP. Patient compliance with SSRIs and gabapentin in painful diabetic neuropathy. Clin J Pain. 2007;23(3):267–9.
5. Dworkin RH, O'Connor AB, Backonja M, Farrar JT, Finnerup NB, Jensen TS, Kalso EA, Loeser JD, Miaskowski C, Nurmikko TJ, Portenoy RK, Rice AS, Stacey BR, Treede RD, Turk DC, Wallace MS. Pharmacologic management of neuropathic pain: evidence-based recommendations. Pain. 2007;132(3):237–51.
6. Scherrer JF, Garfield LD, Lustman PJ, Hauptman PJ, Chrusciel T, Zeringue A, Carney RM, Freedland KE, Bucholz KK, Owen R, Newcomer JW, True WR. Antidepressant drug compliance: reduced risk of MI and mortality in depressed patients. Am J Med. 2011;124(4):318–24.
7. Kvinesdale B, Molin J, Frøland A, Gram LF. Imipramine treatment of painful diabetic neuropathy. JAMA. 1984;251(13):1727–30.
8. Sindrup SH, Gram LF, Brøsen K, Eshøj O, Mogensen EF. The selective serotonin reuptake inhibitor paroxetine is effective in the treatment of diabetic neuropathy symptoms. Pain. 1990;42(2):135–44.
9. Sindrup SH, Ejlertsen B, Frøland A, Sindrup EH, Brøsen K, Gram LF. Imipramine treatment in diabetic neuropathy: relief of subjective symptoms without changes in peripheral and autonomic nerve function. Eur J Clin Pharmacol. 1989;37(2):151–3.
10. Saarto T, Wiffen PJ. Antidepressants for neuropathic pain. Cochrane Database Syst Rev. 2007;17(4):005454.
11. Lance JW, Curran DA. Treatment of chronic tension headache. Lancet. 1964;1(7345):1236–9.
12. Oscarson M. Pharmacogenetics of drug metabolising enzymes: importance for personalised medicine. Clin Chem Lab Med. 2003;41(4):573–80.
13. Kishore-Kumar R, Max MB, Schafer SC, Gaughan AM, Smoller B, Gracely RH, Dubner R. Desipramine relieves postherpetic neuralgia. Clin Pharmacol Ther. 1990;47(3):305–12.
14. Max MB, Kishore-Kumar R, Schafer SC, Meister B, Gracely RH, Smoller B, Dubner R. Efficacy of desipramine in painful diabetic neuropathy: a placebo-controlled trial. Pain. 1991;45(1):3–9; discussion 1–2.
15. Max MB, Lynch SA, Muir J, Shoaf SE, Smoller B, Dubner R. Effects of desipramine, amitriptyline, and fluoxetine on pain in diabetic neuropathy. N Engl J Med. 1992;326(19):1250–6.
16. Roose SP, Laghrissi-Thode F, Kennedy JS, Nelson JC, Bigger Jr JT, Pollock BG, Gaffney A, Narayan M, Finkel MS, McCafferty J, Gergel I. Comparison of paroxetine and nortriptyline in depressed patients with ischemic heart disease. JAMA. 1998;279(4):287–91.
17. Yeragani VK, Pesce V, Jayaraman A, Roose S. Major depression with ischemic heart disease: effects of paroxetine and nortriptyline on long-term heart rate variability measures. Biol Psychiatry. 2002;52(5):418–29.
18. Zhang WH, Wang H, Wang X, Narayanan MV, Stavrovskaya IG, Kristal BS, Friedlander RM. Nortriptyline protects mitochondria and reduces cerebral ischemia/hypoxia injury. Stroke. 2008;39(2):455–62.
19. Raja SN, Haythornthwaite JA, Pappagallo M, Clark MR, Travison TG, Sabeen S, Royall RM, Max MB. Opioids versus antidepressants in postherpetic neuralgia: a randomized, placebo-controlled trial. Neurology. 2002;59(7):1015–21.
20. Gilron I, Bailey JM, Tu D, Holden RR, Jackson AC, Houlden RL. Nortriptyline and gabapentin, alone and in combination for neuropathic pain: a double-blind, randomised controlled crossover trial. Lancet. 2009;374(9697):1252–61.
21. Phillips TJ, Cherry CL, Cox S, Marshall SJ, Rice AS. Pharmacological treatment of painful HIV-associated sensory neuropathy: a systematic review and meta-analysis of randomised controlled trials. PLoS One. 2010;5(12):e14433.
22. Nishishinya B, Urrútia G, Walitt B, Rodriguez A, Bonfill X, Alegre C, Darko G. Amitriptyline in the treatment of fibromyalgia: a systematic review of its efficacy. Rheumatology (Oxford). 2008;47(12):1741–6.
23. Rowbotham MC, Goli V, Kunz NR, Lei D. Venlafaxine extended release in the treatment of painful diabetic neuropathy: a double blind, placebo-controlled study. Pain. 2004;110:697–706.
24. Amr YM, Yousef AA. Evaluation of efficacy of the perioperative administration of venlafaxine or gabapentin on acute and chronic post-mastectomy pain. Clin J Pain. 2010;26:381–5.

25. Quilici S, Chancellor J, Löthgren M, Simon D, Said G, Le TK, Garcia-Cebrian A, Monz B. Meta-analysis of duloxetine vs. pregabalin and gabapentin in the treatment of diabetic peripheral neuropathic pain. BMC Neurol. 2009;9:6.

26. Lunn MP, Hughes RA, Wiffen PJ. Duloxetine for treating painful neuropathy or chronic pain. Cochrane Database Syst Rev. 2009; 7(4):CD007115.

27. Stahl SM, Grady MM, Moret C, Briley M. SNRIs: their pharmacology, clinical efficacy, and tolerability in comparison with other classes of antidepressants. CNS Spectr. 2005;10(9):732–47.

28. Kasper S, Pletan Y, Solles A, Tournoux A. Comparative studies with milnacipran and tricyclic antidepressants in the treatment of patients with major depression: a summary of clinical trial results. Int Clin Psychopharmacol. 1996;11 Suppl 4: 35–9.

29. Attal N, Cruccu G, Baron R, Haanpää M, Hansson P, Jensen TS, Nurmikko T, European Federation of Neurological Societies. EFNS guidelines on the pharmacological treatment of neuropathic pain: 2010 revision. Eur J Neurol. 2010;17(9):1113-e88. Epub 2010 Apr 9. Review.

Anticonvulsant Medications for Treatment of Neuropathic and "Functional" Pain

5

Bruce D. Nicholson

Key Points

- Anticonvulsant therapy is effective for the treatment of neuropathic pain.
- Efficacy is well demonstrated in selected neuropathic pain syndromes.
- Little evidence is available to support generalized use in treatment of neuropathic pain.
- Further research is required to evaluate the utility of anticonvulsant therapy in combination with other drugs.

Introduction

The broad definition of neuropathic pain as articulated by the International Association of Pain, "pain initiated or caused by a primary lesion or dysfunction of the nervous system," unfortunately has done little to guide the clinician when attempting to develop an effective treatment plan that may include an anticonvulsant medication. Current guidelines and indications for use of anticonvulsant therapy primarily utilize a lesion-based approach when recommending treatment for patients suffering from neuropathic pain. However, recent work by Baron and colleagues would suggest that selection of patients based on sensory symptoms and signs rather than strictly by disease etiology has potential benefits in identifying successful therapeutic outcomes [1].

Initial use of anticonvulsant drugs for the etiologic-based treatment of neuropathic pain dates back almost 50 years, with the sequential trials of carbamazepine for the treatment of trigeminal neuralgia [2–4]. From the mid-1960s until the mid-

1990s, only a limited number of clinical trials utilizing anticonvulsants had been completed for the treatment of neuropathic pain. Subsequent to the introduction of gabapentin for the treatment of epilepsy in the mid-1990s, case reports of successful treatment of neuropathic pain began to appear in the medical literature [5, 6]. Several recent reviews of the literature along with meta-analysis of randomized controlled trials (RCT) now support the use of anticonvulsant therapy for first-line treatment of selected neuropathic pain syndromes [7–9]. More recently, fibromyalgia (functional pain) now widely considered to be a neuropathic pain syndrome manifested by widespread pain due to underlying changes in sensory processing has been effectively treated with anticonvulsant therapy [3].

The body of evidence supporting the use of anticonvulsant therapy for the treatment of neuropathic pain as a generalized category is rather limited. The vast majority of clinical trials involving anticonvulsant drugs have been narrowly focused on treatment of specific conditions such as painful peripheral diabetic neuropathy and postherpetic neuralgia [8, 10, 11]. To date, only one trial has been published supporting the use of anticonvulsant therapy for the treatment of neuropathic cancer pain [12]. Of considerable interest is that the literature is devoid of a single trial demonstrating efficacy of anticonvulsant therapy in one of the most common forms of neuropathic pain that being neuropathic low back pain. The following review of anticonvulsant drugs will focus on clinically relevant aspects for the practicing clinician.

Carbamazepine and Oxcarbazepine

Few neuropathic pain conditions are more effectively managed with anticonvulsant therapy than classic trigeminal neuralgia [13, 14]. Consensus guidelines remain clear that carbamazepine is the drug of first choice with initial efficacy of upwards to 80 % and long-term efficacy of 50 % at doses between 200 and 400 mg administered three times a day [14].

B.D. Nicholson, M.D. (✉)
Division of Pain Medicine, Department of Anesthesiology,
Lehigh Valley Health Network, 1240 South Cedar Crest BLVD,
Suite 307, Allentown, PA 18103, USA
e-mail: bruce.nicholson@lvhn.org

Carbamazepine exerts a use-dependent inhibition of sodium channels that leads to a reduction in the frequency of sustained repetitive firing of action potentials in neurons. The effect on pain suppression is hypothesized to occur through both central and peripheral mechanisms. Carbamazepine use in three placebo-controlled studies for treatment trigeminal neuralgia demonstrated a combined numbers needed to treat (NNT) for effectiveness of 1.7 [15].

In a single 2-week placebo-controlled trial involving only 30 participants, carbamazepine demonstrated an NNT of 2.3 for treatment of painful diabetic neuropathy (PDN) [16]. However, several other clinical trials involving various neuropathic pain conditions that include PDN and postherpetic neuralgia (PHN) have failed to demonstrate clinical benefit measured by improvement in pain scores [10].

Unfortunately, problematic issues that may significantly limit the use as well as long-term efficacy include hepatic enzyme induction effects of carbamazepine. This particularly vexing side effect frequently requires close monitoring of other drug activity such as warfarin. Ongoing monitoring of liver function and blood count is recommended as well. The second-generation anticonvulsant oxcarbazepine has a structurally similar sodium channel inhibitor effect as carbamazepine but with significantly fewer complicating side effects. In two relatively small randomized controlled trials, oxcarbazepine was found to be similar to carbamazepine in reduction of number of attacks in patients suffering with trigeminal neuralgia [14]. Titration dosing from 300 mg QD to maximum of 900 mg BID over 5 days is recommended in order to minimize side effects such as dizziness and sedation. One concerning serious side effect is hyponatremia, which may occur in approximately 3 % of individuals taking oxcarbazepine; therefore, monitoring of sodium levels is recommended [10, 15].

Gabapentin and Pregabalin

Gabapentin original synthesized in 1977 as a drug for the treatment of spasticity and subsequently introduced in the mid-1990s for the treatment of epilepsy has garnered over 3,200 citations in the medical literature, with over 1,200 citations in the area of pain [17]. Since 1995, gabapentin has gained approval for the treatment of postherpetic neuralgia in the USA and for the broader indication of peripheral neuropathic pain in many countries outside of the United States [18]. In 2003, a second-generation alpha-2-delta-binding drug pregabalin was introduced in the United States, and FDA approved it for the treatment of epilepsy, postherpetic neuralgia, and painful diabetic peripheral neuropathy and more recently for the treatment of fibromyalgia [19, 20].

Whereas gabapentin and pregabalin both bind to the presynaptic neuronal alpha-2-delta subunit of voltage-gated calcium channels, pregabalin's unique chemical structure confers several clinically important features that distinguish it from gabapentin. Both drugs share the similar characteristics when binding to the alpha-2-delta subunit of voltage-gated calcium channels which results in decreased expression and release of certain neurotransmitters that include substance P, glutamate, and calcitonin-related gene peptide all of which are considered important for induction and maintenance of neuropathic pain states. The suppression of the above-mentioned neuronal peptide activity occurs primarily after tissue or nerve injury has occurred. This unique upregulation of the alpha-2-delta subunit on voltage-gated calcium channels is thought to be required for drug activity, as there is minimal drug effect on activity of normal nerve transmission [21, 22].

Pharmacokinetic characteristic particular to pregabalin that may have clinical benefit over gabapentin includes the linear absorption of pregabalin, which increases proportionally with each dose, resulting in a uniformly linear dose-exposure response across patient populations. On the other hand, the pharmacokinetic profile of gabapentin is considered nonlinear, and bioavailability (approximately 60 % at a dose of 900 mg) is significantly lower and less predictable across patient populations. The amount of gabapentin absorbed is dose dependent, with the proportion of drug absorbed decreasing with increasing dose to the point where only a fraction of the dose is absorbed at relatively higher doses. In single-dose absorption studies, the amount of gabapentin absorbed decreases from 80 % at 100 mg to 27 % at 1,600 mg [18]. On the contrary, pregabalin absorption is independent of dose administered; it is constant and averages >90 % over the dose range of 10–300 mg in single-dose trials [19]. Consequently, this particular pharmacokinetic difference translates into minimal variations between patients in plasma concentrations for pregabalin with dose titration. Whether this has any clinically important, significance remains to be determined, as this has not been measured in any head-to-head trials between gabapentin and pregabalin.

Clinically important characteristics of both gabapentin and pregabalin that simplify the use of these drugs include minimal protein binding and minimal or little drug-drug interaction which importantly includes warfarin. As well, favorable elimination characteristics include minimal metabolism and no CYP 450 interaction for both gabapentin and pregabalin, allowing the clinician to prescribe either drug in a patient who may be taking multiple other medications that may be affected by hepatic enzyme induction. It is particularly important to note clinically that gabapentin and pregabalin do not have any effect on renal function, as quite often this is a misunderstood concept that results in the withdrawal of therapy in patients with renal impairment. However, it is important to take into consideration when dosing both drugs that approximately 95 % of ingested gabapentin and pregabalin is eliminated, unchanged through renal excretion. Therefore, with decreasing creatinine clearance (CC), the dose of drug administered may be decreased proportionally from full-recommended dosing levels when CC is above 60–30 % or less of the normal dose when CC is below 30 [18, 19].

Gabapentin Therapy

Fourteen studies detailing use of gabapentin included the following conditions: two studies in postherpetic neuralgia (PHN), seven studies in painful diabetic neuropathy (PDN), and one each in cancer related neuropathic pain, phantom limb pain, Guillain-Barré syndrome, spinal cord injury pain, and mixed neuropathic pain states [12, 17, 23, 24]. In 2002, gabapentin was the first medication to be granted FDA approval for the treatment of postherpetic neuralgia. RCT results demonstrated in 336 PHN patients that dosing between 1,800 and 3,600 mg/day resulted in a 33–35 % reduction in pain compared to a 7.7 % pain score reduction in the placebo group. Overall, 43.2 % of subjects treated with gabapentin categorized their pain as "much" or "moderately" improved at the end of the study, whereas only 12.1 % in the placebo group experienced any significant improvement [25]. Three trials considered of fair quality conducted over 6–8-week duration at dosing levels varying between 900 and 3,600 mg/day demonstrated mixed results in the same condition [9, 17]. The Cochrane database analysis supports the use of gabapentin for treatment of chronic neuropathic pain and suggests that the numbers needed to treat (NNT) for improvement in all trials with evaluable data is around 5.1. Clinically, it is important to understand that on average, only one in approximately every five patients who receive gabapentin for the treatment of neuropathic pain will report significant improvement [11].

Of clinical importance are the adverse events that occurred more frequently in the gabapentin group compared to those in receiving placebo in decreasing order included somnolence, dizziness, and peripheral edema. The former-mentioned side effect of somnolence may be clinically beneficial in patients suffering from sleep deprivation due to neuropathic pain. The usual starting dose of gabapentin may vary depending on patient tolerance to pharmacotherapy. Therefore, one may start at a very low dose of 100 mg TID of QID titrating to efficacy that is usually seen at an average total daily dose between 900 and 1,800 mg, with occasional dosing to 2,400 mg/day. As mentioned above, asymmetric dosing of gabapentin giving a larger dose of drug at bedtime (600–1,200 mg) to induce somnolence and a lower dose in the morning (300–600 mg) and afternoon (300–600 mg) may help mitigate the somnolence and dizziness side effect profile during the waking hours while improving the sleep-related comorbidity found in up to 80 % of patients suffering with chronic neuropathic pain [9, 26, 27].

Pregabalin Therapy

Pregabalin, a second-generation alpha-2-delta analogue, has demonstrated efficacy in the treatment of postherpetic neuralgia, painful diabetic neuropathy, and central neuropathic pain. In general, the 19 published clinical trials have demonstrated that total daily doses of 150, 300, 450, and 600 mg daily were effective in patients suffering with neuropathic pain. The NNT for at least 50 % pain relief at 600 mg daily dosing compared with placebo were 3.9 for postherpetic neuralgia in five studies, 5.0 for painful diabetic neuropathy in seven studies, and 5.6 for central neuropathic pain in two studies [8, 10, 11, 16].

Seven randomized controlled trials were completed, evaluating the efficacy of pregabalin for treatment of painful diabetic neuropathy (PDN). Dosing ranged between 150 mg/day and a maximum of 600 mg/day with duration of treatment varying from 5 to 13 weeks. Average onset to significant improvement in pain was somewhat related to dosing being 4 days at 600 mg/day and 5 days at 300 mg/day. The longest onset to pain relief occurred in the 150 mg/day treatment group occurring as long as 13 days after start of drug. Analysis of the various dosing schedules for the PDN trials revealed that TID dosing was effective at 150–450 mg/day; however, efficacy in BID dosing was only seen at a total daily dose of 600 mg/day (300 mg BID). Although efficacy was demonstrated across a dosing range of 150–600 mg/day, FDA approval is for total daily dosing of 150–300 mg divided and given TID [28–30].

Three randomized controlled trials varying between 8 and 13 weeks in duration have looked at the efficacy of pregabalin for the treatment of postherpetic neuralgia. Consistent improvement across all three trials was found at dosing strengths between 150 and 600 mg/day. The dosing interval of BID or TID did not seem to affect patient responses at any total dose between 150 and 600 mg/day [20, 31, 32]. Of clinical interest was the varying response in overall pain relief that was targeted at 50 % improvement, but varied depending on the study between 20 and 50 % for the participants.

Two clinical trials involving over 300 patients with central pain found that relatively high doses of pregabalin 600 mg/day were required to achieve even results of minor significance. NNT for 35 % improvement were around 3.5 (2.3–7) and for 50 % improvement around 5.6 (3.5–14), while the discontinuation rates due to lack of efficacy and side effects (all minor) were somewhere around 50 % of participants [8, 11].

Of clinical importance is that consistent across all neuropathic pain trials regardless of condition treated, there was a generalized tendency towards greater improvement in pain relief with increasing dose of drug to a maximum of 600 mg/day. In addition, when compared to placebo on several of the SF-36 subscales, pregabalin demonstrated general improvement [33]. As with gabapentin, the beneficial effect on sleep has been demonstrated with pregabalin therapy in patients suffering with neuropathic pain [31, 34].

In conclusion, when looking at the pregabalin clinical trial data, substantially greater benefit was found at doses between 300 and 600 mg/day administered either BID or TID for the treatment of postherpetic neuralgia and painful diabetic neuropathy and with less but still clinically relevant benefit in central neuropathic pain [33]. Regardless of the pregabalin dose, only a minority of patients will have attained substantial benefit with pregabalin >50 %; however, the majority will demonstrate moderate benefit of between 30 and 50 % reduction in pain [9, 11, 16].

Adverse Events Profile for Gabapentin and Pregabalin

The most common adverse events for both drugs reported in clinical trials by participants were dizziness (22–38 %), somnolence (15–28 %), and peripheral edema (10–15 %). Review of clinical trial side effect data suggest that overall, similar side effects are present for gabapentin but somewhat lower than with pregabalin for dizziness as well as for weight gain. Of importance for the practicing clinician is that the number needed to harm (NNH/safety) for adverse events leading to withdrawal from a clinical trial with gabapentin was 26.1, which suggests a rather high-safety profile [35, 36].

As with gabapentin, the most common side effects with pregabalin therapy included dizziness, reported in 27–46 % of participants with somnolence being reported in 15–25 % of participants. Side effects were most significant with pregabalin aggressive dose escalation to 600 mg daily. Overall, 18–28 % of participants in pregabalin clinical trials discontinued treatment due to adverse events [35].

The current guidelines for dosing of pregabalin recommend a starting dose of 50 mg TID for PDN and 75 mg BID for PHN. However, due to the side effect profile and pharmacokinetic of pregabalin, individualization of treatment is needed to maximize pain relief and minimize adverse events [28, 32]. In the pregabalin study by Stacey and colleagues that utilized flexible verses fixed dosing schedules (150–600 mg/day) in 269 patients with postherpetic neuralgia, flexible dose therapy was demonstrated to be slightly more effective for treatment of allodynia. More importantly, pregabalin was better tolerated at a higher average dosage of 396 mg/day versus 295 mg/day in the fixed dose group. As well, of clinical importance is the onset of measurable reductions in pain that occurred at 1.5 days in the fixed dose group and 3.5 days in the flexible dose group. Reduction in allodynia was present as early as 1 week after onset of therapy. Equally important was the finding that discontinuation rates due to adverse events were more frequent in the fixed dose therapy group [32].

Although weight gain approximately 2–3 kg is relatively unique to pregabalin and has been reported in 4–14 % of participants across multiple studies, few withdrawal-related issues from therapy were seen, that is, <3 % of participants. More importantly, glycemic control was not an issue in diabetic patients as demonstrated by no change in hemoglobin A-1-C levels. A rather unique reported finding was the euphoric effect experienced by approximately 5 % of participants in the generalized anxiety disorder clinical trials with pregabalin. This finding combined with limited evidence suggesting subjective drug "liking" in a study of pregabalin in recreational drug users led the US Drug Enforcement Administration to list pregabalin as a Schedule V drug [19]. However, to date, no current data would suggest that pregabalin presents a significant health-related issue related to drug abuse or misuse.

Combination Drug Therapy

The construct of utilizing drugs from different classes and with different mechanisms of action has long been advocated, although few trials have been published in support of this approach. Meta-analysis of current single-drug therapy trials utilizing anticonvulsants indicates that less than two-thirds of patients suffering with neuropathic pain obtain satisfactory relief [12]. Therefore, combination drug trials may potentially offer greater improvement in various outcome measures related to neuropathic pain syndromes, such as dose-limiting side effects related to therapy, that most likely play a significant role in the low-therapeutic efficacy rates with currently available single-drug treatment protocols.

Gilron and colleagues have demonstrated that when given in combination, gabapentin and nortriptyline seemed to be more efficacious than when given as a single entity for treatment of neuropathic pain. A total of 56 patients, 40 with PDN and 16 with PHN, were randomized in a double-blind, double-dummy crossover-designed study which suggested that combination therapy improved sleep and had a weak effect on SF-36 quality of life outcomes. Of particular interest is the finding that the average dose of each drug was lower in the combination therapy group compared to when monotherapy was utilized [37]. An earlier study by Gilron published in 1995 demonstrated that combination therapy of gabapentin and morphine was superior to gabapentin alone for treatment of neuropathic pain [38]. On the contrary, a recent randomized controlled trial of oxycodone and pregabalin in combination demonstrated no enhanced pain relief. Unfortunately, the trial design required a forced titration of pregabalin to 600 mg/day in the pregabalin/placebo group. This aggressive pregabalin titration approach was thought to result in the high success of pain reduction >50 %, leading to no significant difference compared to the combination of low-dose oxycodone 10 mg/day and pregabalin [27].

Fibromyalgia (Functional Pain)

Fibromyalgia, a chronic pain condition characterized by widespread pain and tenderness, is considered to result from dysfunctional central sensory processing [3]. It is estimated that somewhere around five million Americans suffer from fibromyalgia and manifest symptoms that include widespread allodynia and hyperalgesia clinically identified by anatomical tender points [9]. The central sensitization process underlying this amplified pain perception is thought to result from an imbalance of neurotransmitters involved in pain processing [3]. Several industry-sponsored studies involving over 3,300 participants have demonstrated the efficacy of pregabalin for treatment of symptoms related to fibromyalgia.

The efficacy of pregabalin was demonstrated in clinical trials that utilized the American College of Rheumatology criteria for diagnosis of fibromyalgia. The trials included one 14-week randomized double-blind placebo-controlled multicenter study and one 6-month randomized withdrawal design study. Pregabalin also was shown to be superior to placebo in four randomized double-blind placebo-controlled trials lasting between 8 and 14 weeks for two main efficacy outcome measures that included the visual analogue scale (VAS) for pain and the patient global impression of change (PGIC). The balance between efficacy and side effects has been measured in several short- and long-term open-label safety extension studies [39].

Recommendations from review of these studies would suggest that effective dosing for treatment of fibromyalgia is between a total daily dosage of 300 and 450 mg/day administered BID. The suggested starting dose should be 75 mg BID and increased within 1 week to 150 mg BID based on efficacy and tolerability; importantly, dosing at 150 mg/day was not shown to be superior to placebo. Further up-titration should be considered to a maximum dose of 225 mg BID (total 450 mg/day), again based on individual patient response and tolerability. Dosing above 450 mg/day is not recommended, as patient global impression of change was lower when dosing at 600 mg/day and may have been the result of an increased dose-related side effect burden [40, 41].

On average, individuals with fibromyalgia manifest widespread pain for greater than 3 months and suffer with their symptoms for at least 5 years prior to diagnosis [42, 43]. Therefore, of special interest is the single, 6-month randomized withdrawal study that demonstrated efficacy and durability of pregabalin for the treatment of fibromyalgia. This 6-month study was designed to evaluate the response and durability of pregabalin over placebo therapy in participants whom already had demonstrated at least a 50 % improvement in an open-label run in phase. At the end of study, 68% of the participants administered pregabalin had ongoing therapeutic effect of >30 % pain relief as well as improvement in PGIC scores [39]. The NNT with pregabalin is quite favorable being 3.5 in order to prevent one participant from losing efficacy for treatment of fibromyalgia-related pain symptoms.

In a 12-week randomized placebo-controlled trial, gabapentin at dosages between 1,200 and 2,400 mg/day demonstrated a 51 % response versus 31 % for placebo with improvement of pain. Measures included the Brief Pain Inventory and Fibromyalgia Impact Questionnaire, which demonstrated improvement in symptoms related to fibromyalgia. Of particular interest was that tender point pain thresholds were not improved [42].

Other Anticonvulsant Drugs

Lamotrigine, a sodium channel-blocking AED, has been trialed in several neuropathic pain conditions with conflicting results. In a double-blind, placebo-controlled crossover-design study of 14 patients with trigeminal neuralgia refractory to carbamazepine or phenytoin, lamotrigine was superior to placebo at 400 mg/day [10]. A 14-week long study in HIV painful neuropathy patients, with titration to 300 mg/day, demonstrated benefit compared to placebo [36, 44]. A small 8-week long study in central post-stroke pain patients with titration to 200 mg/day demonstrated pain relief benefit over placebo [45]. Unfortunately, significant side effects including rash, dizziness, and somnolence combined with a painfully slow titration schedule limit the utility of lamotrigine in clinical practice.

The seldom used anticonvulsant sodium valproate has been studied for the treatment of PDN and PHN. Divalproex sodium studied in a randomized placebo-controlled clinical trial has demonstrated benefit at dosing between 800 and 1,600 mg/day. Treatment-limiting side effects were significant and may include nausea (42 %), infection (39 %), alopecia (31 %), and tremor (28 %) as experienced in migraine trials [10].

Lacosamide, a recent addition second-generation voltage-gated sodium channel-blocking agent, has conflicting evidence of efficacy for treatment of painful diabetic neuropathy. After review of phase 2 and phase 3 trial results, both the FDA and the European Medicines Agency rejected the request for approval to treat painful diabetic neuropathy [7].

Various other first-generation drugs such as phenytoin and clonazepam and second-generation drugs including topiramate, tiagabine, and levetiracetam have either not been tested in randomized controlled trial or have been shown not to have benefit in reducing neuropathic pain as in the case of topiramate [9, 10, 12].

Conclusions

As a group, anticonvulsants can be recommended as initial therapy for the treatment of neuropathic pain with significant pain relief of 50 % in approximately 30 % of patients and 30 % relief in 50 % of patients [46]. However, it is important to emphasize that only three peripheral neuropathic pain syndromes including PDN, PHN, and HIV neuropathy have been utilized to validate efficacy and generalized use for the treatment of neuropathic pain. Anticonvulsants, similar to other therapeutic classes of drugs for the treatment of central neuropathic pain, have for the most part demonstrated minimal efficacy. The one exception to this generalization is the 80 % efficacy data for carbamazepine in the treatment of trigeminal neuralgia. The most widely used anticonvulsants gabapentin [47] and pregabalin have been studied extensively and have demonstrated at best moderate efficacy in treatment of peripheral neuropathic pain.

References

1. Baron R, Tolle T, et al. A cross-sectional cohort survey in 2100 patients with painful diabetic neuropathy and postherpetic neuralgia: differences in demographic data and sensory symptoms. Pain. 2009;146:34–40.
2. Blom S. Trigeminal neuralgia: its treatment with a new anticonvulsant drug (G32883). Lancet. 1962;1:829–40.
3. Branco JC. State of the art on fibromyalgia mechanism. Acta Reumatol Port. 2010;35(1):10–5.
4. Rockoff BW, Davis EH. Controlled sequential trials of carbamazepine in trigeminal neuralgia. Arch Neurol. 1966;15:129–36.
5. Mellick LB, Mellick GA. Successful treatment of reflex sympathetic dystrophy with gabapentin. Am J Emerg Med. 1995;13:96.
6. Rosner H, Rubin L, Kestenbaum A. Gabapentin adjuvant therapy in neuropathic pain states. Clin J Pain. 1996;12:56–8.
7. Doworkin R, O'Connor A, et al. Recommendations for the pharmacologic management of neuropathic pain: an overview and literature update. Mayo Clin Proc. 2010;85 Suppl 3:S3–14.
8. Finnerup NB, Sindrup S, Jensen T. The evidence for pharmacological treatment of neuropathic. Pain. 2010;150:573–81.
9. Wiffen P, Collins S, McQuay H, Carroll D, Jadad A, Moore A. Anticonvulsant drugs for acute and chronic pain. Cochrane Database Syst Rev. 2005;20(3):CD001133.
10. Spina E, Perugi G. Antiepileptic drugs: indications of than epilepsy. Epileptic Disord. 2004;6(2):57–75.
11. Finnerup NB, Otto M, et al. Algorithm for neuropathic pain treatment: an evidence based proposal. Pain. 2005;118:289–305.
12. Goodyear-Smith F, Joan Halliwell. Anticonvulsants for neuropathic pain gaps in evidence. Clin J Pain. 2009;25(6):528–36.
13. Campbell FG, Graham JG, Zilkha KJ. Clinical trial of carbamazepine (Tegretol) in trigeminal neuralgia. J Neurol Neurosurg Psychiatry. 1966;29:265–7.
14. Cruccu G, Gronseth G, Alksne J, Argoff C, Brainin M, Burchiel K, et al. AAN-EFNS guidelines on trigeminal neuralgia management. Eur J Neurol. 2008;15:1013–28.
15. Gronseth G, Cruccu G, Alksne J, Argoff C, Brainin M, Burchiel K, et al. Practice parameter: the diagnostic evaluation and treatment of trigeminal neuralgia (an evidence-based review): report of the quality standards subcommittee of the American Academy of Neurology and the European Federation of Neurological Societies. Neurology. 2008;71:1183–90.
16. Zin C, Nissen LM, et al. An update on the pharmacologic management of post herpetic neuralgia and painful diabetic neuropathy. CNS Drugs. 2008;22(5):417–25.
17. Gilron I. Gabapentin and pregabalin for chronic neuropathic and early postsurgical pain: current evidence and future directions. Curr Opin Anaesthesiol. 2007;20:456–72.
18. Neurontin® (gabapentin) [package insert]. New York: Pfizer Inc; 2004.
19. Lyrica™ (pregabalin) capsules [package insert]. New York: Pfizer Inc; 2005.
20. Moore RA, Straube S, Wiffen PJ, Derry S, McQuay HJ. Pregabalin for acute and chronic pain in adults. Cochrane Database Syst Rev. 2009;3 Article No.: CD007076. doi: 10.1002/14651858.CD007076.pub2.
21. Dooley DJ, Taylor CP, et al. Ca^{2+} channel alpha-2-delta ligands; novel modulators of neurotransmission. Trends Pharmacol Sci. 2007;28(2):7582.
22. Taylor CP. Mechanisms of analgesia by gabapentin and pregabalin-calcium channel alpha-2-delta ligands. Pain. 2009;145(1–2):259.
23. Backonja M, Beydoun A, Edwards KR, Schwartz SL, Fonseca V, Hes M, LaMoreaux L, Garofalo E. Gabapentin for the symptomatic treatment of painful neuropathy in patients with diabetes mellitus. JAMA. 1998;280:1831–6.
24. Bennett M, Simpson K. Gabapentin in the treatment of neuropathic pain. Palliat Med. 2004;18:5–11.
25. Rowbotham M, Harden N, Stacey B, Bernstein P, Magnus-Miller L. Gabapentin for the treatment of postherpetic neuralgia. JAMA. 1998;280:1837–42.
26. Serpell M, Neuropathic Pain Study Group. Gabapentin in neuropathic pain syndromes: a randomised, double-blind, placebo-controlled trial. Pain. 2002;99:557–66.
27. Zin C, Nissen L, et al. A Randomized controlled trial of oxycodone vs placebo in patients with postherpetic neuralgia and painful diabetic neuropathy treated with pregabalin. J Pain. 2009;11:1–10.
28. Freynhagen R, Strojek K, et al. Efficacy of pregabalin in neuropathic pain evaluated in a 12-week, randomized, double-blind, multicentre, placebo-controlled trial of flexible- and fixed-dose regimens. Pain. 2005;115:254–63.
29. Lesser H, Sharma U, et al. Pregabalin relieves symptoms of painful diabetic neuropathy: a randomized controlled trial. Neurology. 2004;63:2104–10.
30. Richter RW, Portenoy R, Sharma U, et al. Relief of painful diabetic peripheral neuropathy with pregabalin: a randomized, placebo-controlled trial. J Pain. 2005;6(4):253–60.
31. Sabatowski R, Galvez R, Cherry DA, et al. Pregabalin reduces pain and improves sleep and mood disturbances in patients with postherpetic neuralgia: results of a randomized, placebo-controlled clinical trial. Pain. 2004;109:26–35.
32. Stacey BR, Barrett JA, et al. Pregabalin for postherpetic neuralgia: placebo-controlled trial of fixed and flexible dosing regimens on allodynia and time to onset of pain relief. J Pain. 2008;9(11):1006–17.
33. Siddall PJ, Cousins MJ, et al. Pregabalin in central neuropathic pain associated with spinal cord injury: a placebo-controlled trial. Neurology. 2006;67:1792–800.

34. van Seventer R, Feister HA, et al. Efficacy and tolerability of twice-daily pregabalin for treating pain and related sleep interference in postherpetic neuralgia: a 13-week, randomized trial. Curr Med Res Opin. 2006;22(2):375–84.

35. Killian JM, Fromm GH. Carbamazepine in the treatment of neuralgia. Arch Neurol. 1968;19:129–36.

36. Simpson DM, McArthur JC, et al. Lamotrigine for HIV-associated painful sensory neuropathies: placebo-controlled trial. Neurology. 2003;60:1508–14.

37. Gilron I, Bailey J, et al. Nortriptyline and gabapentin, alone and in combination for neuropathic pain: a double-blind, randomized controlled crossover trial. Lancet. 2009;374:1252–61.

38. Gilron I, Bailey J, et al. Morphine, gabapentin, or their combination for neuropathic pain. N Engl J Med. 2005;352:1324–34.

39. Crofford LJ, Mease PJ, Simpson SL, et al. Fibromyalgia relapse evaluation and efficacy for durability of meaningful relief (FREEDOM): a 6-month, double-blind, placebo-controlled trial with pregabalin. Pain. 2008;136(3):419–31.

40. Arnold LM, Russell IJ, Diri EW, et al. A 14-week, randomized, double-blind, placebo-controlled, monotherapy trial of pregabalin in patients with fibromyalgia. J Pain. 2008;9:792–805.

41. Mease PJ, Russell IJ, Arnold LM, et al. A randomized, double-blind, placebo-controlled, phase III trial of pregabalin in the treatment of patients with fibromyalgia. J Rheumatol. 2008;35(3):502–14.

42. Arnold LM, Goldenberg DL, et al. Gabapentin in the treatment of fibromyalgia: a randomized, double-blind, placebo-controlled, multicenter trial. Arthritis Rheum. 2007;56:1336–44.

43. Wolfe F, Smythe H, et al. The American College of Rheumatology 1990 criteria for the classification of fibromyalgia. Arthritis Rheum. 1990;33(2):160–72.

44. Simpson DM, Olney R, et al. A placebo controlled trial of lamotrigine for painful HIV-associated neuropathy. Neurology. 2000;54:2115–9.

45. Vestergaard K, Andersen G, et al. Lamotrigine for central post-stroke pain: a randomized controlled trial. Neurology. 2001;56:184–90.

46. Chou R, Norris S, Carson S, Chan BKS. Drug class review on drugs for neuropathic pain. 2007. http://www.ohsu.edu/drugeffectiveness/reports/final.cfm. Accessed 2007.

47. Rice AS, Maton S, Postherpetic Neuralgia Study Group. Gabapentin in postherpetic neuralgia: a randomised, double blind, placebo controlled study. Pain. 2001;94:215–24.

NMDA Receptor Antagonists in the Treatment of Pain

6

Yakov Vorobeychik, Channing D. Willoughby, and Jianren Mao

Key Points

- NMDA receptors play a pivotal role in a number of essential physiological functions including neuroplasticity. However, persistent and excessive stimulation of this receptor could be detrimental to the central nervous system, leading to neuronal degenerative changes and neurotoxicity. In this regard, NMDA receptors may play a significant role in the development and maintenance of persistent pathological pain.
- Preclinical evidence suggests that blockade of NMDA receptors would prevent the development of a persistent pain state and effectively reverse signs of a persistent pain. Therefore, NMDA receptor antagonists also would be expected to have a therapeutic role in treating persistent pain states in the clinical setting.
- Many clinical studies demonstrated that NMDA receptor antagonists could be efficacious in the treatment of chronic pain states, particularly neuropathic pain, as

well as in the management of any non-neuropathic opioid-resistant pain due to developing opioid tolerance or opioid-induced hyperalgesia (OIH). Apparent opioid-sparing effects of these drugs also make them an attractive therapy in the acute pain setting. However, some other studies have failed to prove the clinical usefulness of these medications.
- The perioperative use of an NMDA receptor antagonist may lead to the reduction of postoperative pain from a surgical procedure that is more likely to involve central sensitization but may not provide significant pain reduction if the major component of postoperative pain is considered to be nociceptive.
- Side effects of NMDA receptor antagonists, when administered at therapeutic doses, are a primary limiting factor in their use in clinical practice today. Powerful direct competitive NMDA receptor blockers, as well as high-affinity noncompetitive antagonists, exhibit inadequate therapeutic margins for human use when evaluated in clinical trials. An obvious limitation in assessing the role of the NMDA receptor mechanism in clinical pain management has been the lack of highly selective NMDA receptor antagonists suitable for clinical use.
- It may be anticipated that chronic pain treatment can be improved through the use of NMDA receptor antagonists displaying minimal clinical side effects at therapeutic doses.

Y. Vorobeychik, M.D., Ph.D. (✉)
Department of Anesthesiology, Pennsylvania State University Milton S. Hershey Medical Center, 500 University Drive, HU-32, 850, Hershey, PA 17033, USA

Pennsylvania State University College of Medicine, Hershey, PA, USA
e-mail: yvorbeychik@psu.edu

C.D. Willoughby, M.D.
Department of Anesthesiology, Pennsylvania State University Milton S. Hershey Medical Center, 500 University Drive, HU-32, 850, Hershey, PA 17033, USA
e-mail: channingwilloughby@gmail.com

J. Mao, M.D., Ph.D.
Department of Anesthesia, Harvard Medical School, Boston, MA, USA

Department of Anesthesia, Critical Care and Pain Medicine, Massachusetts General Hospital, 15 Parkman St, Boston, MA 02114, USA
e-mail: jmao@partners.org

Introduction

Over the past three decades, the central glutamatergic system, particularly the role of the N-methyl-D-aspartate (NMDA) receptor in the neural mechanisms of persistent pain, has been extensively investigated. Chronic pain can be sustained by way of a central sensitization process involving the NMDA receptor system. A considerable number of clinical trials have also been carried out to evaluate the potential application of

T.R. Deer et al. (eds.), *Treatment of Chronic Pain by Medical Approaches: the AMERICAN ACADEMY of PAIN MEDICINE Textbook on Patient Management*, DOI 10.1007/978-1-4939-1818-8_6,
© American Academy of Pain Medicine 2015

such mechanisms in clinical pain management. Data from the preclinical studies have consistently supported a crucial role of the central glutamatergic system and NMDA receptors in the induction and maintenance of persistent pain resulting from pathological conditions such as inflammation and nerve injury. To date, clinical trials have resulted in mixed conclusions as to the overall effectiveness in treating persistent pain with NMDA receptor antagonists. Nonetheless, NMDA receptor antagonists have been demonstrated as an effective treatment option in the management of chronic pain, particularly for pain which has been refractory to other treatment modalities.

Table 6.1 Common NMDA receptor antagonists

Ketamine
Amantadine
Memantine
Phencyclidine
Dextromethorphan
Methadone[a]

[a]Commonly clinically utilized for opioid agonist properties

NMDA Receptors

The NMDA receptor is a subgroup of a large family of glutamate receptors that utilize excitatory amino acids such as glutamate and aspartate as the endogenous agonist. At least three major families of genes have been identified that encode NMDA receptor subunits, namely, NR1, NR2, and NR3 subunits [1]. Various combinations of NR1 and other NR subunits determine the property of NMDA receptor activity. The NR1 subunit is necessary for the NMDA receptor-coupled channel activity, and other subunits are likely to modulate the properties of such channel activities. Recent studies have examined the NR2B subunit of the NMDA receptor and its effect on modulation of pain, proposing that a positive feedback pathway of this subunit as an explanation for cortical sensitization of chronic pain [2, 3].

A unique characteristic of the NMDA receptor is that this receptor is both voltage- and ligand-gated, such that activation of this receptor requires not only an agonist binding but also cell membrane depolarization. As such, activation of NMDA receptors often involves simultaneous activation of other subtypes of glutamate receptors and/or neuropeptidergic receptors. The NMDA receptor-channel complex can be regulated at multiple sites including glutamate, glycine, and calcium channel sites.

NMDA receptors have been localized in both supraspinal and spinal regions from a number of species including mice, rats, and human subjects. There appears to be a minimal variation of NMDA receptor distributions among different species. At the supraspinal level, NMDA receptor binding has been found in hippocampus, cerebral cortex, thalamus, striatum, cerebellum, and brain stem. At the spinal level, NMDA receptor binding has been demonstrated mainly within the substantia gelatinosa of the dorsal horn with limited, very low-level binding elsewhere in the spinal gray matter [1].

Since most studies show NMDA receptor binding or immunocytochemical labeling in the neuronal somata, the location of NMDA receptors generally is considered to be postsynaptic. However, presynaptic NMDA receptors also have been demonstrated within the terminals of primary afferent fibers using the combined electron microscopic and immunocytochemical technique. The presynaptic NMDA receptors also are likely to be auto-receptors [4]. It is likely that these receptors may have a role in regulating release of excitatory amino acids from presynaptic terminals. NMDA receptors play a pivotal role in a number of essential physiological functions including neuroplasticity. Neuroplasticity takes place in a variety of forms and contributes to such events as memory formation. It is the persistent and excessive stimulation of this receptor that could be detrimental to the central nervous system, leading to neuronal degenerative changes and neurotoxicity [1]. In this regard, NMDA receptors may play a significant role in the development and maintenance of persistent pathological pain following inflammation (inflammatory pain) and/or nerve injury (neuropathic pain).

NMDA Receptors and Pain Mechanisms

Preclinical Studies

Compelling evidence has emerged from preclinical studies that indicate a critical role of NMDA receptors in the neural mechanisms of persistent nociceptive states including neuropathy and inflammation (Table 6.1) [5–10]. These studies reveal several fundamental features of the NMDA receptor involvement in such pain states. First, NMDA receptors are involved in pain states induced by either partial or complete nerve injury or by persistent inflammation. Second, experimental pain states can be prevented and/or reversed by using either experimental (AP5, MK-801) or clinically available (ketamine, amantadine, dextromethorphan) NMDA receptor antagonists. Third, thermal hyperalgesia, mechanical allodynia, and, in some cases, spontaneous pain behaviors were reduced effectively with an NMDA receptor antagonist in experimental persistent pain states.

By and large, preclinical evidence regarding the role of NMDA receptors in persistent pain states is reproducible and reliable. Such preclinical evidence suggests that blockade of NMDA receptors would prevent the development of a persistent pain state in a clinical setting. Because NMDA receptor antagonists also effectively reverse signs of a persistent pain state in preclinical studies, an NMDA receptor antagonist also would be expected to have a therapeutic role in treating persistent pain states in the clinical setting. These are two key hypotheses (the preventive and therapeutic role of an NMDA receptor antagonist) that have been tested in many clinical trials carried out over the last several years.

Clinical Studies

Currently, clinically available NMDA receptor antagonists include ketamine, dextromethorphan, amantadine, and memantine. They bind to the channel site and are considered relatively low-affinity agents. The opioid analgesic methadone is also known to express NMDA receptor antagonistic properties. Unfortunately, direct competitive NMDA receptor blockers that bind to the site of glutamate (e.g., AP5), as well as high-affinity noncompetitive antagonists, all exhibit inadequate therapeutic margins for human use when evaluated in clinical trials [11–15].

The antagonism of NMDA activity and subsequent inhibition of central sensitization offers a valuable pain treatment approach. NMDA antagonists can be efficacious in the treatment of chronic pain states, particularly neuropathic pain, as well as in the management of any non-neuropathic opioid-resistant pain due to developing opioid tolerance or opioid-induced hyperalgesia (OIH). Apparent opioid-sparing effects of these drugs also make them an attractive therapy in the acute pain setting.

In patients with chronic pain states that have been refractory to more standard therapy, particularly neuropathic pain, NMDA receptor antagonists have been frequently utilized. Studies evaluating high-dose IV ketamine in the treatment of complex regional pain syndrome (CRPS) have demonstrated substantial decreases in pain scores and, in some instances, complete resolution of study subjects' pain [16, 17]. There is also some evidence that the use of ketamine at sub-anesthetic doses also improves a multitude of pain parameters in patients with CRPS [15, 18–20]. One particular case series of six patients with CRPS who underwent treatment with the NMDA receptor antagonist memantine for 6 months demonstrated improved pain scores and other markers of disease, including functional MRI changes [21].

In postherpetic neuralgia that has been refractory to more conventional treatment, intravenous ketamine has shown to be an effective therapy in decreasing initial visual analogue scale (VAS) pain scores and offering sustained pain relief 1 year following initial treatment [22]. Several studies have focused upon the use of ketamine in the treatment of phantom limb pain. One such study demonstrated ketamine to be superior to calcitonin in the treatment of persistent phantom limb pain [23]. Yet another study evaluating epidurally administered ketamine with local anesthetic demonstrated improved short-term analgesia and decreased mechanical sensitivity in patients suffering from phantom limb pain condition, further substantiating the role of NMDA receptor antagonism and its inhibition of central sensitization [24]. Memantine has also been evaluated for the treatment of phantom limb pain. While some findings were inconclusive, the overall trend suggests that memantine may serve as a useful adjuvant agent for this disorder [25–28].

NMDA receptor antagonists may play a particularly important role in cancer-related opioid- resistant pain treatment. Utilization of high doses of opioid analgesics may lead to the development of opioid unresponsiveness in oncology patients. OIH, pharmacodynamic, pharmacokinetic, and learned tolerance can all cause decreased opioid efficacy in this patient population [29]. Many studies published during the last decade showed that low to moderate doses of ketamine significantly improve analgesia in patients with opioid refractory cancer pain [30–34]. In dissonance, one systemic review demonstrated lack of suitable randomized trials and insufficient evidence to make recommendations for routine use of ketamine for cancer pain [35]. The most recent work by Kapural et al. failed to prove the use of ketamine as an effective way to lower long-term pain scores in patients taking high-dose opioids in the settings of neuropathic or nociceptive pain [16].

The role of OIH in clinical situations has been demonstrated in some chronic pain patients, many of who were taking "megadoses" of opioid [36–39]. It has been shown that the addition of an NMDA receptor antagonist for the management of patients who have failed to benefit from opioid rotation or other adjunctive treatments may lead to a more favorable clinical outcome. Several publications report the successful use of ketamine for OIH [40–42]. Methadone, with its D-isomer demonstrating NMDA receptor antagonism, is also mechanistically appealing for the treatment of OIH [43–46]. Dextromethorphan has been studied to assess its clinical utility in treating OIH or limiting tolerance with mixed results [47, 48].

Opioid-sparing effects of NMDA receptor antagonists is well established. The combination of NMDA antagonists with opioid and other non-opioid analgesics can act in synergism, providing an optimal multimodal approach to the management of pain. Ketamine has been demonstrated to provide opioid-sparing effects, facilitate postsurgical rehabilitation, and offer decreased postoperative pain in patients following total hip arthroplasty [49]. Likewise, low-dose ketamine administration has been shown to decrease postoperative morphine consumption and improve postoperative analgesia in patients undergoing major abdominal surgery [50]. Amantadine, most known for its antiviral and antiparkinsonian effects, has been shown to lower the morphine dose requirements and VAS pain scores in patients undergoing radical prostatectomy [51].

Discrepancies Between Preclinical and Clinical Studies

A considerable number of clinical studies (both controlled randomized studies and case observations) have been conducted to test the above hypotheses. Clinically available agents, all with the NMDA receptor antagonist properties, were commonly used in these studies. Unlike unequivocal results from the bench studies, however, clinical outcomes of pain relief using NMDA receptor antagonists have varied substantially among different studies.

The role of the NMDA receptor mechanism in persistent pain states is overwhelmingly supported by the data from a large number of preclinical studies, yet outcomes from clinical studies are far less certain. One obvious limitation in assessing the role of the NMDA receptor mechanism in clinical pain management has been the lack of highly selective NMDA receptor antagonists suitable for clinical use.

NMDA Receptor Antagonists and Preemptive Analgesia

The concept of preemptive analgesia suggests that postoperative pain intensity could be enhanced due to the process of central sensitization driven by repeated peripheral nociceptive input and mediated through the NMDA receptor. As such, blocking the establishment of central sensitization preoperatively with a clinically available NMDA receptor antagonist would be expected to prevent the development of postoperative pain hypersensitivity. This potentially beneficial effect would be reflected as diminished pain intensity, hence a lower pain score and/or a reduced consumption of analgesics (such as opioids) in surgical patients who receive perioperative treatment with a clinically available NMDA receptor antagonist. To date, nearly all of the clinical studies examining preemptive analgesia have been conducted along this line of experimental design. Several important issues on this topic deserve some discussion.

Is Postoperative Pain Primarily due to Central Sensitization?

This fundamental question needs to be better addressed for two important reasons. First, although NMDA receptors play a pivotal role in central sensitization, they are not primarily involved in the processing of nociceptive pain. Second, because NMDA receptors do not play a major role in the processing of nociceptive pain, an NMDA receptor antagonist by itself could not function as an effective analgesic. Thus, the perioperative use of an NMDA receptor antagonist alone may not provide significant pain reduction if the major component of postoperative pain is considered to be nociceptive pain. By the same token, one would expect that the reduction of postoperative pain from a surgical procedure that is more likely to involve central sensitization, such as limb amputation, would be better achieved with the perioperative use of an NMDA receptor antagonist.

Is the Study Design Sufficiently Sensitive to Make a Distinction Between the Reduction of Nociceptive Pain and Decreased Pain Hypersensitivity?

It is conceivable that central sensitization would be contributory to postoperative pain if repeated intra- and postoperative nociceptive input is the driving force for the NMDA receptor-mediated cellular and molecular changes underlying the development of neuronal plasticity. In this regard, one might argue that regardless of the relative contribution of nociceptive pain and/or increased pain hypersensitivity, perioperative use of an NMDA receptor antagonist (hence the prevention of pain hypersensitivity) would lead to a reduction of pain scoring and/or sparing of postoperative analgesic use. The issue is whether the clinical trial design is sensitive enough to make such a distinction. Thus, an adequate power of analysis should be considered for clinical studies.

Adverse Effects

Side effects of NMDA receptor antagonists when administered at therapeutic doses are a primary limiting factor in their use in clinical practice today (Table 6.2). They may cause psycho-cognitive issues, sedation, respiratory depression, and cardiostimulatory derangements. Alterations in

Table 6.2 Potential side effects of NMDA antagonists

Psychosocial	Confusion
	Hallucinations
	Delirium
	Anxiety
	Insomnia
Cardiovascular	Arrhythmias
	Hemodynamic instability
Respiratory	Apnea
Gastrointestinal	Nausea/vomiting
	Anorexia
Ocular	Diplopia
	Nystagmus
Musculoskeletal	Myoclonus

body image and mood, feelings of unreality, floating sensation, hallucinations, restlessness, vivid dreams, dissociation, insomnia, fatigue, delirium, confusion, and drowsiness are among the cognitive adverse effects described in the literature [52]. Increased blood pressure and heart rate are the most common cardiovascular complications [40]. NMDA receptor antagonists were found to trigger a dose-dependent neurotoxic reaction in the cingulated and retrosplenial cortices of adult rats when administered as a short-term treatment [53]. Prolonged continuous infusion of intrathecal ketamine has been associated with spinal cord vacuolization [54]. However, most of the mentioned side effects have been reported with intravenous or subcutaneous administration of this NMDA receptor blocker. Oral ketamine produces few adverse effects [55]. Moreover, the incidence of side effects with ketamine's systemic use in combination with opioids is low and does not differ from controls treated with opioids only [56]. Specifically, hallucinations occur in 7.4 %, "pleasant dreams" in 18.3 %, nightmares in 4 %, and visual disturbance in 6.2 % of patients [57]. The overall rate of central nervous system adverse effects in patients receiving low-dose ketamine is about 10 % [58]. It is believed that ketamine may cause psychotomimetic effects by disinhibiting certain excitatory transmitter circuits in the human brain [59]. Some drugs such as benzodiazepines can restore the inhibition to this circuitry, providing a neuroprotective effect and reducing the rate of complications [60]. Therefore, concomitant use of benzodiazepines is recommended during ketamine infusion treatment [61]. Another class of medications, alpha-2 adrenergic agonists, may also protect against neurotoxic, psychotomimetic, and cardiostimulatory side effects of NMDA antagonists and, in the case of neuropathic pain, exert a synergistic analgesic effect [18, 62, 63]. Recent studies focusing upon the neramexane and memantine suggest that NMDA antagonists may be used at therapeutic doses without adverse side effects [64, 65].

Conclusion

In summary, NMDA receptors are likely to play a significant role in the central mechanisms of persistent pain. It is conceivable that the outcome of clinical use of NMDA receptor antagonists may vary significantly depending on pain condition, onset of treatment, dosing regimen, and pain assessment tools. NMDA receptor antagonists are more likely to be helpful in improving pain conditions such as neuropathic pain involving the mechanisms of central sensitization. Thus, it is important to recognize the limitation of using NMDA receptor antagonists in clinical pain management. Recent studies have indicated potential clinical benefits of using agents that target new NMDA receptor sites (e.g., NR2 sub-

unit) [2, 3, 66, 67]. It may be anticipated that chronic pain treatment can be improved through the use of NMDA receptor antagonists displaying minimal clinical side effects at therapeutic doses.

References

1. Mao J. NMDA and opioid receptors: their interactions in antinociception, tolerance, and neuroplasticity. Brain Res Rev. 1999;30:289–304.
2. Hu J, Wang Z, Guo YY, et al. A role of periaqueductal grey NR2B-containing NMDA receptor in mediating persistent inflammatory pain. Mol Pain. 2009;5:71.
3. Zhuo M. Plasticity of NMDA receptor NR2B subunit in memory and chronic pain. Mol Brain. 2009;2:4.
4. Liu J, Wang H, Sheng M, Jan LY, Jan YN, Basbaum AI. Evidence for presynaptic N-methyl-D-aspartate autoreceptors in the spinal cord dorsal horn. Proc Natl Acad Sci USA. 1994;91(18):8383–7.
5. Dickenson AH. A cure for wind-up: NMDA receptor antagonists as potential analgesics. Trends Pharmacol Sci. 1990;11:307–9.
6. Woolf CJ, Thompson SWN. The induction and maintenance of central sensitization is dependent on N-methyl-D-aspartic acid receptor activation: implications for the treatment of post-injury pain hypersensitivity states. Pain. 1991;44:293–9.
7. Woolf CJ, Mannion RJ. Neuropathic pain: aetiology, symptoms, mechanisms, and management. Lancet. 1999;353:1959–64.
8. Dubner R. Neuronal plasticity and pain following peripheral tissue inflammation or nerve injury. In: Bond M, Charlton E, Woolf CJ, editors. Proceedings of 5th world congress on pain. Pain research and clinical management, vol. 5. Amsterdam: Elsevier; 1991. p. 263–76.
9. Mao J, Price DD, Mayer DJ. Mechanisms of hyperalgesia and opiate tolerance: a current view of their possible interactions. Pain. 1995;62:259–74.
10. Chaplan SR, Malmberg AB, Yaksh TL. Efficacy of spinal NMDA receptor antagonism in formalin hyperalgesia and nerve injury evoked allodynia in the rat. J Pharmacol Exp Ther. 1997;280:829–38.
11. Yenari MA, Bell TE, Kotake AN, et al. Dose escalation safety and tolerance study of the competitive NMDA antagonist selfotel (CGS-19755) in neurosurgery patients. Clin Neuropharmacol. 1998;21(1):28–34.
12. Muir KW, Lees KR. Excitatory amino acid antagonists for acute stroke. Cochrane Database Syst Rev. 2003;3:CD001244.
13. Hoyte L, Barber PA, Buchan AM, et al. The rise and fall of NMDA antagonists for ischemic stroke. Curr Mol Med. 2004;4(2):131–6.
14. Wood PL. The NMDA receptor complex: a long and winding road to therapeutics. IDrugs. 2005;8(3):229–35.
15. Harbut RE, Correll GE. Successful treatment of a nine-year case of complex regional pain syndrome type-I (reflex sympathetic dystrophy) with intravenous ketamine-infusion therapy in a warfarin-anticoagulated adult female patient. Pain Med. 2002;3:147–55.
16. Kapural L, Kapural M, Bensitel T, et al. Opioid-sparing effect of intravenous outpatient ketamine infusions appears short-lived in chronic-pain patients with high opioid requirements. Pain Physician. 2010;13:389–94.
17. Goldberg ME, Torjman MC, Schwartzman RJ, et al. Pharmacodynamic profiles of ketamine (R)- and (S)- with 5-day inpatient infusion for the treatment of complex regional pain syndrome. Pain Physician. 2010;13:379–87.
18. Correll EC, Maleki J, Gracely EJ, et al. Subanesthetic ketamine infusion therapy: a retrospective analysis of a novel therapeutic approach to complex regional pain syndrome. Pain Med. 2004;5(3):263–75.

19. Schwartzman RJ, Alexander GM, Grothusen JR, et al. Outpatient intravenous ketamine for the treatment of complex regional pain syndrome: a double-blind placebo controlled study. Pain. 2009;147:107–15.

20. Nama S, Meenan DR, Fritz WT. The use of sub-anesthetic intravenous ketamine and adjuvant dexmedetomidine when treating acute pain from CRPS. Pain Physician. 2010;13:365–8.

21. Sinis N, Birbaumer N, Gustin S, et al. Memantine treatment of complex regional pain syndrome: a preliminary report of six cases. Clin J Pain. 2007;23:237–43.

22. Tsuneyoshi I, Gushiken T, Kanmura Y, Yoshimura N. Changes in pain intensity of post-herpetic neuralgia following intravenous injections of ketamine hydrochloride. J Anesth. 1999;13(1):53–5.

23. Urs E, Neff F, Sveticic G, et al. Chronic phantom limb pain: the effects of calcitonin, ketamine, and their combination on pain and sensory thresholds. Anesth Analg. 2008;106(4):1265–73.

24. Wilson JA, Nimmo AF, Fleetwood-Walker SM, et al. Randomized double blind trail of the effect of pre-emptive epidural ketamine on persistent pain after lower limb amputation. Pain. 2008;135:108–18.

25. Schley M, Topfner S, Wiech K, Schaller HE, Konrad CJ, Schmelz M, Birbaumer N. Continuous brachial plexus blockade in combination with the NMDA receptor antagonist memantine prevents phantom pain in acute traumatic upper limb amputees. Eur J Pain. 2007;11:299–308.

26. Nikolajsen L, Gottrup H, Kristensen AG, Jensen TS. Memantine (a N-methyl-d-aspartate receptor antagonist) in the treatment of neuropathic pain after amputation or surgery: a randomized, double-blinded, cross-over study. Anesth Analg. 2000;91:960–96.

27. Wiech K, Kiefer RT, Topfner S, Preissl H, Braun C, Unertl K, Flor H, Birbaumer N. A placebo-controlled randomized crossover trial of the N-methyl-d-aspartic acid receptor antagonist, memantine, in patients with chronic phantom limb pain. Anesth Analg. 2004;98:408–13.

28. Maier C, Dertwinkel R, Mansourian N, Hosbach I, Schwenkreis P, Senne I, Skipka G, Zenz M, Tegenthoff M. Efficacy of the NMDA-receptor antagonist memantine in patients with chronic phantom limb pain–results of a randomized double-blinded, placebo-controlled trial. Pain. 2003;103:277–83.

29. Chang G, Chen L, Mao J. Opioid tolerance and hyperalgesia. Med Clin North Am. 2007;91(2):199–211.

30. Mercadante S, Arcuri E, Tirelli W, et al. Analgesic effect of intravenous ketamine in cancer patients on morphine therapy. J Pain Symptom Manage. 2000;20:246–52.

31. Good P, Tullio F, Jackson K, et al. Prospective audit of short-term concurrent ketamine, opioid and anti-inflammatory "triple-agent" therapy of episodes of acute on chronic pain. Intern Med J. 2005;35:39–44.

32. Kannan TR, Saxena A, Bhatnagar S, et al. Oral ketamine as an adjuvant to oral morphine for neuropathic pain in cancer patients. J Pain Symptom Manage. 2002;23:60–5.

33. Fitzgibbon EJ, Viola R. Parenteral ketamine as an analgesic adjuvant for severe pain: development and retrospective audit of a protocol for a palliative care unit. J Palliat Med. 2005;8(1):49–57.

34. Lossignol DA, Obiols-Portis M, Body JJ. Successful use of ketamine for intractable cancer pain. Support Care Cancer. 2005;13(3):188–93.

35. Bell RF, Eccleston C, Kalso E. Ketamine as adjuvant to opioids for cancer pain. A qualitative systematic review. J Pain Symptom Manage. 2003;26:867–75.

36. Gardell LR, Wang R, Burgess SE, et al. Sustained morphine exposure induces a spinal dynorphin-dependent enhancement of excitatory transmitter release from primary afferent fibers. J Neurosci. 2002;22(15):6747–55.

37. Gardell LR, King T, Ossipov MH, et al. Opioid receptor-mediated hyperalgesia and antinociceptive tolerance induced by sustained opiate delivery. Neurosci Lett. 2006;396(1):44–9.

38. Mao J. Opioid-induced abnormal pain sensitivity: implications in clinical opioid therapy. Pain. 2002;100(3):213–7.

39. Chu LF, Angst MS, Clark D. Opioid induced hyperalgesia in humans: molecular mechanisms and clinical considerations. Clin J Pain. 2008;24(6):479–96.

40. Okon T. Ketamine: an introduction for the pain and palliative medicine physician. Pain Physician. 2007;10:493–500.

41. Joly V, Richebe P, Guignard B, et al. Remifentanil-induced postoperative hyperalgesia and its prevention with small-dose ketamine. Anesthesiology. 2005;103(1):147–55.

42. Singla A, Stojanovic MP, Chen L, et al. A differential diagnosis of hyperalgesia toxicity, and withdrawal from intrathecal morphine infusion. Anesth Analg. 2007;105(6):1816–9.

43. Vorobeychik Y, Chen L, Bush MC, et al. Improved opioid analgesic effect following opioid dose reduction. Pain Med. 2008;5(6):724–7.

44. Axelrod DJ, Reville B. Using methadone to treat opioid-induced hyperalgesia and refractory pain. J Opioid Manag. 2007;3(2):113–4.

45. Mercandate S, Arcuri E. Hyperalgesia and opioid switching. Am J Hosp Palliat Care. 2005;22:291–4.

46. Chung KS, Carson S, Glassman D, et al. Successful treatment of hydromorphone induced neurotoxicity and hyperalgesia. Conn Med. 2004;68:547–9.

47. Galer BS, Lee D, Ma T, et al. Morphidex (morphine sulfate/dextromethorphan hydrobromide combination) in the treatment of chronic pain: three multicenter, randomized, double-blend, controlled clinical trials fail to demonstrate enhanced opioid analgesia or reduction in tolerance. Pain. 2005;115:284–95.

48. Katz NP. Morphidex (MS:DM) double-blind, multiple-dose studies in chronic pain patients. J Pain Symptom Manage. 2000;19:S42–9.

49. Rémérand F, Le Tendre C, Baud A, et al. The early and delayed analgesic effects of ketamine after total hip arthroplasty: a prospective, randomized, controlled, double-blind study. Anesth Analg. 2009;109(6):1963–71.

50. Zakine J, Samarcq D, Lorne E, et al. Postoperative ketamine administration decreases morphine consumption in major abdominal surgery: a prospective, randomized, double blind, controlled study. Anesth Analg. 2008;106(6):1856–61.

51. Snijdelaar DG, Koren G, Katz J. Effects of perioperative amantadine on postoperative pain and morphine consumption in patients after radical prostatectomy. Anesthesiology. 2004;100:134–41.

52. Fisher K, Coderre TJ, Hagen NA. Targeting the N-methyl-D-aspartate receptor for chronic pain management: preclinical animal studies, recent clinical experience and future research directions. J Pain Symptom Manage. 2000;20(5):358–73.

53. Jevtovic-Todorovic V, Wozniak DF, Benshoff ND, et al. A comparative evaluation of neurotoxic properties of ketamine and nitrous oxide. Brain Res. 2001;895:246–7.

54. Stoltz M, Oehen HP, Gerber H. Histological findings after long-term infusion of intrathecal ketamine for chronic pain: a case report. J Pain Symptom Manage. 1999;18:223–8.

55. Fisher K, Hagen NA. Analgesic effect of oral ketamine in chronic neuropathic pain of spinal origin: a case report. J Pain Symptom Manage. 1999;18:61–6.

56. Visser E, Schug SA. The role of ketamine in pain management. Biomed Pharmacother. 2006;60(7):341–8.

57. Elia N, Tramer MR. Ketamine and postoperative pain – a quantitative systematic review of randomized trials. Pain. 2005;113(1–2):61–70.

58. Subramaniam K, Subramaniam B, Steinbrook RA. Ketamine as adjuvant analgesic to opioids: a quantitative and qualitative systematic review. Anesth Analg. 2004;99(2):482–95.

59. Jevtovic-Todorovic V, Olney JW. Neuroprotective agents. In: Evers AS, Mayes M, editors. Anesthetic pharmacology, physiologic principles and clinical practice. Philadelphia: Churchill Livingstone; 2004. p. 557–72.

60. Farber NB, Kim SH, Dikranian K, et al. Receptor mechanisms and circuitry underlying NMDA antagonist neurotoxicity. Mol Psychiatry. 2002;7:32–43.

61. Prommer E. Ketamine to control pain. J Palliat Med. 2003;6(3): 443–6.

62. Kim SH, Price MT, Olney JW, et al. Excessive cerebrocortical release of acetylcholine induced by NMDA antagonists is reduced by GABAergic and alpha- adrenergic agonists. Mol Psychiatry. 1999;4:344–52.

63. Handa F, Tanaka M, Nishikawa T, et al. Effects of oral clonidine premedication on side effects of intravenous ketamine anesthesia: a randomized, double-blind placebo-controlled study. J Clin Anesth. 2000;12:19–24.

64. Chen S-R, Samoriski G, Pan H-L. Antinociceptive effects of chronic administration of uncompetitive NMDA receptor antago-

nists in a rat model of diabetic neuropathic pain. Neuropharmacology. 2009;57(2):121–6.

65. Hackworth RJ, Tokarz KA, Fowler IA, Wallace SC, Stedje-Larsen ET. Profound pain reduction after induction of memantine treatment in two patients with severe phantom limb pain. Anesth Analg. 2008;107(4):1377–9.

66. Chazot PL. The NMDA receptor NR2B subunit: a valid therapeutic target for multiple CNS pathologies. Curr Med Chem. 2004;11:389–96.

67. Tao YX, Raja SN. Are synaptic MAGUK proteins involved in chronic pain? Trends Pharmacol Sci. 2004;25:397–400.

Role of Muscle Relaxants in the Treatment of Pain

Robert I. Cohen and Carol A. Warfield

Key Points

- Muscle relaxants are a diverse group of medications with limited indications which share few structural similarities and where known, few mechanisms of action.
- There are four different mechanisms by which muscle relaxants are thought to work. Baclofen is active at the GABA-B receptor, tizanidine at the alpha-2 receptor, cyclobenzaprine at small TLRs in spinal microglia, and flupirtine (available in Europe) activates a potassium "M-current" in Kv7 potassium channels.
- As a group, muscle relaxants have a high side effect profile and produce limited benefit.
- FDA indications include treatment of "musculoskeletal disorders" and treatment of "spasticity."
- When used in musculoskeletal disorders such as low back pain, benefit has been established compared with placebo. However, there are few head-to-head trials against active agents suggesting that this group should be utilized as the first-line treatment. At the same time, there is some evidence that these drugs should not be used long term for chronic back pain.
- While evidence of efficacy is poor compared with other classes of drugs, usage of these medications is high, especially among primary care physicians (PCPs) and to a lesser degree by rheumatologists, psychiatrists, and neurologists.

- One of the most commonly prescribed agents, cyclobenzaprine is very closely related to the tricyclic antidepressants and it differs from amitriptyline by only one double bond.
- Carisoprodol is probably the most controversial member of this class which is metabolized by cytochrome P450-CYP2C19 to the barbiturate meprobamate.
- Baclofen is the mainstay for treatment of upper motor neuron syndromes leading to spasticity. Unacceptable sedation at therapeutically effective oral doses makes it desirable to administer this drug intrathecally which minimizes side effects.

Introduction

This chapter is about drugs approved to treat both spastic upper motor neuron conditions like cerebral palsy or multiple sclerosis and drugs that are used to relieve muscle spasm associated with musculoskeletal conditions such as acute non-radicular cervical or low back pain. Unlike other analgesic classes such as opioids and NSAIDS, the muscle relaxant drugs as a group share neither chemical structure nor mechanism of action. For example, two drugs approved to treat spasm, baclofen and tizanidine, work by different mechanisms. The former blocks GABA-B receptors and the latter is an alpha-2 agonist. Cyclobenzaprine, a drug approved for treating spasm-type pain in the low back, except for one double bond, is chemically identical to the tricyclic antidepressant amitriptyline.

If muscle relaxants are dissimilar in structure and mechanism of action, one thing they share as a class is a high side effect profile. Because the evidence for harm is strong and the evidence for benefit is weak, muscle relaxants should not be first-line drugs for musculoskeletal conditions like acute low back pain, and when used, the course should be brief unless there is clear evidence that for a given individual, there is ongoing benefit and lack of significant side effects [1].

R.I. Cohen, M.D., M.A. (Educ) (✉)
Department of Anesthesia, Critical Care and Pain Medicine, Beth Israel Deaconess Medical Center, 330 Brookline Avenue, Boston, MA 02215, USA
e-mail: ricohen@bidmc.hardvard.edu

C.A. Warfield, M.D.
Department of Anesthesia, Critical Care and Pain Medicine, Harvard Medical School, Boston, MA, USA

222, Prides Crossing, MA 01965, USA
e-mail: cwarfiel@bidmc.harvard.edu

T.R. Deer et al. (eds.), *Treatment of Chronic Pain by Medical Approaches: the AMERICAN ACADEMY of PAIN MEDICINE Textbook on Patient Management*, DOI 10.1007/978-1-4939-1818-8_7,
© American Academy of Pain Medicine 2015

While these drugs are not recommended as first-line drugs, in practice, that is frequently how they are used. In a study based on insurance claims of 211,511 patients with low back pain, 69 % were treated with prescription medication with the tendency to prescribe muscle relaxants first; then, on subsequent visits, drugs tended to be prescribed in the following order: NSAIDs, antidepressants, and opioids, with opioids being the last to be prescribed [2].

While there may be a response to the publication of guidelines for best practice, the effect is not necessarily sustained. In 1994, the Agency for Healthcare Research and Quality (AHRQ) published evidence-based guidelines for best practice for low back pain that included recommendations similar to the WHO pain ladder for increased use of acetaminophen and NSAIDs and recommended against the use of muscle relaxant medications. Three years after release of the guidelines, Jackson et al. reviewed a database of ten million patient visits, half in the 3 years before the guidelines were issued and half following release [3]. They report that the AHRQ guidelines had a modest impact on practice, showing increased use of acetaminophen and NSAIDs and decreased use of muscle relaxants. As far as muscle relaxants are concerned, educational efforts have been disappointing due to a lack of sustained effect and repeated efforts at education would seem to be necessary.

Driven by an effort to reduce cost in addition to providing better care, California commissioned an expert physician panel to work with a California Medicaid provider covering more than 100,000 recipients. They identified five overused PCP behaviors, one of which was long-term treatment of back pain with muscle relaxants. Muscle relaxant use decreased significantly after an intervention carried out among 45 primary care physicians where their behaviors were discussed, educational material provided, and ongoing behavior monitored [4]. This is a recent study, and long-term follow-up data is not available to describe whether the educational and monitoring effort will continue and if the behavioral changes in physician prescribing will be sustained.

In the North Carolina Back Pain Project population, more than 1,600 patients with new onset of low back pain had a mean functional recovery in 16 days (8 days median) after their first physician visit. Within this group, half received prescriptions for muscle relaxants. Muscle relaxant use was characterized by younger age, higher proportion of female sex, greater likelihood of being on workers compensation, and an increased history of prior episodes of treatment for low back pain. In terms of return to baseline function, outcome was worse for patients receiving muscle relaxants; however, those who received muscle relaxants also tended to have the highest reported pain intensity and lowest baseline function due to pain interference [5]. A more recent study in the same state surveyed 5,357 households and determined that the rate of prescribing muscle relaxants for low back pain in elders was significantly lower than for younger age groups [6].

While it would seem that muscle relaxants must be very effective based on the extent to which they are prescribed, universally accepted evidence is scarce for muscle relaxants as effective treatment for low back pain. For example, in a recent review, although 17 of 137 studies on medical management of low back pain showed evidence of benefit for opioid and NSAID agents, no study on muscle relaxant treatment of low back pain met their standard for evidence of benefit [7]. Other studies have found muscle relaxants effective for treatment of acute nonspecific low back pain compared to placebo. In a meta-analysis that included 23 high-quality trials of muscle relaxants compared to placebo for low back pain, patients taking active drug were 50 % more likely to have a side effect such as drowsiness, dizziness, or dry mouth (relative risk 1.5). This study showed significant efficacy for acute pain but questioned it for chronic low back pain [8]. A recent review of agents targeting nociceptive and neuropathic pain components mentions that side effects of muscle relaxants outweigh their limited potential benefit as monotherapy for chronic low back pain [9].

Myofascial pain is a muscle pain phenomenon with taught bands (trigger points) that might benefit from muscle relaxants. However, a recent Cochrane review found only two small studies showing efficacy of cyclobenzaprine over clonazepam and placebo [10]. Another soft tissue pain syndrome, fibromyalgia, might also be thought to benefit from muscle relaxant drugs. However, in a recent review comparing medical management of fibromyalgia by various specialties, muscle relaxants were not as commonly used as other analgesic classes, and among muscle relaxants, cyclobenzaprine was the most commonly prescribed. That said, they were prescribed by 35 % of primary care physicians compared to 9, 4, and 3 % of rheumatologists, psychiatrists, and neurologists, respectively [11]. Monotherapy with pregabalin or duloxetine is most common, although 8 % of a recent study group of patients with fibromyalgia are receiving muscle relaxants [12].

Because muscle tension or spasm is brought to mind when discussing tension-type headache, one might find it logical to expect that tension-type headache would respond well to muscle relaxants. However, this has not proved to be the case, even for tizanidine [13]. Compared to migraine, tension-type headache has a higher age of onset, a more even female to male distribution, a greater overall cost, is usually bilateral, and has a pressing-tightening character [13]. Although this type of headache is described in terms of muscular symptoms, the use of muscle relaxants is not indicated for this condition [13].

Metaxalone
C₁₁H₁₅NO₃

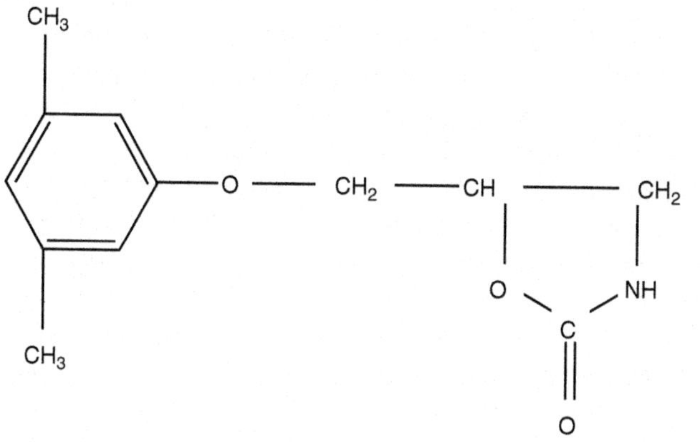

Fig. 7.1 Metaxalone was approved as a muscle relaxant in the 1960s when two small studies suggested benefit in degree of low back spasm over the painful area and decreased pain interference; however, there has been a dearth of recent studies establishing either a mechanism of action or efficacy

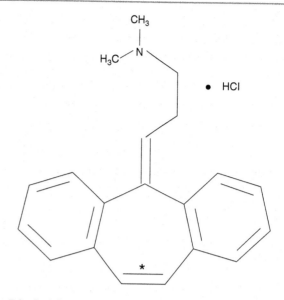

Fig. 7.2 Cyclobenzaprine is one of the most commonly prescribed muscle relaxants, and while the exact mechanism by which it produces a muscle relaxant effect is not known, it may produce inhibition of serotonergic descending systems

Metaxalone

Metaxalone was approved as a muscle relaxant in the 1960s when two small studies suggested benefit in degree of low back spasm over the painful area and decreased pain interference; however, there has been a dearth of recent studies establishing either a mechanism of action or efficacy (Fig. 7.1) [14]. A review of three muscle relaxants, including metaxalone, calls attention to the lack of understanding of the mechanism of action and lower standards for articles reporting on efficacy and safety when these drugs were brought to market in the 1960s and 1970s [14]. Proposed mechanisms for metaxalone included sedation or modulation of signals in polysynaptic fibers sensing passive stretch. Also reviewed were cyclobenzaprine and carisoprodol. Concern was raised for the abuse potential of the latter and thus suggested the former may be safer.

Cyclobenzaprine

Cyclobenzaprine is one of the most commonly prescribed muscle relaxants, and while the exact mechanism by which it produces a muscle relaxant effect is not known, it may produce inhibition of serotonergic descending systems (Fig. 7.2) [15].

Cyclobenzaprine is chemically related to amitriptyline from which it differs by only one double bond. Cyclobenzaprine metabolites also differ from amitriptyline metabolites by only one double bond. When doing forensic testing for the presence of these drugs and their metabolites,

it may be necessary to use advanced techniques, such as high-performance liquid chromatography with ultraviolet detection or gas chromatography with nitrogen-phosphorus detection [16]. Laboratory technology involving high-performance liquid chromatography and tandem mass spectrometry is currently able to rapidly and quantitatively measure the following eight muscle relaxants in human blood: afloqualone, chlorphenesin carbamate, chlorzoxazone, dantrolene, eperisone, methocarbamol, pridinol, and tolperisone [17].

A meta-analysis of studies comparing cyclobenzaprine with placebo showed efficacy to be greatest on day 4 and then declining after the first week. NNT = 3, meaning three patients required treatment for one to show response [18]. In this now 10-year-old paper, a strong recommendation was made for comparing efficacy among active controls such as acetaminophen and NSAIDs which has since been done. A 2010 study shows efficacy for cyclobenzaprine 5 mg TID, but no benefit over an NSAID (ibuprofen 800 mg TID) during a 7-day treatment of acute cervical pain presenting at the emergency department of a large university hospital [19]. In this small study of 61 patients, although findings did not reach statistical significance, pain was more quickly relieved in patients receiving cyclobenzaprine, and the degree of pain intensity relief was greater for cyclobenzaprine compared to ibuprofen and was greatest with a combination of cyclobenzaprine and the NSAID. Cyclobenzaprine is commonly prescribed at a dose of 10 mg TID for muscle spasm with local pain and tenderness, is thought to increase range of motion, and is associated with a high incidence of side effects such as drowsiness and xerostomia. Interestingly, an industry-funded dose ranging study suggests 5 mg TID produces less side effect while maintaining efficacy [20].

Cylobenzaprine, like the related tricyclic antidepressants and also opioids, activates toll-like receptors (TLR) in spinal microglial cells [21]. Glial cell activation can have profound effects modulating pain and affect opioid-induced analgesia and tolerance. A mechanism by which tricyclic antidepressant class drugs including amitriptyline, imipramine, desipramine, cyclobenzaprine, carbamazepine, and oxcarbazepine can potentiate opioid analgesia has been demonstrated in mice [21]. These findings may explain how these drugs function as analgesics in chronic pain syndromes.

Carisoprodol

Regarding the non-tricyclic antidepressant muscle relaxants, one of the most controversial is carisoprodol (Fig. 7.3). Compared to placebo, it demonstrates efficacy for relief from acute muscle spasm and improved functional status at doses of 250 mg QID, although it is usually prescribed at 350 mg QID, a dose associated with a higher incidence of adverse effects [22]. Ralph et al. suggest carisoprodol would be a better drug if prescribed at the lower dose of 250 mg; however, the study was industry-sponsored, and authors disclosed they served on a speaker's bureau for the product [22].

Carisoprodol is metabolized to meprobamate, an anxiolytic and hypnotic with known abuse potential, which also has a longer half-life. Either drug at a sufficient dose can produce mental impairment. An extensive database on non-alcoholic impaired drivers maintained in Norway includes extensive testing of mental function matched with forensic blood testing for drugs including carisoprodol and meprobamate. Impaired drivers admitted to consuming doses of carisoprodol greater than 700 mg and high carisoprodol levels correlated with impairment. Interestingly, Bramness et al. also reported that regular users of carisoprodol did not demonstrate high levels of meprobamate. The study was not designed to identify the mechanism though it was suggested that these patients had developed tolerance for the impairment caused by this active metabolite, while occasional users of carisoprodol who had not yet developed tolerance tended to have higher levels of meprobamate [23]. Metabolism of carisoprodol to meprobamate occurs via the CYP2C19 variant of cytochrome P450 in the liver. If there is variation of the cytochrome P450-CYP2C19 gene, it would be expected to affect meprobamate levels and subsequent side effects. For example, an individual with two CYP2C19 alleles may make more meprobamate and may have increased potential risk for impairment while driving [24].

An extreme case of withdrawal occurred in a patient taking a very high dose of carisoprodol, more than 17 g/day. Some might conclude that if such large doses could be tolerated, carisoprodol may actually have a high therapeutic index. In this case, withdrawal delirium occurred in a patient with back pain due to trauma who purchased large doses of carisoprodol over the internet when her health insurance lapsed. She was noted to be taking very high doses, up to fifty 350 mg tablets per day. She was not overly sedated and probably developed tolerance to the active metabolite, meprobamate. Seven days after deciding to stop, she lost orientation to person, place, and time and reported visual hallucinations, and postural and action tremors were noted on exam. Symptoms of delirium responded to treatment with 2 mg doses of lorazepam [25].

Concern for carisoprodol abuse since the Bramness study has led Norway to reclassify it as class-A (most restricted) led 39 of the United States to restrict its prescribing and led to a drive for the DEA to reclassify carisoprodol as a class-IV drug [26]. A case-control study was done in elderly patients identifying 8,164 cases and as many controls from a population of 1.5 million enrollees in a Medicare Advantage plan offered by a large HMO. Elderly patients receiving muscle relaxants were 1.4 times more likely to suffer a fracture injury, and the authors advised extreme caution be used prescribing muscle relaxants for older adults [27].

As our population ages, increased attention should be given to use and monitoring in elderly patients. Muscle relaxants are not recommended for patients over 65 years of age due to increased risk of injury due to side effects and should specifically to be avoided for elderly patients with bladder outflow obstruction and cognitive impairment [28].

However, while many reports as well as common wisdom advises against the use of muscle relaxants in the elderly, it has recently been suggested that skeletal muscle relaxants may be appropriate in this age group, especially if the patient does not have a high burden of disease and first-line medications were ineffective [29].

Carisoprodol
$C_{12}H_{24}N_2O_4$

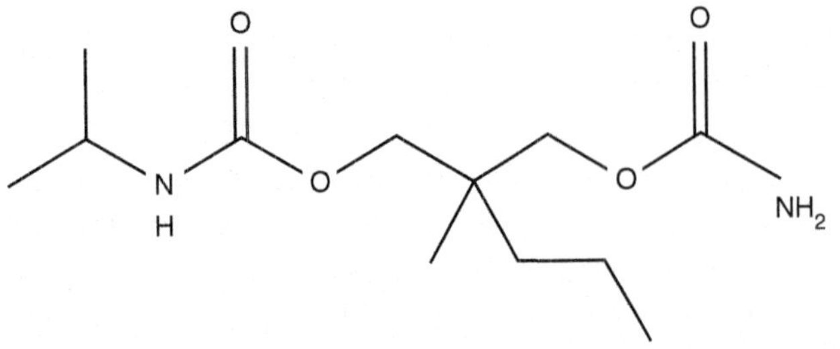

Fig. 7.3 Regarding the non-tricyclic antidepressant muscle relaxants, one of the most controversial is carisoprodol. Compared to placebo, it demonstrates efficacy for relief from acute muscle spasm and improved functional status at doses of 250 mg QID, although it is usually prescribed at 350 mg QID, a dose associated with a higher incidence of adverse effects

Baclofen

The muscle relaxants are a dichotomous group with indications for "skeletal muscle conditions" and for "spasticity" originating in the central nervous system, such as found in upper motor neuron disorders. Spasticity is an active muscle process whereby loss of central modulation causes increased excitability of the stretch reflex such that there is a velocity-sensitive response to limb manipulation [30]. Spasticity results from upper motor neuron pathology with abnormal stretch reflexes that may be the result of changed muscle structure, development of new spinal level collaterals, and/or failure to adequately regulate supraspinal pathways resulting in increased spinal reflex responses [31].

The traditional mainstay of treatment for upper motor neuron spasticity is baclofen, which has been used orally since the 1970s and, more recently, intrathecally (Fig. 7.4). To assess the possible survival advantage of intrathecal baclofen for cerebral palsy patients, 359 patients from Minnesota with intrathecal baclofen pumps were compared with 349 matched controls that were selected from 27,962 Californians with CP who did not have pumps. Interestingly, the survival for those with intrathecal baclofen was somewhat better than their well-matched controls [32].

Whereas benzodiazepines work at GABA-A receptors, increasing chloride ion currents causing cell hyperpolarization and thus inhibiting action potentials, baclofen activates the GABA-B receptor [33]. Designed to mimic GABA, baclofen is basically a GABA molecule with a chlorinated phenol moiety, hence its chemical name p-chlorophenyl-GABA. The only available prescription medicine that activates GABA-B receptors, baclofen has been the drug of choice for the treatment of tetanus, stiff man syndrome, cerebral palsy, and multiple sclerosis. In addition to treatment of spasticity, GABA-B receptor activation may also have a role in treatment of pain, depression and anxiety, drug addiction, and absence epilepsy, and GABA-B receptor antagonism may have a role in treating cognitive impairment [33].

Baclofen as a visceral pain reliever has been studied in sensitized visceral pain models where it appears to have a central site of action in the dorsal horn of the spinal cord at GABA-B receptors and, in a dose response fashion, attenuates both pain behavior and expression of FOS (a nociceptive marker). However, in the dose range that produced the analgesic effect, marked sedation was also observed [34].

In addition to the side effects of its use, in its withdrawal, baclofen may produce respiratory failure, unstable hemodynamics, seizures not responsive to usual treatment, and delirium. Interestingly, delirium is caused by both overdose and rapid withdrawal. If an intrathecal pump fails or needs to be removed due to infection, it is difficult using oral dosing to produce sufficient levels of baclofen in the CSF to prevent these catastrophic effects, and treatment with benzodiazepines, propofol, neuromuscular blocking agents, dantrolene, and tizanidine may be required in an ICU setting [35]. Baclofen and tizanidine withdrawal acutely produced extra-pyramidal signs, delirium, and autonomic dysfunction that were eventually reversed when baclofen was restarted in a sufficient dose [36]. For a clear review of the differential diagnosis of baclofen withdrawal, the reader is referred to a recent case report with an excellent summary chart [37].

Other Muscle Relaxants

Of the muscle relaxants not available in the United States, one that should be mentioned is flupirtine (Fig. 7.5).

Developed in Germany in the 1980s, flupirtine has been described as having many potential analgesic roles, and, equipotent to tramadol, it may also function as a muscle relaxant. Flupirtine activates Kv7 potassium channels, produces an M-current, and dampens hyperexcitable neurons [38]. The Kv7 potassium channel is activated by muscarine and is receiving a great deal of attention recently. There is speculation that further work could lead to new treatments for Alzheimer's disease, seizure disorders, and chronic pain. The subtypes of Kv7 potassium channels regulate the potassium

Baclofen
$C_{10}H_{12}ClNO_2$

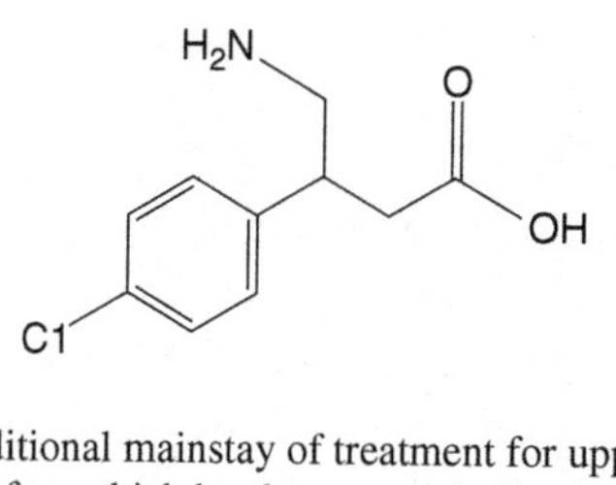

Fig. 7.4 The traditional mainstay of treatment for upper motor neuron spasticity is baclofen, which has been used orally since the 1970s and, more recently, intrathecally

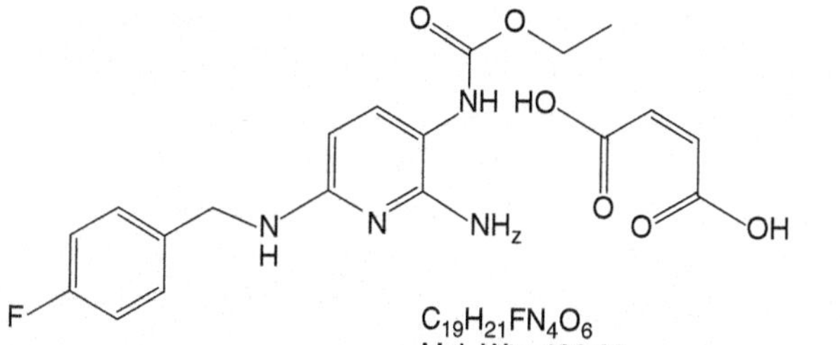

$C_{19}H_{21}FN_4O_6$
Mol. Wt.: 420.39

Fig. 7.5 Of the muscle relaxants not available in the United States, one that should be mentioned is flupirtine. Developed in Germany in the 1980s, flupirtine has been described as having many potential analgesic roles, and, equipotent to tramadol, it may also function as a muscle relaxant

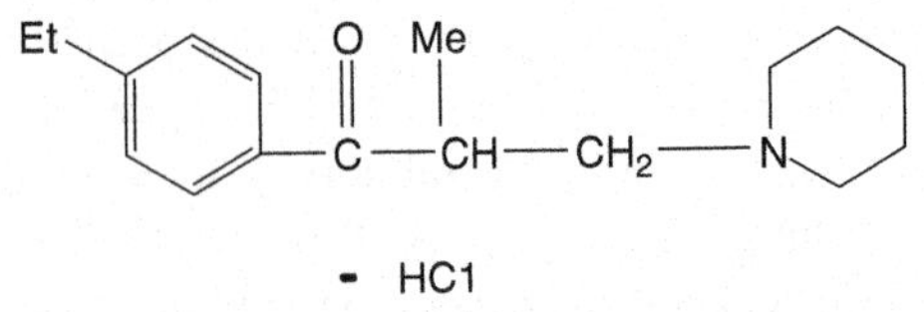

Fig. 7.6 Used to treat painful contracture and spasticity, eperisone inhibits gamma-efferent firing in the spinal cord and produces local vasodilatation and rarely has adverse CNS affects. It has good bioavailability, short onset time, and rapid elimination making it suitable for initial treatment of acute low back pain

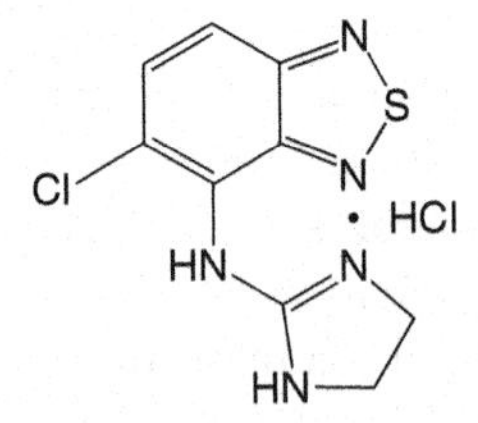

Fig. 7.7 Tizanidine is an alpha-2 agonist which has been shown to have beneficial results in the treatment of muscle spasm

M-current activated by muscarine. Thus, muscarine (or other drugs acting at these sites) can lead to changes in potassium conductance with activation leading to hyperpolarization and blockade leading to increased neuronal activity. The M-current is a low-threshold, non-inactivating voltage-dependent potassium current at the Kv7 channel capable of limiting repetitive firing of neuronal action potentials [39]. Hyperexcitable states such as seizure disorders and chronic pain, including muscle pain and spasm, may respond to channel activators, while blockers at Kv7 channels might increase neuronal activation and provide a treatment of Alzheimer's [39].

Used to treat painful contracture and spasticity, eperisone inhibits gamma-efferent firing in the spinal cord and produces local vasodilatation and rarely has adverse CNS effects (Fig. 7.6). It has good bioavailability, short onset time, and rapid elimination, making it suitable for initial treatment of acute low back pain [40].

While eperisone appears effective for treatment of muscle contracture and chronic low back pain, it is also touted to be free of sedative side effects [41]. Blood flow in low back muscles may increase with eperisone treatment over 4 weeks in comparison with placebo and active physical therapy protocols [42].

Tizanidine

Tizanidine is an alpha-2 agonist which has been shown to have beneficial results in the treatment of muscle spasm (Fig. 7.7). The reader is referred to a major review of the drug class muscle relaxants, Chou et al. [43]. This is an important work and will be given attention in the following paragraphs. The aim of the ambitious 237-page electronic book in the public domain, available at http://www.ncbi.nlm.nih.gov/pubmed/20496453, was to determine among nine muscle relaxants (baclofen, carisoprodol, chlorzoxazone, cyclobenzaprine, dantrolene, metaxalone, methocarbamol, orphenadrine, and tizanidine), whether one or more were superior in efficacy or safety for treatment of muscle spasticity mostly due to multiple sclerosis or for musculoskeletal conditions such as neck and low back pain compared with

the others. Only tizanidine was found to have fair quality evidence for effectiveness in both spasticity and musculoskeletal conditions. Spasticity was evaluated in 59 trials; however, only 18 included an active control, which was sometimes another muscle relaxant. None of the 18 was considered high quality with each containing at least two methodological flaws. For example, there were nine trials comparing baclofen to tizanidine and eight comparing diazepam with tizanidine, baclofen, or dantrolene. Except for one trial comparing clonidine to baclofen, they reported no muscle relaxant trials where the following common adjuvants were used as active controls: clonidine, gabapentin, and other benzodiazepines. There were 5 reviews and 52 trials reviewed for efficacy and safety for muscle relaxant use in musculoskeletal conditions (as opposed to spasticity). Twelve trials used a muscle relaxant as an active control against another muscle relaxant. No active control trials for efficacy or safety for musculoskeletal conditions were found for baclofen, dantrolene, metaxalone, or orphenadrine.

Based on nine head-to-head trials, Chou et al. report that tizanidine and baclofen have similar efficacy for the treatment of spasm including improvement in tone, clonus, and assessments of function and physician and patient preference [43].

Head-to-head trials of muscle relaxants used for musculoskeletal conditions are less common with only two showing carisoprodol or chlorzoxazone, both superior to the active control diazepam, and three showing cyclobenzaprine equivalent to it [43]. Although methodologies were flawed, Chou et al. report that compared to placebo, efficacy has been shown for cyclobenzaprine, carisoprodol, orphenadrine, and tizanidine, while evidence of efficacy is poor for baclofen, chlorzoxazone, dantrolene, methocarbamol, or metaxalone [43].

The Oregon Health & Science University group also reviewed relative risks of treatment including abuse, addiction, and other adverse effects. Used in treatment of spasticity, tizanidine and baclofen have different side effect profiles with the former associated with xerostomia and the latter with weakness [43]. Other muscle relaxants could not be

Diazepam

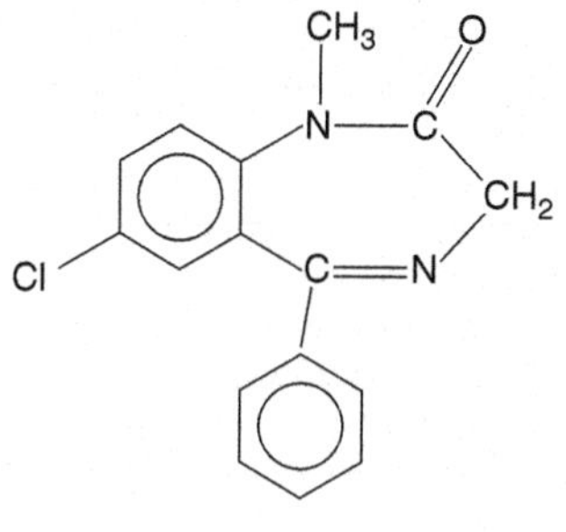

Fig. 7.8 Diazepam. Benzodiazepines have been shown to reduce muscle spasm, especially in the postoperative period but their use is often limited by sedation

compared head to head due to lack of good evidence. Major side effects included hepatic toxicity for dantrolene and tizanidine but not for baclofen, and quantitative comparisons could not be made for serious adverse events such as seizures, withdrawal reaction, and overdose. Frequent adverse events included somnolence, weakness, dizziness, and dry mouth. Abuse and addiction were not evaluated in these studies.

Diazepam

Benzodiazepines have been shown to reduce muscle spasm, especially in the postoperative period but their use is often limited by sedation (Fig. 7.8). This class of drugs is discussed elsewhere in the text.

Dantrolene

Dantrolene appears to work by abolishing excitation/contraction coupling within muscle (Fig. 7.9). While dantrolene has the capacity to reduce muscle spasm and spasticity, its use has been severely limited by its hepatic, cardiovascular, and pulmonary toxicity and by severe CNS side effects including visual disturbances, hallucinations, seizures, and depression. It remains useful as a treatment for malignant hyperthermia.

Orphenadrine

While technically an anticholinergic of the antihistamine class and not a muscle relaxant drug, orphenadrine has been used to treat muscle spasm and pain, but its effectiveness in doing so has not been clearly proven (Fig. 7.10).

Dantrolene
$C_{14}H_{10}N_4O_5$

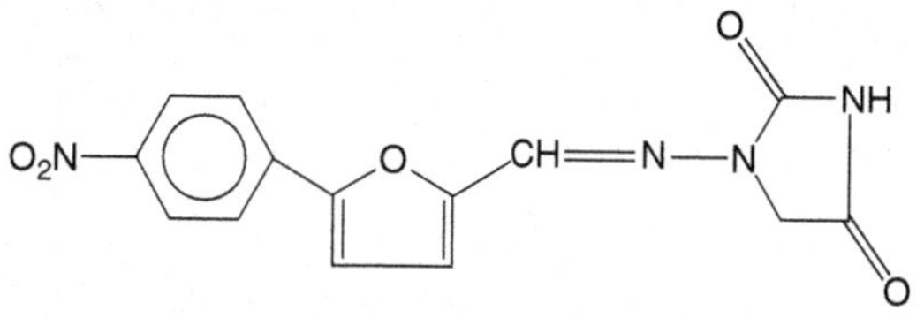

Fig. 7.9 Dantrolene appears to work by abolishing excitation/contraction coupling within muscle

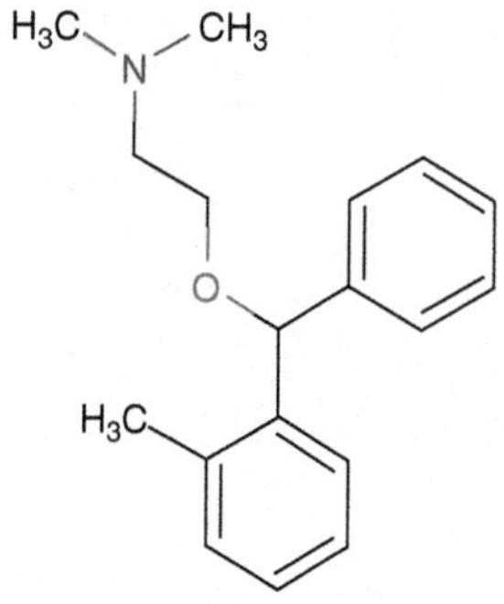

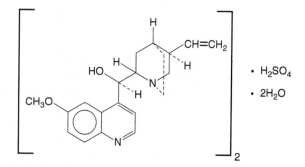

Fig. 7.10 While technically an anticholinergic of the antihistamine class and not a muscle relaxant drug, orphenadrine has been used to treat muscle spasm and pain, but its effectiveness in doing so has not been clearly proven

Quinine
$C_{20}H_{24}N_2O_2 \cdot \frac{1}{2}H_2O_4S \cdot H_2O$

Fig. 7.11 Although not classified as a skeletal muscle relaxant, quinine has long been used to treat muscle cramps

Quinine

Although not classified as a skeletal muscle relaxant, quinine has long been used to treat muscle cramps (Fig. 7.11). An extensive Cochrane review summarizes 23 trials with

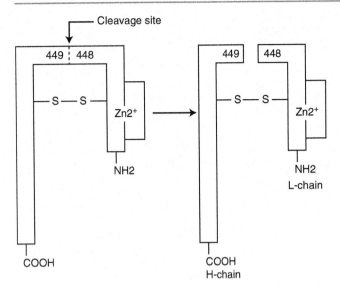

Fig. 7.12 Botulinum toxin type A, but not type B, is helpful for spasticity acting presynaptically at the myoneural junction by inhibiting acetylcholine vesicle release leading to decreased contraction strength and is now considered first-line treatment for spasticity

1,586 participants at daily doses between 200 and 500 mg and concludes there is evidence of moderate quality for reduction in intensity and frequency of cramping pain and that when used for up to 60 days, although there is increase in side effects such as GI symptoms, the serious side effect rate is similar to placebo [44].

Botulinum Toxin

Finally, no discussion of muscle relaxants to treat musculoskeletal conditions and spasticity would be complete without mentioning botulinum toxin. Botulinum toxin type A, but not type B, is helpful for spasticity acting presynaptically at the myoneural junction by inhibiting acetylcholine vesicle release leading to decreased contraction strength and is now considered first-line treatment for spasticity (Fig.7.12) [31]. Further details in the mechanism of action and application of botulinum toxin in treatment of disease are discussed elsewhere in this textbook.

References

1. Chou R. Pharmacological management of low back pain. Drugs. 2010;70(4):387–402.
2. Ivanova JI, et al. Real-world practice patterns, health-care utilization, and costs in patients with low back pain: the long road to guideline-concordant care. Spine J. 2011;11:622–32.
3. Jackson JL, Browning R. Impact of national low back pain guidelines on clinical practice. South Med J. 2005;98(2):139–43.
4. Cammisa C, et al. Engaging physicians in change: results of a safety net quality improvement program to reduce overuse. Am J Med Qual. 2011;26(1):26–33.
5. Bernstein E, Carey TS, Garrett JM. The use of muscle relaxant medications in acute low back pain. Spine. 2004;29(12):1345–51.
6. Knauer SR, Freburger JK, Carey TS. Chronic low back pain among older adults: a population-based perspective. J Aging Health. 2010;22(8):1213–34.
7. Kuijpers T, et al. A systematic review on the effectiveness of pharmacological interventions for chronic non-specific low-back pain. Eur Spine J. 2011;20(1):40–50.
8. van Tulder MW, et al. Muscle relaxants for non-specific low back pain. Cochrane Database Syst Rev. 2003;2:CD004252.
9. Morlion B. Pharmacotherapy of low back pain: targeting nociceptive and neuropathic pain components. Curr Med Res Opin. 2011;27(1):11–33.
10. Kim CS, et al. Teaching internal medicine residents quality improvement and patient safety: a lean thinking approach. Am J Med Qual. 2010;25(3):211–7.
11. McNett M, et al. Treatment patterns among physician specialties in the management of fibromyalgia: results of a cross-sectional study in the United States. Curr Med Res Opin. 2011;27(3):673–83.
12. Dussias P, Kalali AH, Staud RM. Treatment of fibromyalgia. Psychiatry. 2010;7(5):15–8.
13. Bendtsen L, et al. EFNS guideline on the treatment of tension-type headache – report of an EFNS task force. Eur J Neurol. 2010;17(11):1318–25.
14. Toth PP, Urtis J. Commonly used muscle relaxant therapies for acute low back pain- a review of carisoprodol, cyclobenzaprine hydrochloride, and metaxalone. Clin Ther. 2004;26(9):1355–67.
15. Kobayashi H, Hasegawa Y, Ono H. Cyclobenzaprine, a centrally acting muscle relaxant, acts on descending serotonergic systems. Eur J Pharmacol. 1996;311(1):29–35.
16. Lofland JH, Szarlej S, Buttaro T, Shermock S, Jalali S. Cyclobenzaprine hydrochloride is a commonly prescribed centrally acting muscle relaxant which is structurally similar TCAs and differs amitriptyline one double bond. Clin J Pain. 2001;17(1):103–4.
17. Ogawa T, et al. High-throughput and simultaneous analysis of eight central-acting muscle relaxants in human plasma by ultra-performance liquid chromatography-tandem mass spectrometry in the positive and negative ionization modes. Anal Bioanal Chem. 2011;400(7):1959–65.
18. Browning R, Jackson JL, O'Malley PG. Cyclobenzaprine and back pain: a meta-analysis. Arch Intern Med. 2001;161(13):1613–20.
19. Khwaja SM, Minnerop M, Singer AJ. Comparison of ibuprofen, cyclobenzaprine or both in patients with acute cervical strain- a randomized controlled trial. CJEM. 2010;12(1):39–44.
20. Borenstein DG, Korn S. Efficacy of a low-dose regimen of cyclobenzaprine hydrochloride in acute skeletal muscle spasm- results of two placebo-controlled trials. Clin Ther. 2003;25(4):1056–73.
21. Hutchinson MR, et al. Evidence that tricyclic small molecules may possess toll-like receptor and myeloid differentiation protein 2 activity. Neuroscience. 2010;168(2):551–63.
22. Ralph L, et al. Double-blind, placebo-controlled trial of carisoprodol 250-mg tablets in the treatment of acute lower-back spasm. Curr Med Res Opin. 2008;24(2):551–8.
23. Bramness JG, Skurtveit S, Morland J. Impairment due to intake of carisoprodol. Drug Alcohol Depend. 2004;74(3):311–8.
24. Musshoff F, Stamer UM, Madea B. Pharmacogenetics and forensic toxicology. Forensic Sci Int. 2010;203(1–3):53–62.
25. Ni K, Cary M, Zarkowski P. Carisoprodol withdrawal induced delirium – a case study. Neuropsychiatr Dis Treat. 2007;3(5):679–82.
26. Fass JA. Carisoprodol legal status and patterns of abuse. Ann Pharmacother. 2010;44(12):1962–7.
27. Golden AG, et al. Risk for fractures with centrally acting muscle relaxants: an analysis of a national Medicare advantage claims database. Ann Pharmacother. 2010;44(9):1369–75.
28. Fick DM. Updating the beers criteria for potentially inappropriate medication use in older adults: results of a US consensus panel of experts. Arch Intern Med. 2003;163(22):2716–24.

29. Billups SJ, Delate T, Hoover B. Injury in an elderly population before and after initiating a skeletal muscle relaxant. Ann Pharmacother. 2011;45(4):485–91.

30. Nielsen JB, Crone C, Hultborn H. The spinal pathophysiology of spasticity – from a basic science point of view. Acta Physiol. 2007;189(2):171–80.

31. Simon O, Yelnik A. Managing spasticity with drugs. Eur J Phys Rehabil Med. 2010;46(3):401–10.

32. Krach LE, et al. Survival of individuals with cerebral palsy receiving continuous intrathecal baclofen treatment: a matched-cohort study. Dev Med Child Neurol. 2010;52(7):672–6.

33. Bowery NG. GABAB receptor: a site of therapeutic benefit. Curr Opin Pharmacol. 2006;6(1):37–43.

34. Liu LS, Shenoy M, Pasricha PJ. The analgesic effects of the GABA(B) receptor agonist, baclofen, in a rodent model of functional dyspepsia. Neurogastroenterol Motil. 2011;23(4):356–61.

35. Ross JC, et al. Acute intrathecal baclofen withdrawal: a brief review of treatment options. Neurocrit Care. 2011;14(1):103–8.

36. Karol DE, Muzyk AJ, Preud'homme XA. A case of delirium, motor disturbances, and autonomic dysfunction due to baclofen and tizanidine withdrawal: a review of the literature. Gen Hosp Psychiatry. 2011;33(1):84.e1–2.

37. Ross JC, et al. Acute intrathecal baclofen withdrawal: a brief review of treatment options. Neurocrit Care. 2010;14(1):103–8.

38. Devulder J. Flupirtine in pain management: pharmacological properties and clinical use. CNS Drugs. 2010;24(10):867–81.

39. Miceli F, et al. Molecular pharmacology and therapeutic potential of neuronal Kv7-modulating drugs. Curr Opin Pharmacol. 2008;8(1):65–74.

40. Melilli B, et al. Human pharmacokinetics of the muscle relaxant, eperisone hydrochloride by liquid chromatography-electrospray tandem mass spectrometry. Eur J Drug Metab Pharmacokinet. 2011;36(2):71–8.

41. Pham JC, et al. ReCASTing the RCA: an improved model for performing root cause analyses. Am J Med Qual. 2010;25(3):186–91.

42. Dull DL, Fox L. Perception of intimidation in a perioperative setting. Am J Med Qual. 2010;25(2):87–94.

43. Chou R, Peterson K. Drug class review on skeletal muscle relaxants: final report. Portland: Oregon Health & Science University; 2005.

44. El-Tawil S, et al. Quinine for muscle cramps. Cochrane Database Syst Rev. 2010;(12):CD005044.

Topical Analgesics

Charles E. Argoff, Manpreet Kaur, and Kelly Donnelly

Key Points

- Topical analgesics differ from systemic analgesics especially because the systemic concentration of the analgesic is likely to be low compared to systemic analgesics.
- Do not confuse topical analgesics with transdermal analgesics that use the skin as a means for the analgesic to achieve a systemic concentration.
- Even though the site of action of a topical analgesic may be within the peripheral nervous system, there may be central nervous system effects of the topical analgesic.
- Topical analgesics are often more tolerable than systemic analgesics.
- There is significant evidence for the potential clinical benefit of topical analgesics for a broad range of chronic pain conditions including various neuropathic as well as non-neuropathic states.

Introduction

Topical analgesics differ from systemic analgesics by exhibiting analgesia without significant systemic absorption as compared to systemic analgesics, which require systemic absorption for their analgesic activity. Topical analgesics are frequently confused with transdermal agents; however, they

C.E. Argoff, M.D. (✉)
Neurology/Comprehensive Pain Center, Albany Medical College,
4 Loudon Lane North, Loudonville, NY 12211, USA

Comprehensive Pain Center, Albany Medical Center,
Albany, NY, USA
e-mail: cargoff@nycap.rr.com

M. Kaur, M.D. • K. Donnelly, DO
Department of Neurology, Albany Medical Center,
47 New Scotland Avenue, Albany, NY 12208, USA
e-mail: kaurm@mail.amc.edu; donnelk1@mail.amc.edu

differ from transdermal analgesics (e.g., transdermal fentanyl patch) because systemic absorption of a transdermal agent is required for clinical benefit. There is a variety of mechanism of actions of specific topical analgesics. Topical analgesics have been studied in acute pain as well as in various types of chronic pain including both non-neuropathic and neuropathic pain types. The results of many of these studies are described in this chapter. New data that suggest that topical analgesics which were assumed almost by definition, to act peripherally, may affect central pain processing are also discussed.

Background and Scientific Foundation

Pain, by definition, does not occur without the activation of relevant brain areas, and indeed, this fact has certainly been clearly established over the past few decades. At the same time, scientific advances have pointed to a significant role of the peripheral nervous system (PNS) in initiating and maintaining acute and chronic painful conditions; thus, it is not surprising that even though topical analgesics are believed to exert their principle analgesic activity peripherally, multiple chronic pain syndromes have been shown to be responsive to certain topical analgesics. In addition, while there are certain painful conditions such as central poststroke pain or spinal cord injury pain in which almost exclusively, the mechanisms of the pain lie entirely within the brain and/or central nervous system (CNS), other pain syndromes including those which we commonly encounter as clinicians including postherpetic neuralgia (PHN), chronic low back pain (CLBP), and osteoarthritis (OA) ultimately likely result from both peripheral as well as CNS mechanisms. The designation of a medication as a topical analgesic has been made when the analgesic is applied locally and directly to the painful areas and whose primary site of action is local to the site of analgesic application. The term "topical analgesic" should not be confused with the term "transdermal analgesic" which in contrast to a topical analgesic requires a systemic analgesic concentration to be effective. Be aware that not infrequently in the authors' experiences, analgesics have been inappropriately considered as "topical" agents even when formal pharmacological studies to demonstrate a lack of systemic activity and/or systemic drug concentration had not been completed.

Nociception, the activation of specialized nerve endings by mechanical, thermal, and/or chemical stimuli, is not equivalent to pain, yet interfering with nociception can possibly result in a person experiencing less pain. Consequently, even though the mechanism of action of a topical analgesic may largely be within the peripheral nervous system and thus on nociceptive mechanisms, this peripheral effect may actually lead to a reduction of central pain mechanisms and thus pain as well. Put another way, since the pain experience requires the brain receiving and processing pain-related information, if less such information from the PNS presents to the CNS for central processing, it is certainly possible that fewer central mechanisms will be activated and thus less pain experienced. This chapter reviews the use of topical analgesics in the treatment of various painful conditions and provides an update to previously published similar reviews [1–3].

The clinical effectiveness of any analgesic or, for that matter, any medication may be diminished by that medication's adverse effect profile, toxicities, and drug-drug interaction. The risk and severity of significant adverse effects and drug-drug interactions are less than for the same medication given systemically [4]. This may be especially important when considering what type of nonsteroidal anti-inflammatory (NSAID) agent to use for a given patient as will be discussed further below. Localized drug effects such as rash or unpleasant skin sensations have been described but are not generally experienced [5]. Additionally, since the use of a topical analgesic does not result in a significant systemic concentration of the analgesic, the use of a topical analgesic does not produce significant systemic accumulation of the specific analgesic. Of the FDA-approved topical analgesics, the 5 % lidocaine patch (Lidoderm®) has been one of the most extensively studied. It might help to illustrate some of the above principles by focusing briefly on this preparation. The tolerability and safety of daily, 24 h/day, use of four lidocaine 5 % patches has been specifically studied. The results demonstrate that there were no significant systemic side effects experienced and plasma lidocaine levels remained below those that have been associated with cardiac abnormalities. Similar safety and tolerability was noted regardless of whether or not the subject used the patch for 12- or 24-h daily [6]. In a separate investigation, patients with a history of chronic low back pain were treated safely with four lidocaine 5 % patches every 24 h for extended periods [5]. No significant dermal reactions were experienced in either of these reports [6, 7].

In addition to the potential for dermal sensitivity, other adverse effects may be associated with the use of specific topical analgesic that is, in general, specific to the particular chemical entity in the preparation. For example, upon application of topical capsaicin, severe burning at the site of application may occur in the overwhelming majority of treated patients. This effect may in fact lead to a reduced effectiveness of this type of topical analgesic because although this drug when applied topically in its currently available forms does not result in significant systemic accumulation or in any life-threatening outcomes, and even though the incidence of burning may decrease with repeated use, the frequent occurrence of this side effect may negatively impact upon patient compliance and, as a result, may potentially hinder the patient's ability to benefit from it [8]. However, as will be discussed below, the 8 % capsaicin patch (Qutenza®), now FDA approved for the treatment of PHN, was generally well tolerated in the clinical trials completed, leading to its approval.

The fact that drug-drug interactions may be minimized when using topical analgesics may be of enormous importance for a patient who must use systemic medications concurrently for additional medical conditions. This is a point that has been emphasized in recent guidelines for the pharmacotherapeutic management of persistent pain in older adults [9]. Consider, for example, an 82-year-old person who suffers from hypertension, coronary artery disease, and type 2 diabetes mellitus. Consider that this person requires analgesic treatment for his knee OA. He is using a total of six other medications for his other chronic medical conditions. Assuming that comparable or even better pain relief is experienced, the use of a topical medication in this setting may offer several advantages over a systemic agent due to the lack of drug-drug interactions [10]. The use of a topical analgesic in place of or in addition to a systemic analgesic may have an additional advantage in that the use of a topical analgesic does not typically require dose titration, making these relatively simple medications to use.

Not all "topical" analgesics are prescribed as commercially available, FDA-approved agents. When prescribing a topical analgesic, one must distinguish between those which are FDA (or other similar agency in non-US countries) approved, commercially available, and with consistent manufacturing standards/quality control and those that may be manufactured on an individualized basis by a specialized compounding pharmacy. Many of the "topical" analgesics currently in use are not commercially available products, and for many years, health-care providers have ordered other so-called topical agents from compounding pharmacies. Often the preparations prescribed are combinations of medications put into a single product. This chapter will only review the use of those topical agents which are commercially available or for which there is clear evidence that they were manufactured in a dependable manner. To the best of our knowledge, for many compounding pharmacies, no matter the good intentions of the prescriber or pharmacy, there is no proof of quality control or consistency from one batch to another as would be required for an FDA-approved product. The reader might nevertheless appreciate that compounded, noncommercially available agents are prescribed as topical agents quite often, likely in an attempt to help a patient for whom other perhaps FDA-approved measures have not yielded effective results. For example, in a survey of members of the American Society of Regional Anesthesia and Pain Medicine, 27 % of the survey responders indicated that they prescribed such an agent, and 47 % of the responders reported that they felt that their patient responded positively to the prescribed agent(s) [11].

There appears to be increasing interest in the commercial development of new topical analgesics. As will be discussed below in more detail, recently, three topical NSAIDs and one high-concentration capsaicin preparation have been FDA approved, and in addition, opioids, local anesthetics, antidepressants, glutamate receptor antagonists, alpha-adrenergic receptor agonists, adenosine, cannabinoids, cholinergic receptor agonists, gabapentinoids, prostanoids, bradykinin, ATP, biogenic amines, and nerve growth factor are each being considered as potential topical analgesics [12].

Not surprisingly, the mechanism of action of each topical analgesic depends upon the specific analgesic. For example, the mechanism of action of capsaicin-containing topical analgesics appears through their agonist activity at the transient receptor potential vanilloid receptor 1 (TRPV1) on A-delta and C-fibers [13, 14]. This results in the release of substance P as well as calcitonin gene-related peptide (CGRP). With the older preparations, therapeutic responses to capsaicin were generally achieved only with repeated topical application; however, as will be summarized below, the more recently FDA-approved 8 % capsaicin patch has been shown to provide analgesic benefit for up to 12 weeks following a single 1-h application [15]. It has been suggested that reduced peripheral as well as central excitability with resulting less pain through reduced afferent input is the outcome of the depletion of substance P in C-fibers [8, 13, 15]. Histopathological examination results of human nerve biopsies as well as animal experiments have suggested that application of capsaicin may lead to nerve fiber degeneration in the skin underneath the site of application. This neurodegenerative effect of capsaicin has been hypothesized to be one of its mechanisms of pain relief [16]. In contrast, the mechanism of action of a topical NSAID is probably related to the inhibition of prostaglandin synthesis and associated anti-inflammatory effect; however, because the anti-inflammatory effect is not always proportional to the amount of pain relief experienced, additional mechanisms of action

might also be important to consider [17]. The combination of different topical therapies may be synergistic, and as an example, the antinociceptive effects of topical morphine have been shown to be enhanced by a topical cannabinoid in a recent study in rats in which the radiant tail-flick test was utilized [18]. No similar human studies have thus far been published. The analgesic action of local anesthetic agents based upon currently available data appears to be related to the ability of these agents to suppress the activity of peripheral sodium channels within sensory afferents and subsequent pain transmission; however, other mechanisms of action are under investigation. Reduced expression of messenger ribonucleic acid (mRNA) for specific sodium channel subtypes following local anesthetic use has been reported as well [1, 5]. Several local anesthetic-containing analgesics which may be considered topical agents are currently commercially available. Although use of the 5 % lidocaine patch is associated with an *analgesic* effect without creating *anesthetic* skin, in contrast, the use of EMLA® cream (eutectic mixture of local anesthetics, 2.5 % lidocaine/2.5 % prilocaine) or the FDA-approved Synera™ patch (lidocaine 70 mg/tetracaine 70 mg) may create both analgesia as well as anesthesia when applied topically. In certain clinical settings, for example, venipuncture, lumbar puncture, intramuscular injections, and circumcision, this property of EMLA® or Synera™ may actually be desirable. In other clinical situations, it might not be [5]. Choosing which topical analgesic to use clearly depends upon the clinical setting in which the medication is being used. A mechanism of action of the lidocaine 5 % patch as a topical agent which is unrelated to the active medication is that the patch itself may reduce the allodynia experienced by those afflicted by neuropathic pain states such as PHN through the patch's ability to protect the skin [1].

The development of tricyclic antidepressants as topical analgesics is novel and is under investigation. These agents as a group are known to have multiple mechanisms of action including sodium channel blockade; the potential clinical benefit of their ability to block sodium channels when topically applied is being actively investigated at this time [19, 20]. In fact, in the United States, there is currently one commercially available topical antidepressant, Zonalon® (doxepin hydrochloride) cream. While it is indicated for use by the FDA for the short-term treatment of adult patients with pruritis associated with atopic dermatitis or lichen simplex chronicus, there have been sporadic anecdotal reports of use of this agent in an "off-label" manner as a topical analgesic [21]. Other topical agents including topical opioids, glutamate receptor antagonists, and cannabinoids have potential as topical analgesics as well. Certain studies of some of these agents will be commented upon further below.

Clinical Examples

What follows is a summary of the clinical uses of topical agents based upon the painful disorder for which they are being used and/or for some FDA approved.

Neuropathic Pain

Without a doubt, clinical trial data provide varying levels of evidence for the use of certain topical analgesics in the treatment of neuropathic pain, and various published reviews of the treatment of neuropathic pain have emphasized the role of these agents [22–24].

Local Anesthetics

The lidocaine 5 % patch is FDA approved for the treatment of PHN. In fact, this agent was the first medication approved by the FDA for PHN. Clinical trials of PHN patients which led to the FDA approval demonstrated that use of the lidocaine 5 % patch by patients compared to use of placebo patches resulted in statistically significant more pain reduction and was in addition safe and well-tolerated [25, 26]. After the FDA approval of this drug for PHN, an open-label study was completed that was designed to examine the effect, if any, of the lidocaine 5 % patch on various quality of life measures. A total of 332 patients with PHN were studied, and a validated pain assessment tool, the Brief Pain Inventory (BPI), utilized. As many as three lidocaine 5 % patches, 12 h each day, were utilized by enrolled patients; the BPI was completed daily over 4 weeks. There were 204/332 (67 %) of the patients reported reduced pain intensity following repeated lidocaine 5 % patch application by the end of the first week of the study. Pain intensity reduction was noted by the second week of patch use in over 40 % of the remaining patients. Seventy percent of enrolled patients experienced notable improvement by the study's conclusion [27]. In a separate randomized open-label study in which use of the 5 % lidocaine patch was compared to the use of pregabalin (Lyrica®) for PHN, the 5 % lidocaine patch was determined to be at least as effective as pregabalin for pain relief in PHN patients with a favorable safety profile. Furthermore, in this study, for patients who were unresponsive to either the lidocaine 5 % patch or pregabalin as monotherapy, combining the use of these agents provided additional efficacy and was well tolerated by such patients [28].

Patients with neuropathic pain states other than PHN have also been treated with the lidocaine 5 % patch in various studies. In Europe, a randomized, double-blind, placebo-controlled trial studied the efficacy of the lidocaine 5 % patch in the treatment of "focal" neuropathic pain syndromes such as mononeuropathies, intercostal neuralgia, and ilioin-guinal neuralgia. Trial results suggested that when the lidocaine 5 % patch is added to other pharmacotherapeutic regimens, the 5 % lidocaine patch can reduce ongoing pain as well as allodynia as quickly as in the first 8 h of use but also over a period of 7 days [29]. The results of another smaller open-label study of 16 patients with various chronic neuropathic pain conditions (post-thoracotomy pain, complex regional pain syndrome, postamputation pain, painful diabetic neuropathy, meralgia paresthetica, postmastectomy pain, neuroma-related pain) demonstrated that the lidocaine 5 % patch provided pain relief without significant side effects in 81 % of these patients [30]. It is worthy to note that according to the study's authors, patients enrolled in this study, prior to the use of the lidocaine 5 % patch, had experienced suboptimal outcomes with numerous other agents commonly prescribed for the treatment of neuropathic pain. Several other noncontrolled studies of patients with painful diabetic neuropathy who were treated with the lidocaine 5 % patch have been completed. These studies allowed patients to use as many as four lidocaine 5 % patches for as long as 18 h/day. Considered together as a group, these studies reported pain reduction for the majority of patients and good tolerability of this medication [31–34]. In a 3-week single center, open-label study of the lidocaine 5 % patch in patients with painful idiopathic sensory polyneuropathy, noted over the treatment period, significant improvements in both pain and quality of life measures were noted [35].

Changes in the quality of the pain of patients with PHN treated with the lidocaine 5 % patch compared to placebo were examined in a multicenter, randomized, vehicle-controlled study of 150 PHN patients who were treated with either actual or placebo lidocaine 5 % patches (up to three lidocaine 5 % or vehicle patches for 12 h each day). The use of the lidocaine 5 % patch but not the vehicle patch was associated with reduced intensity of certain neuropathic pain qualities utilizing the Neuropathic Pain Scale (NPS). The results additionally demonstrated that some of the qualities of neuropathic pain (deep, sharp, and burning) which were reduced had previously been assumed not to be related to peripheral but to central nervous system mechanisms. The authors of this study proposed that their results suggested that peripheral mechanisms of neuropathic pain might also indeed play a role in the development of these neuropathic pain qualities [36]. Also of great interest are the results of a functional brain MRI study of patients with PHN who were treated with the 5 % lidocaine patch for various time periods. Depending upon the length of application, brain activity for the spontaneous pain of PHN appeared to be modulated by treatment with this medication, again suggesting that a peripherally acting agent may have an impact on central pain mechanisms [37].

EMLA® cream is another local anesthetic preparation (the eutectic mixture of 2.5 % lidocaine and 2.5 % prilocaine).

It is indicated as a topical anesthetic for use on normal intact skin for analgesia, but it is not FDA approved for any specific neuropathic pain disorder. Regardless, it is worth noting that several studies of the use of the eutectic preparation of 2.5 % lidocaine and 2.5 % prilocaine cream in the treatment of PHN have been completed. In a randomized, controlled study of PHN patients, treatment with the eutectic preparation of 2.5 % lidocaine and 2.5 % prilocaine cream did not result in significant differences between the treated and placebo groups [38]. In two studies, each of which was uncontrolled and thus less rigorously designed, the results were more encouraging suggesting that use of the eutectic preparation of 2.5 % lidocaine and 2.5 % prilocaine cream might relieve the pain associated with PHN [39, 40].

Capsaicin

There has been great interest in using capsaicin in a number of neuropathic pain disorders such as diabetic neuropathy, painful HIV neuropathy, PHN, and postmastectomy pain, but past available strengths of capsaicin (0.025 % and 0.075 %) had yielded disappointing results with the treatment being poorly tolerated, regimens poorly adhered to, and not enough pain relief experienced [41]. In contrast, examining the results of a higher-strength capsaicin preparation, notable analgesia had been reported by patients with painful HIV neuropathy receiving a 7.5 % topical capsaicin cream. The patients, to be able to tolerate this medication, required concurrent treatment with epidural anesthesia [42]. At the 2004 Annual Scientific Meeting of the American Academy of Neurology, two open-label studies, one in patients with PHN and one in patients with painful HIV-associated distal symmetrical polyneuropathy, reported notable pain relief for the majority of patients following the single application of a high-concentration (8 %) capsaicin patch. The duration of pain relief lasted as long as 48 weeks (PHN) [15, 43]. A review of the published randomized trials involving the use of topical capsaicin in the treatment of either neuropathic or musculoskeletal pain syndromes concluded that "although topically applied capsaicin has moderate to poor efficacy in the treatment of chronic musculoskeletal or neuropathic pain, it may be useful as an adjunct or sole therapy for a small number of patients who are unresponsive to, or intolerant of, other treatments" [44]. Recently, the 8 % capsaicin patch (Qutenza®) has received FDA approval for the treatment of PHN. In studies leading to its FDA approval, it was shown to be more effective in reducing pain intensity than an active, lower concentration capsaicin product that served as placebo, and it was generally well tolerated. It has also been studied in other neuropathic pain states such as painful HIV neuropathy with favorable outcome as well [45–49].

A novel study comparing the analgesic effect of a topical preparation containing either 3.3 % doxepin alone or 3.3 % doxepin combined with 0.075 % capsaicin to placebo in patients with various different chronic neuropathic pain problems demonstrated that each treatment resulted in equal degrees of analgesia and each was superior to placebo [50].

Other Agents

There has been interest in the use of topical tricyclic antidepressants in the treatment of neuropathic pain with clinical trials completed. In each two such studies, the preparation tested was a combination of amitriptyline 2 % and ketamine 1 %. The results of one of these, a double-blind, randomized, placebo-controlled study involving 92 patients with diabetic neuropathy, PHN, postsurgical, or posttraumatic neuropathic pain, were no difference in pain relief among the four treatment groups (placebo, amitriptyline 2 % alone, ketamine 1 % alone, or combination amitriptyline 2 %/ketamine 1 %) [51]. In a separate open-label study by the same group, 28 patients with neuropathic pain for 6–12 months were treated with the combination topical analgesic amitriptyline 2 %/ketamine 1 %. The investigators reported that on average, patients experienced 34 % pain reduction [52]. In another open-label study by the same group, the benefit of a combination of topical amitriptyline and ketamine for neuropathic pain also demonstrated encouraging results; however, no controlled study has yet been published [53]. Noncontrolled studies of topical ketamine, one in patients with PHN and one in patients with complex regional pain syndrome type 1, have suggested that topical ketamine may be an effective topical analgesic; however, serum ketamine levels were not measured in either study [54]. There is one report that suggests that the topical application of geranium oil may provide temporary relief from PHN [55].

Case Example: A 35-year-old female with complex regional pain syndrome type 2 following a traumatic injury to her left peroneal nerve presents to your office for evaluation and treatment. She is married with two children and is currently working part-time as an accountant. She is utilizing several medications and complains of severe, burning pain and hypersensitivity to anything that touches her left leg and foot, with a visual analogue scale score of 6/10. The pain is continuous but worst at night. She has achieved 30 % pain relief taking both duloxetine and pregabalin at maximally tolerated doses. She has failed a trial of both spinal as well as peripheral nerve stimulation and had previously benefitted only temporarily from sympathetic nerve blocks. Should this person be treated as well with a topical analgesic, even in an "off-label" manner? If so, which and what evidence do we use in making this decision? We think it would be reasonable to attempt such treatment providing the patient was fully informed of the "off-label" use, the potential benefits and risk of the prescribed agent, and the evidence for its use and of course the patient was to be properly monitored.

Soft Tissue Injuries and Osteoarthritis

Soft tissue injuries and osteoarthritis are each an example of musculoskeletal pain states. The use of topical analgesics for these heterogeneous conditions has been actively studied, and in fact, since 2007, the FDA has approved three topical NSAIDs. The diclofenac sodium gel 1 % (Voltaren gel 1 %) was FDA approved for use in treating pain associated with OA in joints that can be managed with topical treatment such as the knees and hands. The diclofenac epolamine topical patch (Flector® patch) has been FDA approved for the topical treatment of acute pain due to minor strains, sprains, and contusions. The diclofenac sodium topical solution (Pennsaid) has been FDA approved for the treatment of the signs and symptoms of OA of the knee [56]. Additional information about these more recently FDA-approved agents as well as other topical therapies for these conditions is reviewed below.

NSAIDs

Outside of the US, other topical NSAIDs have been studied. The use of a topical ketoprofen patch (100 mg) was superior to placebo in reducing pain after 1 week of treatment in a 14-day randomized, placebo-controlled study of 163 patients with an ankle sprain [57]. A similar ketoprofen preparation has been studied in patients with tendonitis in a randomized, double-blind, placebo-controlled study. Results were positive in favor of the active treatment, and the treatment was in general, except for skin irritation, well tolerated [58]. In a child with Sever's disease, a common cause of heel pain in athletic children, ketoprofen gel has been used as adjunctive therapy to physical therapy with reported benefit [59]. In a randomized, controlled study of a diclofenac patch in 120 individuals experiencing acute pain following a "blunt" injury, use of the patch was well tolerated as well as significantly better than placebo in reducing the pain associated with this injury [60]. In two separate studies (one open-label and one multicenter, randomized, controlled study), each completed by different investigators, of pain associated with acute sports injuries, a diclofenac patch was found to be effective in providing pain relief and well tolerated. On average, patients experienced 60 % pain relief in the open-label study [61, 62]. An open-label study of patients with "soft tissue pain" concluded that topical flurbiprofen was associated with greater pain reduction than oral diclofenac with fewer adverse effects reported [63]. In another controlled study, the use of topical ibuprofen cream in the management of acute ankle sprains was found to be superior to placebo in reducing pain [64]. In a controlled study of ketoprofen gel in the management of acute soft tissue pain, the gel was found to be more effective than placebo in providing pain relief [65]. A topical formulation of 5 % ibuprofen gel was examined in a placebo-controlled study in patients with painful soft tissue injuries. Patients received either the 5 % ibuprofen gel ($n = 40$) or placebo gel ($n = 41$) for a maximum of 7 days. Pain intensity levels as well as limitations of physical activity were assessed daily. A significant difference ($p < 0.001$) in pain reduction as well as improvement in physical activities for those patients who received the active gel compared to placebo recipients was noted [66]. An additional study of a similar population of patients completed by the same investigators resulted in similar outcomes [67]. A recent Cochrane Database review has concluded that topical NSAIDs can provide good levels of pain relief without the systemic adverse effects of oral NSAIDs for the treatment of acute musculoskeletal pain [68].

There has also been interest in studying the use of topical analgesics in the treatment of osteoarthritis in addition to soft tissue injuries, and in fact, multiple recent reviews of this subject have been recently published [69–72]. A diclofenac patch has been studied in a randomized, double-blind, controlled study in patients with osteoarthritis of the knee, and the results have demonstrated that this patch may be safe and effective for this condition [73]. A randomized, controlled study comparing the use of topical diclofenac solution to oral diclofenac for the treatment of osteoarthritis of the knee concluded that use of this topical diclofenac solution in patients with osteoarthritis of the knee produced symptom relief which was equivalent to oral diclofenac while resulting in significantly reduced incidence of diclofenac-related gastrointestinal complaints [74]. A recently published long-term study with this preparation has confirmed the safety of this preparation during the study period [75]. In a study of patients with pain in the temporomandibular joint, a group of patients received diclofenac solution applied topically several times daily, and a second group received oral diclofenac. No significant difference was demonstrated with respect to pain relief between the two groups; however, there were significantly fewer gastrointestinal side effects experienced by the patients receiving the diclofenac topical solution [76]. Other topical NSAID trials include a placebo-controlled trial that has demonstrated the efficacy of topical diclofenac gel 1.16 % for patients with osteoarthritis of the knee and a randomized, controlled study demonstrating benefit from the application of a topical diclofenac solution compared to placebo after 6 weeks of treatment for patients with painful osteoarthritis of the knee [77, 78]. More than one meta-analysis of this topic has been completed. A meta-analysis examining the use of topical NSAIDs in the treatment of osteoarthritis concluded that there was evidence that topical NSAIDs are superior to placebo during the first 2 weeks of treatment only. This meta-analysis concluded as well that available evidence suggested that topical NSAIDs were inferior to oral NSAIDs during the first week of treatment [79]. Another meta-analysis examining the evidence for the use of topical NSAIDs for chronic musculoskeletal pain also concluded that topical NSAIDs are effective and safe in treating chronic musculoskeletal conditions for 2 weeks [80]. Yet another meta-analysis of the use of topical NSAIDs for osteoarthritis suggested that of the four studies which had been completed in which a topical NSAID was compared to placebo or vehicle lasting 4 weeks or more for patients with osteoarthritis of the knee, pain relief did occur for a longer duration than placebo, but not all preparations had uniform results [81].

One should recognize that topical salicylates are used by patients in nonprescription preparations. A meta-analysis examining the effects of topical salicylates in acute and chronic pain concluded that based on the sparse data available that use of topically applied rubefacients containing salicylates based upon available trials of musculoskeletal and arthritic pain resulted in moderate to poor efficacy. The authors emphasized that efficacy estimates for rubefacients were at present unreliable due to a lack of appropriate clinical trials [82]. A randomized, controlled study completed in Germany with another topical NSAID, eltenac, examined its effect compared to placebo in 237 patients with osteoarthritis of the knee. Demonstrated efficacy and safety of the use of topical eltenac in the treatment of osteoarthritis of the knee compared to placebo were concluded by the authors [83]. In a separate study, topical eltenac gel was compared to oral diclofenac and placebo in patients with osteoarthritis of the knee. While both therapies were found to be superior to placebo with respect to analgesia, as reported in the meta-analysis above, the incidence of gastrointestinal side effects was notably lower in the group treated with topical eltenac gel compared to those treated with oral diclofenac [84]. Multiple other additional studies have demonstrated that topical diclofenac may be effective in reducing the pain associated with various types of degenerative joint disease [85–87].

Other topical agents have been studied in these conditions as well. No benefit of 0.025 % capsaicin cream over vehicle (not active) cream in a randomized, double-blind study of 30 patients with pain in the temporomandibular joint has been noted [88]. A topical cream containing glucosamine sulfate, chondroitin sulfate, and camphor for osteoarthritis of the knee showed a significant reduction of pain in the treatment group after 8 weeks compared to the placebo group in a randomized, controlled study [89].

A recently published case series reported the potential benefit of "topical" morphine in the management of chronic osteoarthritis-related pain; however, since the report emphasized that morphine or its metabolites were identifiable in the urine of treated patients, it is unclear how truly "topical" this preparation was [90].

Case Report: Consider a 67-year-old female with osteoarthritis of both knees and severe hypertension and esophageal reflux, who may be considered to be an inappropriate candidate for an oral NSAID, who has had little to no response to opiates, injection therapy, and /or physical therapy and is not a candidate for knee replacement. Might she be a candidate for a topical analgesic?

Low Back and Myofascial Pain

Far fewer studies regarding the use of topical analgesics for low back pain or myofascial pain have been published. The results of a double-blind, placebo-controlled study comparing topical capsaicin to placebo in 154 patients with chronic low back pain indicated that 60.8 % of capsaicin-treated patients compared with 42.1 % of placebo patients experienced 30 % pain relief after 3 weeks of treatment ($p < 0.02$) [91]. Other studies have been published in abstract form only – two are novel since they both involve the use of a local anesthetic in conditions not typically thought of as response to such and will be considered here. A multicenter, open-label study involving treatment of 120 patients with acute (<6 weeks), subacute (<3 months), short-term chronic (3–12 months), or long-term chronic (>12 months) low back pain with the 5 % lidocaine patch was completed. During the 6-week study period, participants applied four lidocaine 5 % patches to areas of maximal low back pain every 24 h. Initial evaluation suggests that the majority of patients experience moderate or greater degree of pain relief. Significant positive changes in quality of life indicators on this scale have been noted as well as demonstrated by the use of the NPS in this study [7]. An open-label study of patients with chronic myofascial pain was presented at the 2002 Scientific Meeting of the American Pain Society; 16 patients with chronic myofascial pain were treated with the lidocaine 5 % patch. After 28 days of treatment, statistically significant improvements were noted for average pain, general activity level, ability to walk, ability to work, relationships, sleep, and overall enjoyment of life in approximately 50 % of the patients studied [91].

Other Uses of Topical Analgesics

Although only small numbers of patients have been studied, it is interesting to note other conditions in which topical analgesics have been used. Topical analgesic of various types including opiates may be helpful in reducing pain associated with pressure ulcers or dressing changes [92–97]. A topical analgesic may help to treat postoperative pain and reduce the need for systemic analgesics. Controlled studies have demonstrated the benefit of the eutectic mixture of local anesthetics, 2.5 % lidocaine/2.5 % prilocaine cream in the reduction of pain associated with circumcision and venipuncture as well as for the pain associated with breast cancer surgery [5, 98]. More than one study has suggested that either ketamine or morphine may be used topically for mucositis-associated pain following chemotherapy or radiation therapy in patients with head and neck carcinomas [99, 100]. Topical opiates have been reported to reduce pain for two children with epidermolysis bullosa who were treated successfully with topical opiates [101]. An interesting report notes that the analgesic effect of menthol, an ingredient common to many over-the-counter analgesic preparations, may in part be as the result of activation of kappa-opioid receptors [102]. Burn pain has been reported to be treated effectively with a topical loperamide preparation [103]. Two randomized, controlled studies – one involving postoperative pain (diclofenac patch) and one involving wound pain treatment (capsicum plaster topically applied at acupuncture sites) – have been published as well [104, 105]. Central neuropathic itch has been treated successfully with the lidocaine 5 % patch according to a single case report [106]. Two other novel approaches to studying topical analgesia are worth mentioning. The results of an enriched enrollment study in which an open-label initial study led to the randomization of responders in a placebo-controlled study of the use of either a 4 % amitriptyline/2 % ketamine cream, 2 % amitriptyline/1 % ketamine cream, or placebo for patients with PHN demonstrated that after 3 weeks of treatment, the average daily pain intensity was lowest in patients receiving the higher concentration combination cream compared to the lower concentration combination or placebo ($p = 0.026$ high-concentration cream vs. placebo). Plasma levels of either drug were detected in fewer than 10 % of those patients receiving active treatment [107]. An open-label study of the use of a 0.25 % capsaicin topical agent in a lidocaine-containing vehicle in 25 patients with painful diabetic polyneuropathy and seven patients with PHN demonstrated pain relief in the majority of patients who were studied [108, 109].

Future Directions and Summary

The use of topical analgesics should be considered for a variety of painful conditions. The number of FDA-approved topical agents has grown recently. Off-label use of available therapies requires careful consideration of the potential risks as well benefits and deserves further study. Since topical analgesic use is generally associated with a better side effect profile than orally, transdermally, parenterally, or intrathecally administered analgesics, this should be considered when developing a pharmacologic treatment regimen for an individual patient. Further large, well-designed studies including comparative trials with nontopical analgesics are needed to further understand the role of topical analgesics in the management of acute and chronic pain.

References

1. Argoff CE. New analgesics for neuropathic pain: the lidocaine patch. Clin J Pain. 2000;16 Suppl 2:S62–5.
2. Argoff CE. Topical treatments for pain. Curr Pain Headache Rep. 2004;8:261–7.
3. Argoff CE, Khan KR. Chapter 17: Topical analgesics for neuropathic pain. In: Rice A, Howard R, Justins D, Miaskowski C, editors. Clinical pain management. 2nd ed. London: Hodder Arnold. 2008.
4. Argoff CE. Targeted topical peripheral analgesics in the management of pain. Curr Pain Headache Rep. 2002;7(1):34–8.
5. Galer BS. Topical medications. In: Loeser JD, editor. Bonica's management of pain. Philadelphia: Lippincott-Williams & Wilkins; 2001. p. 1736–41.
6. Gammaitoni AR, Alvarez NA. 24-hour application of the lidocaine patch 5% for 3 consecutive days is safe and well tolerated in healthy adult men and women. Abstract PO6.20. In: Presented at the 54th Annual American Academy of Neurology Meeting, Denver, 13–20 Apr 2002.
7. Argoff C, Nicholson B, Moskowitz M, et al. Effectiveness of lidocaine patch 5% (Lidoderm®) in the treatment of low back pain. In: Presented at the 10th world congress on pain, San Diego, 17–22 Aug 2002.
8. Watson CPN. Topical capsaicin as an adjuvant analgesic. J Pain Symptom Manage. 1994;9:425–33.
9. American Geriatrics Society Panel on Pharmacological Management of Persistent Pain in Older Adults. Pharmacological management of persistent pain in older persons. J Am Geriatr Soc. 2009;57(8):1331–46.
10. Gammaitoni AR, Davis MW. Pharmacokinetics and tolerability of lidocaine 5% patch with extended dosing. Ann Pharmacother. 2002;36:236–40.
11. Ness TJ, Jones L, Smith H. Use of compounded topical analgesics – results of an internet survey. Reg Anesth Pain Med. 2002;27(3):309–12.
12. Sawynok J. Topical and peripherally acting analgesics. Pharmacol Rev. 2003;55:1–20.
13. Robbins W. Clinical applications of capsaicinoids. Clin J Pain. 2000;16 Suppl 2:S86–9.
14. Bley KR. Recent developments in transient receptor potential vanilloid receptor 1 agonist-based therapies. Expert Opin Investig Drugs. 2004;13(11):1445–56. Review.
15. Backonja M, Malan P, Brady S, et al. One-hour high concentration capsaicin applications provide durable pain relief in initial and repeat treatment of postherpetic neuralgia. In: Presented at the 2004 Annual Scientific Meeting of the American Academy of Neurology, San Francisco, 2004.
16. Rowbotham MC. Topical analgesic agents. In: Fields HL, Liebeskind JC, editors. Pharmacologic approaches to the treatment of chronic pain: new concepts and critical issues. Seattle: IASP Press; 1994. p. 211–27.
17. Cashman JN. The mechanism of action of NSAIDs in analgesia. Drugs. 1996;52 suppl 5:13–23.
18. Yesilyurt O, Dogrul A, Gul H, et al. Topical cannabinoid enhances topical morphine antinociception. Pain. 2003;105(1–2):303–8.
19. Sawynok J, Esser MJ, Reid AR. Antidepressants as analgesics: an overview of central and peripheral mechanisms of action. J Psychiatry Neurosci. 2001;26(1):21–9.

20. Gerner P, Kao G, Srinivasa V, et al. Topical amitriptyline in health volunteers. Reg Anesth Pain Med. 2003;28(4):289–93.
21. Physicians desk reference. 55th edn. Montvale: Medical Economics Company; 2002.
22. Sawynok J. Topical analgesics in neuropathic pain. Curr Pharm Des. 2005;11(23):2995–3004.
23. Attal N, Crucci G, Haanpaa M, et al. EFNS guidelines on pharmacological treatment of neuropathic pain. Eur J Neurol. 2006;13(11):1153–69.
24. Rowbotham MC. Pharmacologic management of complex regional pain syndrome. Clin J Pain. 2006;22(5):425–9.
25. Rowbotham MC, Davies PS, Verkempinck C, et al. Lidocaine patch: double-blind controlled study of a new treatment method for post-herpetic neuralgia. Pain. 1996;65:39–44.
26. Galer BS, Rowbotham MC, Perander J, et al. Topical lidocaine patch relieves post-herpetic neuralgia more effectively than vehicle patch: results of an enriched enrollment study. Pain. 1999;80:533–8.
27. Katz NP, Davis MW, Dworkin RH. Topical lidocaine patch produces a significant improvement in mean pain scores and pain relief in treated PHN patients: results of a multicenter open-label trial. J Pain. 2001;2:9–18.
28. Rehm S, Binder A, Baron R. Post-herpetic neuralgia: 5% lidocaine medicated plaster, pregabalin or a combination of both? A randomized, open clinical effectiveness study. Curr Med Res Opin. 2010;26(7):1607–19.
29. Meier T, Wasner G, Faust M, et al. Efficacy of lidocaine patch 5% in the treatment of focal peripheral neuropathic pain syndromes: a randomized, double-blind, placebo-controlled study. Pain. 2003;106:151–8.
30. Devers A, Galer BS. Topical lidocaine patch relieves a variety of neuropathic pain conditions: an open-label study. Clin J Pain. 2000;16(3):205–8.
31. Data on file. Chadds Ford: Endo Pharmaceuticals, Inc.
32. Hart-Gouleau S, Gammaitoni A, Galer BS, et al. Open-label study of the effectiveness and safety of the lidocaine patch 5 % (Lidoderm®) in patients with painful diabetic neuropathy. In: Presented at the 10th world congress on pain, San Diego, 17–22 Aug 2002.
33. Galer BS, Jensen MP. Development and preliminary validation of a pain measure specific to neuropathic pain: the neuropathic pain scale. Neurology. 1997;48:332–8.
34. Barbano RL, Herrmann DN, Hart-Gouleau S, et al. Effectiveness, tolerability and impact on quality of life of lidocaine patch 5% in diabetic polyneuropathy. Arch Neurol. 2004;61(6):914–8.
35. Herrmann DN, Barbano RL, Hart-Gouleau S, et al. An open-label study of the lidocaine patch 5% in painful polyneuropathy. Pain Med. 2005;6(5):379–84.
36. Galer BS, Jensen MP, Ma T, et al. The lidocaine patch 5% effectively treats all neuropathic pain qualities: results of a randomized, double-blind, vehicle-controlled, 3-week efficacy study with use of the neuropathic pain scale. Clin J Pain. 2002;18:297–301.
37. Geha PY, Baliki MN, Chialvo DR, et al. Brain activity for spontaneous pain of post herpetic neuralgia and its modulation by lidocaine patch therapy. Pain. 2007;128(1–2):88–100.
38. Lycka BA, Watson CP, Nevin K, et al. EMLA® cream for the treatment of pain caused by post-herpetic neuralgia: a double-blind, placebo-controlled study. In: Proceedings of the annual meeting of the American Pain Society, 1996:A111(abstract).
39. Attal N, Brasseur L, Chauvin M, et al. Effects of single and repeated applications of a eutectic mixture of local anesthetics (EMLA®) cream on spontaneous and evoked pain in post-herpetic neuralgia. Pain. 1999;81:203–9.
40. Litman SJ, Vitkun SA, Poppers PJ. Use of EMLA® cream in the treatment of post-herpetic neuralgia. J Clin Anesth. 1996;8:54–7.
41. Rains C, Bryson HM. Topical capsaicin: a review of its pharmacological properties and therapeutic potential in post-herpetic neuralgia,

diabetic neuropathy, and osteoarthritis. Drugs Aging. 1995;7:317–28.
42. Robbins WR, Staats PS, Levine J, et al. Treatment of intractable pain with topical large-dose capsaicin: preliminary report. Anesth Analg. 1998;86:579–83.
43. Simpson D, Brown S, Sampson J, et al. A single application of high-concentration capsaicin leads to 12 weeks of pain relief in HIV-associated distal symmetrical polyneuropathy: results of an open label trail. In: Presented at the 2004 Annual Scientific Meeting of the American Academy of Neurology, San Francisco, 2004.
44. Mason L, Moore RA, Derry S, et al. Systematic review of topical capsaicin for the treatment of chronic pain. BMJ. 2004;328(7446):991–6.
45. Backonja MM, Malan TP, Vanhove GF, et al. NGX-4010, a high concentration patch, for the treatment of post herpetic neuralgia: a randomized, double-blind, controlled study with an open-label extension. Pain Med. 2010;11(4):600–8.
46. Backonja M, Wallace MS, Blonsky ER, et al. NGX-4010, a high-concentration capsaicin patch, for the treatment of post herpetic neuralgia: a randomised, double-blind study. LancetNeurol. 2008;7(12):1106–12.
47. Wallace M, Pappagallo M. Qutenza®: a capsaicin 8% patch for the management of post herpetic neuralgia. Expert Rev Neurother. 2011;11(1):15–27.
48. Simpson DM, Brown S, Tobias J, et al. Controlled trial of high-concentration capsaicin patch for treatment of painful HIV neuropathy. Neurology. 2008;70(24):2305–13.
49. Phillips TJ, Cherry CL, Cox S, et al. Pharmacological treatment of painful HIV-associated sensory neuropathy: a systematic review and meta-analysis of randomised controlled trials. PLoS One. 2010;5(12):e14422. Epub2010 Dec 28.
50. McCleane G. Topical application of doxepin hydrochloride, capsaicin and a combination of both produces analgesia in chronic neuropathic pain: a randomized, double-blind, placebo-controlled study. Br J Clin Pharmacol. 2000;49(6):574–9.
51. Lynch ME, Clark AJ, Sawynok J, et al. Topical 2% amitriptyline and 1% ketamine in neuropathic pain syndromes: a randomized, double-blind, placebo-controlled trial. Anesthesiology. 2005;103(1):140–6.
52. Lynch ME, Clark AJ, Sawynok J, et al. Topical amitriptyline and ketamine in neuropathic pain syndromes: an open-label study. J Pain. 2005;6(10):644–9.
53. Lynch ME, Clark AJ, Sawynok J. A pilot study examining topical amitriptyline, ketamine, and a combination of both in the treatment of neuropathic pain. Clin J Pain. 2003;19(5):323–8.
54. Quan D, Wellish M, Gilden DH. Topical ketamine treatment of postherpetic neuralgia. Neurology. 2003;60(8):1391–2.
55. Greenway FL, Frome BM, Engels TM, et al. Temporary relief of postherpetic neuralgia pain with topical geranium oil. Am J Med. 2003;115(7):586–7.
56. Barthel HR, Axford-Gatley RA. Topical non-steroidal anti-inflammatory drugs for osteoarthritis. Postgrad Med. 2010;122(6):98–106.
57. Mazieres B, Rouanet S, Velicy J, et al. Topical ketoprofen patch (100 mg) for the treatment of ankle sprain: a randomized, double-blind, placebo-controlled study. Am J Sports Med. 2005;33(4):515–23.
58. Mazieres B, Rouanet S, Guillon Y, et al. Topical ketoprofen patch in the treatment of tendonitis: a randomized, double blind, placebo controlled study. J Rheumatol. 2005;32(8):1563–70.
59. White RL. Ketoprofen gel as an adjunct to physical therapy management of a child with Sever disease. Phys Ther. 2006;86(3):424–33.
60. Predel HG, Koll R, Pabst H, et al. Diclofenac patch for topical treatment of acute impact injuries: a randomized, double blind, placebo controlled, multicenter study. Br J Sports Med. 2004;38(3):318–23.
61. Galer BS, Rowbotham MC, Perander J, et al. Topical diclofenac patch significantly reduces pain associated with minor sports injuries:

results of a randomized, double-blind, placebo-controlled, multicenter study. J Pain Symptom Manage. 2000;19:287–94.

62. Jenoure P, Segesser B, Luhti U, et al. A trial with diclofenac HEP plaster as topical treatment in minor sports injuries. Drugs Exp Clin Res. 1993;19:125–31.

63. Marten M. Efficacy and tolerability of a topical NSAID patch (local action transcutaneous flurbiprofen) and oral diclofenac in the treatment of soft-tissue rheumatism. Clin Rheumatol. 1997;16:25–31.

64. Campbell J, Dunn T. Evaluation of topical ibuprofen cream in the treatment of acute ankle sprains. J Accid Emerg Med. 1994;11: 178–82.

65. Airaksinen O, Venalainen J, Pietilainen T. Ketoprofen 2.5% gel versus placebo gel in the treatment of acute soft tissue injuries. Int J Clin Pharmacol Ther Toxicol. 1993;31:561–3.

66. Machen J, Whitefield M. Efficacy of a proprietary ibuprofen gel in soft tissue injuries: a randomized, double-blind, placebo-controlled study. Int J Clin Pract. 2002;56(2):102–6.

67. Whitefield M, O'Kane CJ, Anderson S. Comparative efficacy of a proprietary topical ibuprofen gel and oral ibuprofen in acute soft tissue injuries: a randomized, double-blind study. J Clin Pharm Ther. 2002;27(6):409–17.

68. Massey T, Derry S, Moore RA, et al. Topical NSAIDs for acute pain in adults. Cochrane Database Syst Rev. 2010;6:CD007402.

69. Brewer AR, McCarberg B, Argoff CE. Update on the use of topical NSAIDs for the treatment of soft tissue and musculoskeletal pain: a review of recent data and current treatment options. Phys Sportsmed. 2010;38(2):62–70.

70. Stanos SP. Topical agents for the management of musculoskeletal pain. J Pain Symptom Manage. 2007;33(3):342–55.

71. Harovtiunian S, Drennan DA, Lipman AG. Topical NSAID therapy for musculoskeletal pain. Pain Med. 2010;11(4):535–49.

72. Baraf HS, Gloth FM, Barthel HR, et al. Safety and efficacy of topical diclofenac sodium gel for knee osteoarthritis in elderly and younger patients; pooled data from three randomized, double-blind, parallel-group, placebo-controlled, multicenter trials. Drugs Aging. 2011;28(1):27–40.

73. Bruhlmann P, Michel BA. Topical diclofenac patch in patients with knee osteoarthritis: a randomized, double-blind, controlled clinical trial. Clin Exp Rheumatol. 2003;21(2):193–8.

74. Tugwell PS, Wells GA, Shainhouse JZ. Equivalence study of a topical diclofenac solution (pennsaid) compared with oral diclofenac in symptomatic treatment of osteoarthritis of the knee: a randomized, controlled trial. J Rheumatol. 2004;31(10):2002–12.

75. Shainhouse JZ, Grierson LM, Naseer Z. A long-term open label study to confirm the safety of topical diclofenac solution containing dimethyl sulfoxide in the treatment of the osteoarthritic knee. Am J Ther. 2010;17(6):566–76.

76. Di Rienzo BL, Di Rienzo BA, D'Emilia E, et al. Topical versus systemic diclofenac in the treatment of temporo-mandibular joint dysfunction symptoms. Acta Otorhinolaryngol Ital. 2004;24(5):279–83.

77. Niethard FU, Gold MS, Solomon GS, et al. Efficacy of topical diclofenac diethylamine gel in osteoarthritis of the knee. J Rheumatol. 2005;32(12):2384–92.

78. Baer PA, Thomas LM, Shainhouse Z. Treatment of osteoarthritis of the knee with a topical diclofenac solution: a randomized, controlled, 6 week trial (ISRCTN53366886). BMC Musculoskelet Disord. 2005;6:44.

79. Lin J, Zhang W, Jones A, et al. Efficacy of topical non-steroidal anti-inflammatory drugs in the treatment of osteoarthritis: meta-analysis of randomized controlled trials. BMJ. 2004;329(7461):324–8.

80. Mason L, Moore RA, Edwards JE, et al. Topical NSAIDS for chronic musculoskeletal pain: a systematic review and meta-analysis. BMC Musculoskelet Disord. 2004;5:28.

81. Biswal S, Medhi B, Pandhi P. Longterm efficacy of topical nonsteroidal anti-inflammatory drugs in knee osteoarthritis: metaanalysis of randomized placebo-controlled clinical trials. J Rheumatol. 2006;33(9):1841–4.

82. Mason L, Moore RA, Edwards JE, et al. Systematic review of topical rubefacients containing salicylates for the treatment of acute and chronic pain. BMJ. 2004;328:995.

83. Ottillinger B, Gomor B, Michel BA, et al. Efficacy and safety of eltenac gel in the treatment of knee osteoarthritis. Osteoarthritis Cartilage. 2001;9(3):273–80.

84. Sandelin J, Harilainen A, Crone H, et al. Local NSAID gel (eltenac) in the treatment of osteoarthritis of the knee. A double-blind study comparing eltenac with oral diclofenac and placebo gel. Scand J Rheumatol. 1997;26:287–92.

85. Dreiser RL, Tisne-Camus M. DHEP plasters as a topical treatment of knee osteoarthritis: a double-blind placebo-controlled study. Drugs Exp Clin Res. 1993;19:107–15.

86. Galeazzi M, Marcolongo R. A placebo-controlled study of the efficacy and tolerability of a nonsteroidal anti-inflammatory drug, DHEP plaster in inflammatory peri- and extra-articular rheumatological diseases. Drugs Exp Clin Res. 1993;19:107–15.

87. Gallachia G, Marcolongo R. Pharmacokinetics of diclofenac hydroxyethylpyrrolidine (DHEP) plasters in patients with monolateral knee joint effusion. Drugs Exp Clin Res. 1993;19:95–7.

88. Winocur E, Gavish A, Halachmi M, et al. Topical application of capsaicin for the treatment of localized pain in the temporomandibular joint area. J Orofac Pain. 2000;14(1):31–6.

89. Cohen M, Wolfe R, Mai T, et al. A randomized, double blind placebo-controlled trial of a topical crème containing glucosamine sulfate, chondroitin sulfate and camphor for osteoarthritis of the knee. J Rheumatol. 2003;30(3):523–8.

90. Wilken M, Ineck JR, Rule AM. Chronic arthritis pain management with topical morphine:case series. J Pain Palliat Care Pharmacother. 2005;19(4):39–44.

91. Keitel W, Frerick H, Kuhn U, et al. Capsicum pain plaster in chronic non-specific low back pain. Arzneimittelforschung. 2001;51:896–903.

92. Lipman AG, Dalpiaz AS, London SP. Topical lidocaine patch therapy for myofascial pain. Abstract 782. In: Presented at the Annual Scientific Meeting of the American Pain Society, Baltimore, 14–17 Mar 2002.

93. Briggs M, Nelson EA. Topical agents or dressings for pain in venous leg ulcers. Cochrane Database Syst Rev. 2003;1: CD001177.

94. Flock P. Pilot study to determine the effectiveness of diamorphine gel to control pressure ulcer pain. J Pain Symptom Manage. 2003;25(6):547–54.

95. Zeppetella G, Ribeiro PJ. Analgesic efficacy of morphine applied topically to painful ulcers. J Pain Symptom Manage. 2003;25(6): 555–8.

96. Gallagher RE, Arndt DR, Hunt KL. Analgesic effects of topical methadone: a report of four cases. Clin J Pain. 2005;21(2):190–2.

97. Vernassiere C, Cornet C, Trechot P, et al. Study to determine the efficacy of topical morphine on painful chronic skin ulcers. J Wound Care. 2005;14(6):289–93.

98. Ashfield T. The use of topical opioids to relieve pressure ulcer pain. Nurs Stand. 2005;19(45):90–2.

99. Fassoulaki A, Sarantopoulos C, Melemeni A, et al. EMLA reduces acute and chronic pain after breast surgery for cancer. Reg Anesth Pain Med. 2000;25(4):35–355.

100. Cerchietti LC, Navigante AH, Bonomi MR, et al. Effect of topical morphine for mucositis-associated pain following concomitant chemoradiotherapy for head and neck carcinoma. Cancer. 2002;95(10):2230–6.

101. Slatkin NE, Rhiner M. Topical ketamine in the treatment of mucositis pain. Pain Med. 2003;4(3):298–303.

102. Watterson G, Howard R, Goldman A. Peripheral opiates in inflammatory pain. Arch Dis Child. 2004;89(7):679–81.

103. Galeotti N, DeCesare Mannelli L, Mazzanti G, et al. Menthol: a natural analgesic compound. Neurosci Lett. 2002;322(3):145–8.

104. Ray SB. Loperamide: a potential topical analgesic for the treatment of burn pain. J Burn Care Res. 2006;27(1):121–2.

105. Alessandri F, Lijoi D, Mistrangelo E, et al. Topical diclofenac patch for postoperative wound pain in laparoscopic gynecologic surgery: a randomized study. J Minim Invasive Gynecol. 2006;13(3):195–200.

106. Kim KS, Nam YM. The analgesic effects of capsicum plaster at the Zusanli point after abdominal hysterectomy. Anesth Analg. 2006;103(3):709–13.

107. Sandroni P. Central neuropathic itch: a new treatment option? Neurology. 2002;59:778–9.

108. Lockhart E. Topical combination of amitriptyline and ketamine for post herpetic neuralgia. J Pain. 2004;3 suppl 1:82.

109. Bernstein J, Phillips S, Group T. A new topical medication for the adjunctive relief of painful diabetic neuropathy and postherpetic neuralgia. J Pain. 2004;5(3 suppl 1):82.

Sleep Aids

Howard S. Smith

Key Points

- Insomnia relates to complaints of inadequate sleep (e.g., problems falling asleep, problems with staying asleep [sleep duration], and/or quality of sleep) and may need treatment especially if it is associated with significant patient distress and/or daytime sleepiness.
- Treatment for insomnia may require nonpharmacologic approaches as well as pharmacologic approaches.
- Medications that are FDA approved for the treatment of insomnia include benzodiazepines, "Z-drugs," and melatonin receptor agonists.
- "Z-drugs" (e.g., zaleplon, zolpidem, zopiclone, eszopiclone) may have less potential for rebound insomnia and withdrawal symptoms than benzodiazepines, but they still have a significant potential for abuse.

Introduction

Sleep is one of the most universal biological processes in existence. Depriving an organism of sleep altogether can be extremely detrimental and may even lead to death [1]. Sleep is therefore considered necessary for life, but why this is so remains unclear. Sleep is subdivided into rapid eye movement (REM) sleep, which is characterized by high-frequency electroencephalogram (EEG) recordings and muscle atonia [2], and non-REM (slow-wave) sleep, characterized by low-frequency EEG recordings and body rest [3].

While the cholinergic and monoaminergic systems act to promote wakefulness in conjunction with the orexins, there are other neuronal groups that act to promote sleep. The primary population of sleep-promoting neurons is located in the preoptic area, specifically the ventrolateral preoptic area of the hypothalamus (VLPO). Thus, multiple mediators can be targeted in efforts to combat insomnia and/or promote sleep/sedation (e.g., acetylcholine, norepinephrine, gamma-aminobutyric acid, histamine, serotonin, adenosine dopamine, melatonin, orexin).

Insomnia is a condition of perceived inadequate sleep, with patients typically presenting with difficulty falling asleep, difficulty maintaining sleep, or poor quality sleep [4]. To manage insomnia successfully, pharmacological treatments for insomnia may be required to reduce sleep latency, increase sleep maintenance, and improve sleep quality. In addition, such treatments should enable normal wakening with no subsequent impairment of daytime function and minimal risk of dependence.

Sivertsen et al. studied insomnia symptoms and the use of health-care services and medications and concluded that insomnia symptoms represent a significant public health concern, being independently associated with substantially elevated use of health-care services, medications, and alcohol overuse [5].

Kyle and colleagues concluded from the relatively small literature that insomnia impacts on diverse areas of health-related quality of life (HRQoL), and that both pharmacological and nonpharmacological interventions can produce, to varying degrees, improvements in domains spanning physical, social, and emotional functioning [6].

Insomnia Assessment

The following questions can serve as the initial assessment regarding sleep [7]: What time do you normally go to bed at night and wake up in the morning? Do you often have trouble falling asleep at night? About how many times do you wake up at night? If you do wake up during the night,

H.S. Smith, M.D., FACP, FAAPM, FACNP (✉)
Department of Anesthesiology, Albany Medical College,
Albany Medical Center, 47 New Scotland Avenue,
Albany, NY 12159, USA
e-mail: smithh@mail.amc.edu

T.R. Deer et al. (eds.), *Treatment of Chronic Pain by Medical Approaches: the AMERICAN ACADEMY of PAIN MEDICINE Textbook on Patient Management*, DOI 10.1007/978-1-4939-1818-8_9,
© American Academy of Pain Medicine 2015

do you usually have trouble falling back asleep? Does your bed partner say (or are you aware) that you frequently snore, gasp for air, or stop breathing—kick, thrash about, eat, punch, or scream during sleep? Are you sleepy or tired during much of the day? Do you unintentionally doze off during the day? Do you usually take one or more naps during the day?

The ISI, developed by Morin, is a seven-item Likert-type self-rating scale designed to assess the subjective perception of the severity of insomnia [8]. The scale contains items that measure the symptoms and associated features and impacts of insomnia, including difficulty falling asleep, difficulty maintaining sleep, early morning awakening, satisfaction with sleep, concerns about insomnia, and functional impacts of insomnia.

Treatment for Insomnia

The treatment for insomnia may involve pharmacologic as well as nonpharmacologic approaches.

Nonpharmacologic Approaches to Insomnia

Sleep Hygiene and Sleep Education

Sleep hygiene refers to the general rules of behavioral practices and environmental factors that are consistent with good quality sleep. When defined broadly, it includes guidelines for general health practices (e.g., diet, exercise, substance use), environmental factors (e.g., light, temperature, noise), as well as sleep-related behavioral practices (e.g., regularity of sleep schedule, pre-sleep activities, efforts to try to sleep) [9]. The International Classification of Sleep Disorders even includes the diagnostic category "inadequate sleep hygiene," which is designated for the sleep disruption associated with poor sleep hygiene practices [10]. In addition, poor sleep-related habits leading to conditioned arousal in bed are considered to be one of the major etiological factors of psychophysiological insomnia [10]. Poor sleep hygiene practices have been considered to be a contributing factor to insomnia [9].

Previous studies have shown that sleep hygiene alone is not a sufficient treatment for insomnia [11–14]. Interventions aimed to reduce physiological or cognitive arousal (e.g., relaxation training, cognitive restructuring) and stimulus control instructions to reduce conditioned arousal with bedtime cues may be indicated to generate better results.

Behaviors and habits that may impair sleep include the following [7]: frequent daytime napping, spending too much time in bed, insufficient daytime activities, late-evening exercises, insufficient bright-light exposure, excess caffeine, evening alcohol consumption, smoking in the evening, late, heavy dinner, watching television or engaging in other stimulating activities at night, anxiety and anticipation of poor sleep, clock watching, and environmental factors, such as the room being too warm, too noisy, or too bright; pets on the bed or in the bedroom; and active or noisy bed partners.

The following are helpful instructions for using stimulus control and practicing good sleep hygiene [7]: develop a sleep ritual, such as maintaining a 30-min relaxation period before bedtime or taking a hot bath 90 min before bedtime; make sure the bedroom is restful and comfortable; go to bed only if you feel sleepy; avoid heavy exercise within 2 h of bedtime; avoid sleep-fragmenting substances, such as caffeine, nicotine, and alcohol; avoid activities in the bedroom that keep you awake. Use the bedroom only for sleep and sex; do not watch television from bed or work in bed; sleep only in your bedroom; if you cannot fall asleep, leave the bedroom and return only when sleepy; maintain stable bedtimes and rising times. Arise at the same time each morning, regardless of the amount of sleep obtained that night, and avoid daytime napping. If you do nap during the day, limit it to 30 min and do not nap, if possible, after 2 p.m.

Relaxation Therapy

The goal of relaxation therapy is to guide individuals to a calm, steady state when they wish to go to sleep. The methods used include progressive muscle relaxation (tensing and then relaxing each muscle group), guided imagery, diaphragmatic breathing, meditation, and biofeedback [15].

Cognitive Behavioral Therapy

Vitiello et al. performed randomized controlled trial of cognitive behavioral therapy for insomnia (CBT-I) in patients with osteoarthritis and comorbid insomnia [16]. CBT-I subjects reported significantly improved sleep and significantly reduced pain after treatment. Control subjects reported no significant improvements. One-year follow-up found maintenance of improved sleep and reduced pain for both the CBT-I group alone and among subjects who crossed over from control to CBT-I, suggesting that improving sleep, per se, in patients with osteoarthritis may result in decreased pain [16].

Sivertsen and colleagues performed a randomized double-blind placebo-controlled trial examining short- and long-term clinical efficacies of cognitive behavioral therapy (CBT) and pharmacological treatment in older adults experiencing chronic primary insomnia [17]. Participants receiving CBT improved their sleep efficiency from 81.4 % at pretreatment to 90.1 % at 6-month follow-up compared with a decrease from 82.3 to 81.9 % in the zopiclone group, suggesting that interventions based on CBT may be superior to zopiclone treatment both in short- and long-term management of insomnia in older adults [17]. This agrees with the findings of Dolan et al. [18] and of a similar study which found temazepam equal to CBT in the short term but inferior to CBT in the long term [19]. Three meta-analyses [12, 14, 20]

Table 9.1 Conclusions from the Agency for Healthcare Research and Quality Evidence Report/technology assessment regarding the manifestations and management of chronic insomnia [23]

Evidence exists to support that:

Chronic insomnia is associated with older age.

Benzodiazepines and nonbenzodiazepines are effective in the management of chronic insomnia. However, benzodiazepines, nonbenzodiazepines, and antidepressants pose a risk of harm.

Benzodiazepines have a greater risk of harm than nonbenzodiazepines.

Melatonin is effective in the management of chronic insomnia in subsets of the chronic insomnia population, and there is no evidence that melatonin poses a risk of harm.

Relaxation therapy and cognitive behavioral therapy are effective in the management of chronic insomnia in subsets of the chronic insomnia population.

have concluded that 70–80 % of middle-aged adults with insomnia benefit from interventions based on CBT. Irwin et al. performed a meta-analysis and concluded that behavioral interventions were more effective in middle-aged adults versus older adults in improving both total sleep time and sleep efficiency [20]. Morin et al. conducted a prospective, randomized controlled trial involving 2-stage therapy for 160 adults with persistent insomnia [21]. Participants received CBT alone or CBT plus 10 mg/day (taken at bedtime) of zolpidem for an initial 6-week acute therapy, followed by extended 6-month therapy. The best long-term outcome was obtained with patients treated with combined therapy initially, followed by CBT alone, as evidenced by higher remission rates at the 6-month follow-up compared with patients who continued to take zolpidem during extended therapy [21].

Acupuncture

Cao and colleagues performed a systematic review of randomized controlled trials (RCTs) of acupuncture for treatment of insomnia [22]. They found that acupuncture appears to be effective in treatment of insomnia; however, further large, rigorous designed trials are warranted [22].

Pharmacologic Approaches to Insomnia

In 2005, the Agency for Healthcare Research and Quality released its Evidence Report/Technology Assessment (see Table 9.1) [23]. Several nutritional or herbal products are sold for the treatment of insomnia (e.g., valerian root, melatonin, hops, chamomile, St. John's wort). Only valerian and melatonin have demonstrated some benefit in promoting sleep. Melatonin, however, can cause sleep disruption, daytime fatigue, headaches, and dizziness at higher doses, while valerian root can cause residual daytime sedation and, in rare instances, hepatotoxicity [24].

Common drug classes used to treat insomnia, but not FDA approved for that use, include antihistamines (e.g., diphenhydramine), antidepressants (e.g., amitriptyline, doxepin, trazodone), atypical antipsychotics (quetiapine), and sedatives (e.g., chloral hydrate). These drug classes are used due to their sedative properties.

FDA-Approved Pharmacologic Therapies for Management of Insomnia

The FDA-approved therapies for the management of insomnia are classified as sedative-hypnotic agents. These sedative hypnotics can be categorized into three groups: benzodiazepines, nonbenzodiazepine selective GABA agonists, and melatonin receptor agonists (see Table 9.2).

Benzodiazepines

The first benzodiazepine, chlordiazepoxide (discovered serendipitously by Leo Sternbach in 1955), is a fusion of a benzene ring and a diazepine ring. Benzodiazepines such as chlordiazepoxide (Librium) and diazepam (Valium) were first developed as sedatives in the 1960s and rapidly gained popularity essentially replacing barbiturates as the sedatives of choice for "sleeping pills" [25]. Benzodiazepines could be acting on receptors directly within the VLPO to promote sleep, or they could be acting more globally to facilitate inhibitory GABA transmission [26]. The $\alpha 1$ subunit of the GABAA receptor is especially important for benzodiazepine-induced sedation. Mice with mutations in the $\alpha 1$ subunit are insensitive to the sedative effects of the traditional benzodiazepine diazepam but maintain sensitivity to its anxiolytic, myorelaxant, and motor-impairing functions, indicating that the sedating effects of benzodiazepines are primarily mediated by actions on the $\alpha 1$ subunit [27].

Nonbenzodiazepine Selective GABA Agonists

The $GABA_A$ receptor is a pentameric molecule composed of a combination of one or more specific subunit types. Although 19 different subunits are known to exist, the majority of $GABA_A$ receptors in the central nervous system consist of $\alpha_{(1-6)}$, $\beta_{(1-3)}$, and $\gamma_{(1-3)}$ subunits [28]. The interaction of benzodiazepines with multiple $GABA_A$ receptor subunits containing $\alpha_{(1-3,5)}$ is thought to elicit the variety of effects seen with these agents such as anxiolysis, amnesia, muscle relaxation, sedation, and anticonvulsant activity [28]. The theoretical advantage of having a selective α_1 subunit agonist of the GABA receptor is that sedating effects are achieved while avoiding other effects thought to be mediated by the other α subunits to which benzodiazepines bind.

In contrast to benzodiazepines, the nonbenzodiazepine sedative hypnotics (i.e., zolpidem, eszopiclone, zopiclone, zaleplon) are more selective for the $GABA_A$ receptors with

Table 9.2 Food and Drug Administration–approved drugs for insomnia

Drugs	Adult dose (mg)	Half-life (h)	Onset (min)	Peak effect (h)
BzRAs				
Estazolam	(1, 2)	10–24	15–60	0.5–1.6
(*ProSom*™)	0.5–2			
Flurazepam	(15, 30)	47–100	15–20	3–6
(*Dalmane*™)	15–30			
Quazepam	(15)	P: 25–41	15–60	15–3
(*Doral*™)	7.5–15 (max. 30)	AM: 40–114 (2-oxoquazepam-[2 h] *N*-desalkyl-2-oxoquazepam [40–114 h])		
Temazepam	(17.5, 15, 22.5, 30)	6–16	15–60	1.5–3
(*Restoril*™)	7.5–30			
Triazolam	(0.125, 0.25)	1.5–5.5	15–30	1.7–5
(*Halcion*™)	0.125–0.25 (max. 0.5)			
Non–BzRAs				
Eszopiclone	(1, 2, 3)	6	30	1
(*Lunesta*™)	1–2 (max. 3)	(9 in elderly)		
Zaleplon	(5, 10)	1	Rapid	1
(*Sonata*™, *Starnoc*™)	5–10 (max. 20)			
Zopiclone	(5, 7.5)	~5–6	30	1–2
(*Imovane*™)	5–15	(5–10 in elderly)		
Zolpidem tartrate IR	(5, 10)	~2.5	15–30	1–3
(*Ambien*™)	5–20			
Zolpidem tartarate ER	(6.25, 12.5)	~3	30	1.5–4
(*Ambien CR*™)	6.25–12.5			
Melatonin receptor agonist				
Ramelton	(8)	P: 0.5–2.6	30	0.5–1.5
(*Rozerem*™)	8½ h before bedtime	AM: 2–5 (M-II)		

Abbreviations: *P* parent drug, *AM* active metabolite, *BzRAs* benzodiazepines, *Non-BzRAs* nonbenzodiazepines, *IR* immediate release, *ER* extended release, *CR* controlled release, *()* dosage forms

the α_1-receptor subunit [29]. Indiplon is a novel pyrazolopyrimidine, nonbenzodiazepine γ-aminobutyric acid (GABA) agonist with a high affinity and selectivity for the α1 subunit associated with sedation for the treatment of insomnia [29]. Petroski and colleagues [30] showed indiplon to be at least nine times more selective for α_1 as compared to α_2, α_3, and α_5 subunits [30]; a greater degree of selectivity for α_1, over the α_2 and α_3 subunits, was greater for indiplon as compared to zolpidem, zopiclone, and zaleplon.

"Z-DRUGS"

Initial nonbenzodiazepine selective GABA agonists are often referred to as the "Z-drugs" because they include zolpidem (Ambien), zaleplon (Sonata), zopiclone (Imovane), and eszopiclone (Lunesta). Zaleplon and zolpidem have much higher efficacy at benzodiazepine receptors containing the α1 subunit compared with other types of α subunits, whereas traditional benzodiazepines (e.g., triazolam) lack this specificity [31].

Zaleplon

It appears that zaleplon binds preferentially to alpha 1-containing GABAA receptors [32] and may be considered alpha 1-selective, and so zaleplon's effects are likely mediated via the alpha 1 receptor and are predominantly sedative in nature [30]. Zaleplon has a short T_{max} and the shortest $t_{1/2}$ of the current Z-drugs (see Table 9.2), explaining its fast onset and the fastest offset of action. Zolpidem IR has a longer $t_{1/2}$ than zaleplon, resulting in a longer duration of action. Zolpidem CR consists of a two-layer tablet: The outer layer dissolves quickly, while the second layer dissolves slowly to maintain plasma zolpidem concentrations above those seen for the IR formulation, particularly at 3–6 h post-dose [33].

Zolpidem

Zolpidem was the first subtype-selective GABAA receptor agonist and has the highest affinity at the alpha 1 subtype of all the nonbenzodiazepine GABAA receptor modulators.

Zolpidem will activate alpha 2 and alpha 3 receptors, though at considerably higher concentrations than those that activate the alpha 1 subtype.

Zopiclone

Zopiclone shows relatively high binding affinity for the alpha 1 over the alpha 3 receptor subtype [34], and zopiclone also binds to the alpha 5 receptor with high affinity [35]. Sivertsen et al. examined polysomnographic parameters and sleep apnea and periodic limb movement disorder (PLMD) in chronic users of zopiclone compared with aged-matched drug-free patients with insomnia versus "good sleepers" [36]. Forty-one percent of the patients treated pharmacologically for insomnia also had sleep apnea. There were no differences between the zopiclone and insomnia group on any of the polysomnography parameters, and a similar pattern was found for data based on sleep diaries [36]. This study suggests that the sleep of chronic users of zopiclone is no better than that of drug-free patients with insomnia [36].

Zopiclone is a racemic mixture of (S)- and (R)-isomers, with stereoselective PK profiles [37, 38] and clinical outcomes [39]. Racemic zopiclone has the longest T_{max} of the Z-drugs, and plasma concentrations of the more active enantiomer, (S)-zopiclone, remain below the sleep-inducing threshold (of 10 ng/ml) for more than half an hour after administration [40]. Racemic zopiclone has a longer $t_{1/2}$ than either zaleplon or zolpidem, suggesting a longer duration of action. However, this means that (S)-zopiclone plasma concentrations may not fall below the sleep-inducing threshold until more than 9 h after racemic zopiclone dosing. An additional consideration is the duration of effects of zopiclone's active metabolite, (S)-desmethylzopiclone (SDMZ), and the less active enantiomer, (R)-zopiclone. Measurable plasma concentrations of both SDMZ and (R)-zopiclone are present 8 h after zopiclone dosing and could contribute to unwanted next-day residual effects [41].

Eszopiclone

Eszopiclone is the pure (S)-enantiomer of racemic zopiclone [42] and was licensed in the USA in December 2004. Although eszopiclone is the isolated (S)-enantiomer of zopiclone, this study revealed notable differences in the pharmacodynamic effects of eszopiclone compared with racemic (R, S)-zopiclone. The pattern of eszopiclone binding at alpha 1, alpha 2, alpha 3, and alpha 5 subtypes is similar (although not identical) to that of zopiclone, but the binding affinities of eszopiclone are all higher than those seen with zopiclone. Eszopiclone's potency is greatest at alpha 5 receptors, followed by alpha 2 and alpha 3 receptors, but it is still a very potent drug at the alpha 1 receptor subtype with an EC50 of the same order of magnitude as zaleplon and zopiclone. Eszopiclone is particularly efficacious at alpha 2 and 3 receptors, with the highest efficacy of the nonbenzodiazepine GABAA modulators when examined in the same study [35].

Melatonin Receptor Agonists (MRAs)

Melatonin is an endogenous neuromodulator synthesized by the pineal gland, and its secretion is regulated by the suprachiasmatic nucleus (SCN), the circadian pacemaker of the brain [43]. The SCN receives light signals from the retina, which are transmitted to the dorsal medial hypothalamus (DMH), which acts as a relay center for signals to regions involved in sleep and wake maintenance [e.g., VLPO, locus coeruleus (LC)]. Melatonin acts largely through MT1 receptors in the SCN to suppress firing of SCN neurons, thereby disinhibiting the sleep-promoting neurons in the VLPO [43]. Secretion of melatonin is low during the day and high at night, and the onset of melatonin secretion coincides with the onset of nightly sleepiness. Exogenous melatonin crosses the blood–brain barrier, and various over-the-counter melatonin preparations are used to treat insomnia, jet lag, shift-work-related sleepiness, and delayed phase syndrome, with various degrees of effectiveness [44]. Melatonin, ramelteon (Rozerem), and agomelatine (Valdoxan) are all agonists for melatonin 1 (MT1) and melatonin 2 (MT2) receptors [43]. Ramelteon has an affinity for both receptors that is 3–16 times greater than melatonin, and it has a longer half-life. Agomelatine also has a high affinity for melatonin receptors, in addition to acting as an antagonist at serotonin 5-HT2C receptors to decrease anxiety as well as promote sleep. Both MT1 and MT2 play a role in sleep induction; MT1 activation suppresses firing of SCN neurons, and MT2 receptors are involved in entraining circadian rhythms.

The administration of melatonin (MEL) during the daytime, i.e., out of the phase of its endogenous secretion, can facilitate sleep [45]; however, if the treatment goal is to maintain daytime sleep for ~8 h, then fast-release oral MEL with its short elimination half-life (~40 min) may be more appropriate [46]. Aeschbach et al. show in healthy subjects that transdermal delivery of MEL during the daytime can elevate plasma MEL and reduce waking after sleep onset, by promoting sleep in the latter part of an 8-h sleep opportunity [46].

Antihistamines

Antihistaminergics exert their sedative effects by antagonizing the H1 receptors in the brain. The H1 antagonist cyproheptadine (Periactin) is effective at increasing slow-wave sleep and REM sleep in rats [47], whereas the H1 antagonists diphenhydramine (Benadryl) and chlorpheniramine (Chlor-Trimeton) decrease sleep latency but have no effect on amount of sleep. In humans, diphenhydramine initially increases subjective sleepiness and reduces latency to sleep compared with placebo, but after 4 days of administration, this effect is abolished, indicating tolerance to its effects [48].

Antidepressants/Atypical Antipsychotics

The effects of antidepressants on sleep are diverse, even within a class of medications. Sedation and drowsiness are common side effects of the TCAs (e.g., desipramine (Norpramin), imipramine (Tofranil), and amitriptyline (Elavil)). Amitriptyline increases drowsiness and shortens sleep latency compared with placebo, whereas imipramine actually increases sleep latency and decreases total sleep time. MAOIs and SSRIs (e.g., fluoxetine (Prozac), sertraline (Zoloft), and citalopram (Celexa)) can cause insomnia and decreased sleep efficiency. The TCAs which seem to be utilized most commonly to help combat insomnia include amitriptyline and doxepin. Notably, all these classes of antidepressants suppress REM sleep to some degree and have significant anticholinergic effects while doxepin has significant antihistaminergic effects. Cyclobenzaprine (an agent traditionally viewed as a muscle relaxant but structurally very similar to amitriptyline) has been used to help combat insomnia by some clinicians.

Trazodone (Desyrel) is an antidepressant that is also commonly prescribed for insomnia [49]. Trazodone acts as both a weak serotonin (5-HT) reuptake inhibitor and as an antagonist at $5-HT_{2A}$ and $5-HT_{2C}$, α_1-adrenergic, and histamine H_1 receptors [50]. Trazodone has been shown to suppress REM sleep; however, its effects on sleep latency, sleep duration, and number of wakenings are controversial.

Schwartz et al. attempted to compare the effectiveness and tolerability of two hypnotic agents, trazodone (Desyrel) (50–100 mg) and zaleplon (Sonata) (10–20 mg), on psychiatric inpatients with insomnia. Schwartz and colleagues suggested that in their pilot study, it appeared that trazodone may be a better agent to promote longer, deeper subjective quality sleep for psychiatric inpatients with insomnia in terms of effectiveness. However, tolerability was much better with zaleplon as daytime residual side effects were less [51]. Meta-chlorophenylpiperazine (mCPP) is a synthetic drug that was identified for the first time in 2004 in Sweden as an illicit recreational drug and is also a metabolite of trazodone [52]. mCPP has stimulant and hallucinogenic effects similar to those of 3,4-methylenedioxymethamphetamine (MDMA) and has the potential to lead to the development of serotonergic syndrome when interacting with certain agents [53].

Cankurtaran and colleagues compared the effectiveness of mirtazapine and imipramine on multiple distressing symptoms (e.g., pain, nausea) and other symptoms, e.g., sleep disturbances and also depressive and anxiety symptoms [54]. For initial, middle, and late insomnia, only the mirtazapine group showed improvements, suggesting that mirtazapine is effective for helping to resolve insomnia [54].

If antidepressants are used to address insomnia, sedating ones should be preferred over activating agents such as serotonin reuptake inhibitors. In general, drugs lacking strong cholinergic activity should be preferred over agents with strong cholinergic activity (e.g., amitriptyline). Drugs blocking serotonin 5-HT2A or 5-HT2C receptors should be preferred over those whose sedative property is caused largely by histamine receptor blockade (e.g., doxepin). However, sometimes these "nonpreferred" agents (which tend to be very sedating) appear to address insomnia the best. The dose should be as low as possible (e.g., as an initial dose: doxepin 25 mg, mirtazapine 15 mg, trazodone 50 mg, trimipramine 25 mg) [55]. Regarding the lack of substantial data allowing for evidence-based recommendations, we are facing a clear need for well-designed, long-term, comparative studies to further define the role of antidepressants versus other agents in the management of insomnia. Atypical antipsychotic agents which have been utilized (largely because of their sedative effects) in patients that also have chronic insomnia with relatively little data include olanzapine, quetiapine, and clozapine [56].

Alpha 2-Delta Ligands

The use of gabapentin has been evaluated for sleep on healthy persons, patients with seizure, or alcoholic patients [57–60]. All of these studies, though not on persons with primary insomnia, showed generally beneficial effects of sleep and increased slow-wave sleep. Lo and colleagues studied 18 patients with primary insomnia who received gabapentin treatment for at least 4 weeks [61]. All patients received polysomnography, a biochemical blood test, and neuropsychological tests before and after the treatment period. They found that gabapentin enhances slow-wave sleep in patients with primary insomnia [61]. It also improves sleep quality by elevating sleep efficiency and decreasing spontaneous arousal. The results suggest that gabapentin may be beneficial in the treatment of primary insomnia [61]. Hindmarch and colleagues assessed the effects of pregabalin compared with alprazolam and placebo on aspects of sleep in healthy volunteers using a randomized, double-blind, placebo- and active-controlled, 3-way crossover study design [62]. Although there were no differences between the active treatments, both pregabalin and alprazolam reduced rapid eye movement sleep as a proportion of the total sleep period compared with placebo. Pregabalin also significantly reduced the number of awakenings of more than 1 min in duration [62]. Leeds Sleep Evaluation Questionnaire ratings of the ease of getting to sleep and the perceived quality of sleep were significantly improved following both active treatments, and ratings of behavior following awakening were significantly impaired by both drug treatments [62].

Sympatholytics

Sedation and fatigue are among the most common side effects in patients taking βAR antagonists, α1AR antagonists, and clonidine, an agonist for α2AR inhibitor autoreceptors that attenuates NE release. Interestingly, prazosin is used to alleviate nightmares in posttraumatic stress disorder patients [63], potentially by acting as a dual anxiolytic and sedative. Twenty-two veterans with posttraumatic stress disorder (PTSD) were assessed for trauma-related nightmares and nonnightmare distressed awakenings (NNDA) before and after treatment with the alpha-1 adrenoreceptor antagonist prazosin at an average bedtime dose of 9.6 mg/day. Ratings combining frequency and intensity dimensions of trauma-related nightmares decreased from 3.6 to 2.2, NNDA from 5.2 to 2.1, and sleep difficulty from 7.2 to 4.1 per week [64]. Tizanidine (an alpha 2 agonist traditionally viewed as a muscle relaxant/antispasticity agent) has been used by some clinicians to help combat insomnia.

Barbiturates

Gamma-hydroxybutyrate (GHB) is not a barbiturate; it is a euphoric, prosocial, and sleep-inducing drug that binds with high affinity to its own GHB receptor site and also more weakly to GABA (B) receptors [65]. GHB is only available from one pharmacy and has been used for patients with severe intractable sleep disturbances who also have fibromyalgia.

In addition to its established efficacy for the treatment of cataplexy and EDS, nightly sodium oxybate administration significantly reduces measures of sleep disruption and significantly increases slow-wave sleep in patients with narcolepsy [66].

Potential Future Sleep Aids

Accumulating evidence supports a role for 5-HT2A antagonism in the treatment of sleep maintenance insomnias [67]. Indeed, several selective 5-HT2A inverse agonists have entered clinical development for the treatment of insomnia; these include eplivanserin, volinanserin, pruvanserin, and nelotanserin [68].

In healthy human volunteers, nelotanserin was rapidly absorbed after oral administration and achieved maximum concentrations 1 h later. All doses (up to 40 mg) of nelotanserin significantly improved measures of sleep consolidation, including decreases in the number of stage shifts, number of awakenings after sleep onset, microarousal index, and number of sleep bouts, concomitant with increases in sleep bout duration [69].

EVT 201 is considered a partial $GABA_A$ receptor agonist because it produces a lower maximal potentiation of $GABA_A$ receptors than a full agonist [70]. It has an elimination half-life of 3–4 h and an active metabolite with similar affinity and elimination characteristics but lower intrinsic activity [71]. Compared to placebo, EVT 201 1.5 and 2.5 mg increased total sleep time (TST), reduced wake after sleep onset, and reduced latency to persistent sleep [72].

Orexin Receptor Modulators

Almorexant (ACT-078573) is an orally active dual orexin receptor antagonist that is being developed for the treatment of primary insomnia [73]. Hoever and colleagues enrolled 70 healthy male subjects in a double-blind, placebo- and active-controlled study [74]. Population pharmacokinetic/pharmacodynamic modeling suggested that doses of ~500 mg almorexant and 10 mg zolpidem are equivalent with respect to subjectively assessed alertness [74].

Conclusion

The approach to insomnia/sleep disturbances is challenging and like the approach to patients with pain involves a multidimensional assessment with a history and physical examination as well as perhaps with other testing to develop a working diagnosis. Treatment approaches should begin with nonpharmacologic approaches and if necessary also involve pharmacologic approaches. An interdisciplinary team and sleep medicine specialist should be involved in complex and poorly responsive cases. A step-ladder approach may be helpful to health-care providers unfamiliar with sleep disturbance issues (Fig. 9.1) [75].

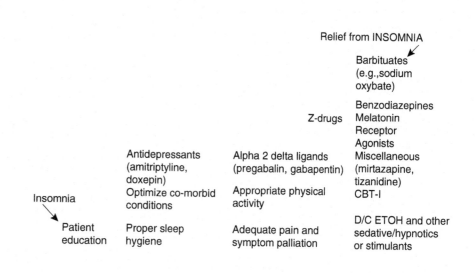

Fig. 9.1 Insomnia relief ladder

References

1. Rechtschaffen A, Bergmann BM, Everson CA, et al. Sleep deprivation in the rat. X. Integration and discussion of the findings. Sleep. 1989;12:68–87.
2. Remy P, Doder M, Lees A, et al. Depression in Parkinson's disease: loss of dopamine and noradrenaline innervation in the limbic system. Brain. 2005;128:1314–22.
3. Stenberg D. Neuroanatomy and neurochemistry of sleep. Cell Mol Life Sci. 2007;64:1187–204.
4. Roth T. Insomnia: definition, prevalence, etiology, and consequences. J Clin Sleep Med. 2007;3:S7–10.
5. Sivertsen B, Krokstad S, Mykletun A, Overland S. Insomnia symptoms and use of health care services and medications: the HUNT-2 study. Behav Sleep Med. 2009;7:210–22.
6. Kyle SD, Morgan K, Espie CA. Insomnia and health-related quality of life. Sleep Med Rev. 2010;14:69–82.
7. Joshi S. Non-pharmacological therapy for insomnia in the elderly. Clin Geriatr Med. 2008;24:107–19.
8. Morin CM. Insomnia: psychological assessment and management. New York: Guildford Press; 1993.
9. Yang CM, Lin SC, Hsu SC, Cheng CP. Maladaptive sleep hygiene practices in good sleepers and patients with insomnia. J Health Psychol. 2010;15:147–55.
10. AmericanAcademy of SleepMedicine. International classification of sleep disorders: diagnostic and coding manual. 2nd ed. Westchester: American Academy of Sleep Medicine; 2005.
11. Morin CM, Bootzin RR, Buysse DJ, et al. Psychological and behavioral treatment of insomnia: update of the recent evidence (1998–2004). Sleep. 2006;29:1398–414.
12. Morin CM, Culbert JP, Schwartz SM. Nonpharmacological interventions for insomnia: a meta-analysis of treatment efficacy. Am J Psychiatry. 1994;151:1172–80.
13. Morin CM, Hauri PJ, Espie CA, et al. Nonpharmacologic treatment of chronic insomnia. An American Academy of Sleep Medicine review. Sleep. 1999;22:1134–56.
14. Murtagh DR, Greenwood KM. Identifying effective psychological treatments for insomnia: a meta-analysis. J Consult Clin Psychol. 1995;63:79–89.
15. Manber R, Kuo TF. Cognitive-behavioral therapies for insomnia. In: Lee-Chiong TL, Sateia MJ, Carskadon MA, editors. Sleep medicine. Philadelphia: Hanley & Belfus; 2002. p. 177–85.
16. Vitiello MV, Rybarczyk B, Von Korff M, Stepanski E. Cognitive behavioral therapy for insomnia improves sleep and decreases pain in older adults with co-morbid insomnia and osteoarthritis. J Clin Sleep Med. 2009;5:355–62.
17. Sivertsen B, Omvik S, Pallesen S, et al. Cognitive behavioral therapy vs zopiclone for treatment of chronic primary insomnia in older adults: a randomized controlled trial. JAMA. 2006;295:2851–8.
18. Dolan DC, Taylor DJ, Bramoweth AD, Rosenthal LD. Cognitive-behavioral therapy of insomnia: a clinical case series study of patients with co-morbid disorders and using hypnotic medications. Behav Res Ther. 2010;48:321–7.
19. Morin CM, Colecchi C, Stone J, et al. Behavioral and pharmacological therapies for late-life insomnia: a randomized controlled trial. JAMA. 1999;281:991–9.
20. Irwin MR, Cole JC, Nicassio PM. Comparative meta-analysis of behavioral interventions for insomnia and their efficacy in middle-aged adults and in older adults 55+ years of age. Health Psychol. 2006;25:3–14.
21. Morin CM, Vallières A, Guay B, et al. Cognitive behavioral therapy, singly and combined with medication, for persistent insomnia: a randomized controlled trial. JAMA. 2009;301:2005–15.
22. Cao H, Pan X, Li H, Liu J. Acupuncture for treatment of insomnia: a systematic review of randomized controlled trials. J Altern Complement Med. 2009;15:1171–86.
23. Buscemi N, Vandermeer B, Friesen C, et al. Manifestations and management of chronic insomnia in adults. AHRQ publication no. 05-E021-2. 2008. Available at: www.ahrq.gov/downloads/pub/evidence/pdf/insomnia/insomnia.pdf. Accessed 27 May 2008.
24. Ramakrishnan K, Scheid DC. Treatment options for insomnia. Am Fam Physician. 2007;76:517–26.
25. Wafford KA, Ebert B. Emerging anti-insomnia drugs: tackling sleeplessness and the quality of wake time. Nat Rev Drug Discov. 2008;7:530–40.
26. Mitchell HA, Weinshenker D. Good night and good luck: norepinephrine in sleep pharmacology. Biochem Pharmacol. 2010; 79:801–9.
27. Rudolph U, Crestani F, Benke D, et al. Benzodiazepine actions mediated by specific gamma-aminobutyric acid(A) receptor subtypes. Nature. 1999;401:796–800.
28. Möhler H, Fritschy JM, Rudolph U. A new benzodiazepine pharmacology. J Pharmacol Exp Ther. 2002;300(1):2–8.
29. Foster AC, Pelleymounter MA, Cullen MJ, et al. In vivo pharmacological characterization of indiplon, a novel pyrazolopyrimidine sedative hypnotic. J Pharmacol Exp Ther. 2004;311:547–59.
30. Petroski RE, Pomeroy JE, Das R, et al. Indiplon, is a high-affinity positive allosteric modulator with selectivity for $\alpha 1$ subunit-containing $GABA_A$ receptors. J Pharmacol Exp Ther. 2006;317:369–77.
31. Sanger DJ. The pharmacology and mechanisms of action of new generation, non-benzodiazepine hypnotic agents. CNS Drugs. 2004;18:9–15.
32. Wegner F, Deuther-Conrad W, Scheunemann M, et al. GABAA receptor pharmacology of fluorinated derivatives of the novel sedative-hypnotic pyrazolopyrimidine indiplon. Eur J Pharmacol. 2008;580:1–11.
33. Weinling E, McDougall S, Andre F, et al. Pharmacokinetic profile of a new modified release formulation of zolpidem designed to improve sleep maintenance. Fundam Clin Pharmacol. 2006; 20:397–403.
34. Sanna E, Busonero F, Talani G, et al. Comparison of the effects of zaleplon, zolpidem, and triazolam at various GABAA receptor subtypes. Eur J Pharmacol. 2002;451:103–10.
35. Brunello N, Cooper J, Bettica P, et al. Differential pharmacological profiles of the GABAA receptor modulators zolpidem, zopiclone, eszopiclone, and (S)-desmethylzopiclone. In: Abstract Presented at the World Psychiatric Association International Congress (WPA), Florence; 2009.
36. Sivertsen B, Omvik S, Pallesen S, et al. Sleep and sleep disorders in chronic users of zopiclone and drug-free insomniacs. J Clin Sleep Med. 2009;5:349–54.
37. Fernandez C, Maradeix V, Gimenez F, et al. Pharmacokinetics of zopiclone and its enantiomers in Caucasian young healthy volunteers. Drug Metab Dispos. 1993;21:1125–8.
38. Fernandez C, Alet P, Davrinche C, et al. Stereoselective distribution and stereoconversion of zopiclone enantiomers in plasma and brain tissues in rats. J Pharm Pharmacol. 2002;54:335–40.
39. McMahon LR, Jerussi TP, France CP. Stereoselective discriminative stimulus effects of zopiclone in rhesus monkeys. Psychopharmacology (Berlin). 2003;165:222–8.
40. Fernandez C, Martin C, Gimenez F, Farinotti R. Clinical pharmacokinetics of zopiclone. Clin Pharmacokinet. 1995;29:431–41.
41. Carlson JN, Haskew R, Wacker J, et al. Sedative and anxiolytic effects of zopiclone's enantiomers and metabolite. Eur J Pharmacol. 2001;415:181–9.
42. Najib J. Eszopiclone, a nonbenzodiazepine sedative-hypnotic agent for the treatment of transient and chronic insomnia. Clin Therapy. 2006;28:491–516.

43. Pandi-Perumal SR, Srinivasan V, Spence DW, Cardinali DP. Role of the melatonin system in the control of sleep: therapeutic implications. CNS Drugs. 2007;21:995–1018.

44. Reiter RJ, Tan DX, Manchester LC, et al. Medical implications of melatonin: receptor-mediated and receptor-independent actions. Adv Med Sci. 2007;52:11–28.

45. Wyatt JK, Dijk DJ, Ritz-De Cecco A, et al. Sleep facilitating effect of exogenous melatonin in healthy young men and women is circadian-phase dependent. Sleep. 2006;29:609–18.

46. Aeschbach D, Lockye Jr B, Dijk D-J, et al. Use of transdermal melatonin delivery to improve sleep maintenance during daytime. Clin Pharmacol Ther. 2009;864:378–82.

47. Tokunaga S, Takeda Y, Shinomiya K, et al. Effects of some H1-antagonists on the sleep–wake cycle in sleep-disturbed rats. J Pharmacol Sci. 2007;103:201–6.

48. Richardson GS, Roehrs TA, Rosenthal L, et al. Tolerance to day-time sedative effects of H1 antihistamines. J Clin Psychopharmacol. 2002;22:511–5.

49. Mendelson WB. A review of the evidence for the efficacy and safety of trazodone in insomnia. J Clin Psychiatry. 2005;66:469–76.

50. Morin AK, Jarvis CI, Lynch AM. Therapeutic options for sleep maintenance and sleep-onset insomnia. Pharmacotherapy. 2007; 27:89–110.

51. Schwartz T, Nihalani N, Virk S, et al. A comparison of the effectiveness of two hypnotic agents for the treatment of insomnia. Int J Psychiatr Nurs Res. 2004;10:1146–50.

52. Ellenhorn MJ, Schonwald S, Ordog J, et al. Ellenhorn's medical toxicology: diagnosis and treatment of human poisoning. 8th ed. Baltimore: Williams and Wilkins; 2006.

53. m-chlorophénylpipérazine nouvelle identification. Observatoire Francxais des Drogues et des Toxicomanies web site. 2006. Available at: http://www.drogues.gouv.fr/IMG/pdf/note_mCPP. pdf. Accessed 14 Mar 2006.

54. Cankurtaran ES, Ozalp E, Soygur H, et al. Mirtazapine improves sleep and lowers anxiety and depression in cancer patients: superiority over imipramine. Support Care Cancer. 2008;16:1291–8.

55. Wiegand MH. Antidepressants for the treatment of insomnia: a suitable approach? Drugs. 2008;68:2411–7.

56. Miller DD. Atypical antipsychotics: sleep, sedation, and efficacy. J Clin Psychiatry. 2004;6:3–7.

57. Foldvary-Schaefer N, De Leon Sanchez I, Karafa M, et al. Gabapentin increases slow-wave sleep in normal adults. Epilepsia. 2002;43:1493–7.

58. Ehrenberg B. Importance of sleep restoration in co-morbid disease: effect of anticonvulsants. Neurology. 2000;54:S33–7.

59. Karam-Hage M, Brower KJ. Gabapentin treatment for insomnia associated with alcohol dependence [comment]. Am J Psychiatry. 2000;157:151.

60. Bazil CW, Battista J, Basner RC. Gabapentin improves sleep in the presence of alcohol. J Clin Sleep Med. 2005;1:284–7.

61. Lo HS, Yang CM, Lo HG, et al. Treatment effects of gabapentin for primary insomnia. Clin Neuropharmacol. 2010;33:84–90.

62. Hindmarch I, Dawson J, Stanley N. A double-blind study in healthy volunteers to assess the effects on sleep of pregabalin compared with alprazolam and placebo. Sleep. 2005;28:187–93.

63. Dierks MR, Jordan JK, Sheehan AH. Prazosin treatment of nightmares related to posttraumatic stress disorder. Ann Pharmacother. 2007;41:1013–7.

64. Thompson CE, Taylor FB, McFall ME, et al. Nonnightmare distressed awakenings in veterans with posttraumatic stress disorder: response to prazosin. J Trauma Stress. 2008;21:417–20.

65. van Nieuwenhuijzen PS, McGregor IS, Hunt GE. The distribution of gamma-hydroxybutyrate-induced Fos expression in rat brain: comparison with baclofen. Neuroscience. 2009;158:441–55.

66. Black J, Pardi D, Hornfeldt CS, Inhaber N. The nightly administration of sodium oxybate results in significant reduction in the nocturnal sleep disruption of patients with narcolepsy. Sleep Med. 2009;10:829–35.

67. Monti JM, Jantos H. Effects of the serotonin 5-HT2A/2C receptor agonist DOI and of the selective 5-HT2A or 5-HT2C receptor antagonists EMD 281014 and SB-243213, respectively, on sleep and waking in the rat. Eur J Pharmacol. 2006;553:163–70.

68. Teegarden BR, Al Shamma H, Xiong Y. 5-HT2A inverse-agonists for the treatment of insomnia. Curr Top Med Chem. 2008;8: 969–76.

69. Al-Shamma HA, Anderson C, Chuang E, et al. Nelotanserin, a novel selective human 5-hydroxytryptamine2A inverse agonist for the treatment of insomnia. J Pharmacol Exp Ther. 2010;332: 281–90.

70. Kemp JA, Baur R, Sigel E. EVT 201: a high affinity, partial positive allosteric modulator of GABAA receptors with preference for the a1-subtype. Sleep. 2008;31:A34.

71. Boyle J, Stanley N, Hunneyball I, et al. A placebo controlled, randomised, double-blind, 5 way cross-over study of 4 doses of EVT 201 on subjective sleep quality and morning after performance in a traffic noise model of sleep disturbance. Sleep. 2007;30:A262.

72. Walsh JK, Salkeld L, Knowles LJ, et al. Treatment of elderly primary insomnia patients with EVT 201 improves sleep initiation, sleep maintenance, and daytime sleepiness. Sleep Med. 2010; 11:23–30.

73. Neubauer DN. Almorexant, a dual orexin receptor antagonist for the treatment of insomnia. Curr Opin Investig Drugs. 2010;11: 101–10.

74. Hoever P, de Haas S, Winkler J, et al. Orexin receptor antagonism, a new sleep-promoting paradigm: an ascending single-dose study with almorexant. Clin Pharmacol Ther. 2010;87:593–600.

75. Smith HS, Barkin RL, Barkin SJ, et al. Personalized pharmacotheraphy for treatment approaches focused at primary insomnia. AM J Ther. 2011 May;18(3):227–40.

Clinical Use of Opioids

Andrea Trescot

Key Points

- Opioids are extremely useful but potentially dangerous broad-spectrum analgesics.
- Understanding the pharmacology and metabolism of opioids may help predict effectiveness and potential side effects of opioids.
- Opioid use may differ when used for specific indications, such as cancer pain, acute versus chronic pain, and pediatric or geriatric population.

Introduction

Opioids are compounds that work at specific receptors in the brain to provide analgesia. Originally extracted from the sap of the poppy plant, opioids may be naturally occurring, semi-synthetic, or synthetic, and their clinical activity is a function of their affinity for the opioid receptors in the brain. Opioids are useful for a wide variety of painful conditions, including acute pain, cancer pain, and chronic pain, as well as cough suppression and air hunger. However, opioid use is associated with a significant risk of addiction potential, which limits their use and contributes to the current "opioid phobia." In this chapter, we will discuss the history, pharmacology, clinical uses, and future directions.

History

Opioids have been used for their euphoric and analgesic properties for thousands of years. Records show that around 3400 BC [1], the opium poppy was cultivated in lower

A. Trescot, M.D. (✉)
Algone Pain Center, 4 Oceanside Circle, St. Augustine,
FL 32080, USA
e-mail: drtrescot@gmail.com

Mesopotamia by the Sumerians who referred to it as *Hul Gil*, the "joy plant." In 1817, a German pharmacist, Friedrich Wilhelm Adam Serturner, isolated morphine from opium [2]. After ingesting the crystals, Serturner discovered that the compound induced a dreamlike state; thus, he named the compound "morphium" after Morpheus, the Greek god of dreams [3]. Joseph Louis Gay-Lussac coined the term "morphine" later when he translated Serturner's article from German to French [4]. Morphine is only one of 24 alkaloids found within the resin of the opium poppy plant (*Papaver somniferum*) and comprises approximately 10 % of the total opium extract.

Opioid Receptors

"Opiates" are naturally occurring compounds derived from the poppy. The term "opioid" is now used broadly to describe any compound that exerts activity at an opioid receptor [5]. The opioid receptors were first discovered in 1972 [6], and the first endogenous opioid, or "endorphin," was identified in 1975 [7]. Multiple opioid receptors have now been identified, including *Mu*, *Kappa*, and *Delta* [8]. *Mu* receptors are found primarily in the brainstem, ventricles, and medial thalamus, and activation of these receptors can result in supraspinal analgesia, respiratory depression, euphoria, sedation, decreased gastrointestinal motility, and physical dependence. *Kappa* receptors are found in the limbic system, brainstem, and spinal cord and are felt to be responsible for spinal analgesia, sedation, dyspnea, dependence, dysphoria, and respiratory depression. *Delta* receptors are located largely in the brain itself and are thought to be responsible for psychomimetic and dysphoric effects.

These opioid receptors are G-linked proteins within the membranes of cells; when activated, the receptor releases a protein, which migrates within the cell, activating Na/K channels or influencing enzymes within the cell or influencing nuclear gene transcription (Fig. 10.1) [9]. Presynaptic opioid

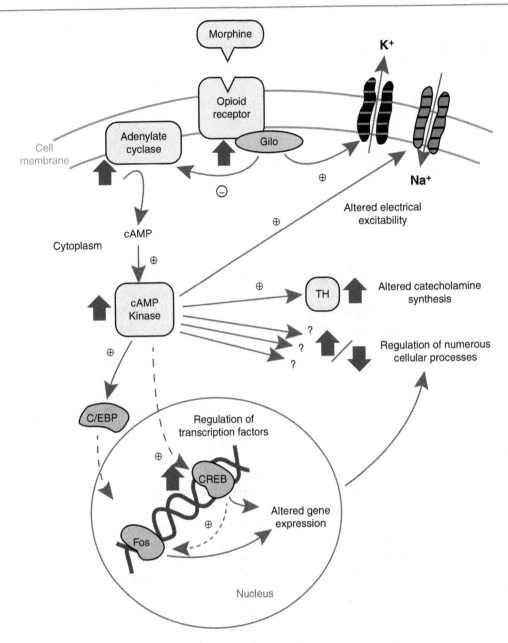

Fig. 10.1 Intracellular opioid actions (With permission from Trescot et al. [5])

receptors inhibit neurotransmitter release of compounds such as acetylcholine, norepinephrine, serotonin, and substance P. The inhibition of an inhibitory neuron may then result in excitation (Fig. 10.2) [9].

The dopaminergic system in the ventral tegmental area (VTA) is the site of the natural reward centers of the brain, and GABA neurons usually inhibit these dopaminergic systems. Opioids inhibit the presynaptic receptors on these GABA neurons, which increases the release of dopamine, which is intensely pleasurable. These are the same areas of the brain associated with other drugs of abuse such as alcohol, nicotine, and benzodiazepines (Fig. 10.3) [10].

Opioid Genetics

Each opioid receptor has a different activity, as well as a different receptor affinity (which is genetically controlled). For example, OPRM1, the gene that encodes the mu receptor, is polymorphic, and approximately 20–30 % of the population has heterozygous changes in the alleles, associated with altered sensitivities to pain [11]. Different opioids also have different relative affinity for each receptor, so that the same opioid may have very different effects on different people, and the same person might have different effects from different opioids.

There is now considerable evidence suggesting genetic variability in the ability of individuals to metabolize and respond to drugs. All opioid drugs are substantially metabolized, mainly by the cytochrome P450 system as well as to a lesser degree the UDP-glucuronosyltransferase system (UGTs). Activity of these enzymes depends on whether patient is homozygous for nonfunctioning alleles (poor metabolizer or PM), has at least one functioning allele (extensive metabolizer or EM), or has multiple copies of a functional allele (ultrarapid metabolizer UM) [12].

As a result, the morphine dose needed for postoperative pain relief after similar surgery may vary fivefold between individuals, and the dose needed at a defined stage of cancer pain varies threefold [13]. As another example, CYP 450 2D6 is a critical enzyme involved in the metabolism of a variety of opioids described below; activity of this enzyme is highly variable, and there may be as much as a 10,000-fold difference among individuals [14]. Approximately 8–10 % of Caucasians but up to 50 % of people of Asian descent have an inactive form of this enzyme [15]. As discussed below, hydrocodone is metabolized to hydromorphone via CYP 2D6; in one study [16], the metabolism of hydrocodone to hydromorphone was eight times faster in EMs than in PMs. Medications may also interfere with enzyme activity; in this same study, quinidine, a potent CYP2D6 inhibitor, reduced the excretion of hydromorphone, resulting in plasma levels five times higher in EMs than PMs.

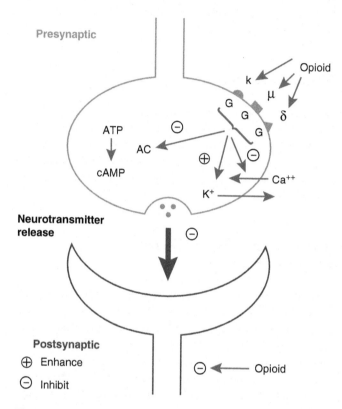

Fig. 10.2 Opioid receptors, pre- and postsynaptic (With permission from Trescot et al. [5])

Opioid Side Effects

Opioids are well known to cause a variety of side effects, most commonly nausea and vomiting, constipation, sedation, and respiratory depression [17]. These side effects can be significant, and some patients avoid opioids even in the face of significant pain, in an effect to limit such side effects, which may act as a significant barrier to adequate pain relief [18].

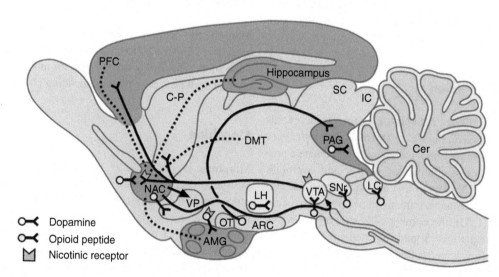

Fig. 10.3 Opioid activity sites (With permission from Trescot et al. [5])

Constipation

Constipation is the most common adverse effect from opioids, occurring in 40–95 % of patients treated with opioids [19], and is caused by opioid receptor stimulation in the gut. The subsequent decrease in GI motility results in increased fecal fluid absorption, resulting in hard, dry stools. It is essential that prophylactic treatment be instituted on the initiation of opioid treatment since this, of all the side effects of opioids, does not resolve over time.

Nausea

Nausea has been reported to occur in up to 25 % of patients treated with opioids [20]. Mechanism for this nausea may include direct stimulation of the chemotactic trigger zone (CTZ), reduced gastrointestinal motility leading to gastric distention, and increased vestibular sensitivity [21].

Pruritus

Two to ten percent of patients on opioids will develop pruritus [18], which results from a direct release of histamine and not usually an antigen/antibody reaction. It is therefore better considered an adverse reaction than an allergic reaction and is usually treated symptomatically with antihistamines such as diphenhydramine.

Sedation and Cognitive Dysfunction

The incidence of sedation can vary from 20 to 60 % [22]; it is usually associated with an initiation or increase in opioids and is usually transient. Cognitive dysfunction can be confounded by the presence of infection, dehydration, metabolic abnormalities, or advanced disease [23].

Respiratory Depression

A significant proportion of patients taking long-term opioids develop central apnea during sleep. Teichtahl and colleagues [24] examined ten patients in a methadone maintenance program and performed a clinical assessment and overnight polysomnography. They found that all ten patients had evidence of central sleep apnea, with six patients having a central apnea index (CAI) [the number of central apnea events per hour] [25] greater than 5, and four patients with a CAI greater than 10. In a larger follow-up study of 50 patients taking long-term methadone, 30 % of the patients had a CAI greater than 5, and 20 % had a CAI greater than 10 [26].

Endocrine Effects

Endorphins appear to be primarily involved in the regulation of gonadotropins and ACTH release [27]. Amenorrhea developed in 52 % female patients on opioids for chronic pain [28], while the testosterone levels were subnormal in 74 % of males on sustained-release oral opioids [29]. These effects are more profound with IV or intrathecal opioids than oral opioids [30].

Immunologic Effects

Acute and chronic opioid administration can cause inhibitory effects on antibody and cellular immune responses, natural killer cell activity, cytokine expression, and phagocytic activity. Chronic administration of opioids decreases the proliferative capacity of macrophage progenitor cells and lymphocytes [31].

Relationship Between Side Effects and Sex or Ethnicity

Several studies suggest that sex and ethnic differences exist to explain the differences seen in side effect profiles. Women have, for instance, been found to be more sensitive to the respiratory effects of morphine [32] and more often have nausea and emesis with opioids [33]. Varying levels of opioid metabolites due to genetic differences in CYP 450 isoenzymes and glucuronidation between ethnic groups [34] may explain the variety of responses seen to similar doses of medications (see section "Opioid Metabolism").

Opioid Metabolism

Many of the positive effects, as well as the side effects of opioids, can be traced to their metabolites, and knowledge of these metabolites may help to explain many of the puzzling clinical scenarios seen by the practicing physician.

Morphine

Morphine is metabolized by glucuronidation, producing morphine-6-glucuronide (M6G) and morphine-3-glucuronide (M3G) in a ratio of 6:1. M6G is believed to be responsible for some additional analgesic effects of morphine [35]. M3G, on the other hand, is believed to potentially lead to hyperalgesia [36], with increased pain, agitation, and myoclonus. Morphine is also metabolized in small amounts to codeine and hydromorphone. For instance, in one study, hydromorphone was present in 66 % of morphine consumers without aberrant drug behavior [37]; this usually occurs with doses higher than 100 mg/day.

Codeine

It is believed that the analgesic activity from codeine occurs from metabolism of codeine to morphine by CYP2D6. Because of the great heterogeneity in the CYP2D6 enzyme, with both fast metabolizers and slow metabolizers, codeine may not be an effective drug in all populations. Recently, the FDA has issued a Public Health Advisory [38] regarding a serious side effect in nursing infants whose mothers are apparent CYP2D6 ultrarapid metabolizers, who, while taking codeine, had rapid and higher levels of morphine in the breast milk, with subsequent potentially fatal neonate respiratory depression.

Although codeine is often referred to as a "weak" analgesic, in a cancer pain study comparing 25 mg of hydrocodone (a "strong" analgesic) to 150 mg of codeine (a "weak" analgesic), 58 % of the codeine patients obtained relief compared to 57 % of the hydrocodone patients [39].

Hydrocodone

Hydrocodone is similar in structure to codeine and is a weak mu receptor agonist, but the CYP2D6 enzyme demethylates it into hydromorphone, which has much stronger mu binding [16]. Like codeine, it has been proposed that hydrocodone is a prodrug. In other words, patients who are CYP2D6 deficient, or patients who are on CYP2D6 inhibitors, may not produce the hydromorphone metabolites and may have less than expected analgesia.

Oxycodone

Oxycodone has activity at multiple opiate receptors including the kappa receptor, which gives it a unique anti-sedative effect ("perky Percocet"). It undergoes extensive hepatic metabolism by glucuronidation to noroxycodone (which has less than 1 % of the analgesia potency of oxycodone) and by CYP2D6 to oxymorphone [40]. Because oxycodone is dependent on the CYP2D6 pathway for clearance, it is possible that drug–drug interactions can occur with 2D6 inhibitors.

Oxymorphone

Although oxycodone has activity at multiple receptors, its metabolite oxymorphone is a pure mu agonist. Oxymorphone is about ten times more potent than morphine. It has limited

protein binding and is not affected by CYP2D6 or CYP3A4, which decreases the risk of drug–drug interactions [41]. Oxymorphone has a reduced histamine effect and may be of use in patients who complain of headache or itching with other opioids [42].

Hydromorphone

Hydromorphone is a hydrogenated ketone of morphine [43]. Like morphine, it acts primarily on mu opioid receptors and to a lesser degree on delta receptors. While hydromorphone is 7–10 times more potent than morphine in single-dose studies [44], the oral and parenteral steady-state equivalence is 1:5, while the equivalence of chronic infusions may be as little as 1:3.5 [45]. It is highly water-soluble, which allows for very concentrated formulations, and in patients with renal failure, it may be preferred over morphine. Hydromorphone is metabolized primarily to hydromorphone-3-glucuronide (H3G), which, similar to the corresponding M3G, is not only devoid of analgesic activity but also evokes a range of dose-dependent excited behaviors including allodynia, myoclonus, and seizures in animal models [46].

Methadone

Methadone is a synthetic mu opioid receptor agonist medication. It is a racemic mixture of two enantiomers; the R form is more potent, with a tenfold higher affinity for opioid receptors (which accounts for virtually all of its analgesic effect), while S-methadone is the NMDA antagonist. The inherent NMDA antagonistic effects make it potentially useful in severe neuropathic and "opioid-resistant" pain states. The S isomer also inhibits reuptake of serotonin and norepinephrine, which should be recognized when using methadone in combination with SSRIs and TCAs. Although it has traditionally been used to treat heroin addicts, its flexibility in dosing, use in neuropathic pain, and cheap price have led to a recent increase in its use. Unfortunately, a lack of awareness of its metabolism and potential drug interactions, as well as its long half-life, has led to a dramatic increase in the deaths associated with this medication.

Methadone is unrelated to standard opioids, leading to its usefulness in patients with "true" morphine allergies. Methadone is metabolized in the liver and intestines and excreted almost exclusively in feces, an advantage in patients with renal insufficiency or failure.

The metabolism of methadone is always variable. Methadone is metabolized by CYP3A4 primarily and CYP2D6 secondarily; CYP2D6 preferentially metabolizes the R-methadone, while CYP3A4 and CYP1A2 metabolize both enantiomers. CYP1B2 is possibly involved, and a newly proposed enzyme CYP2B6 may be emerging as an important intermediary metabolic transformation [47]. CYP3A4 expression can vary up to 30-fold, and there can be genetic polymorphism of CYP2D6, ranging from poor to rapid metabolism. The initiation of methadone therapy can induce the CYP3A4 enzyme for 5–7 days, leading to low blood levels initially, but unexpectedly high levels may follow about a week later if the medication has been rapidly titrated upward. A wide variety of substances can also induce or inhibit these enzymes [48]. The potential differences in enzymatic metabolic conversion of methadone may explain the inconsistency of observed half-life.

Methadone has no active metabolites and therefore may result in less hyperalgesia, myoclonus, and neurotoxicity than morphine. It may be unique in its lack of profound euphoria, but its analgesic action (4–8 h) is significantly shorter than its elimination half-life (up to 150 h), and patient self-directed redosing and a long half-life may lead to the potential of respiratory depression and death.

Methadone also has the potential to cause cardiac arrhythmias, specifically prolonged QTc intervals and/or torsade de pointes under certain circumstances. Congenital QT prolongation, high methadone levels (usually over 60 mg/day), and conditions that increase QT prolongation (such as hypokalemia and hypomagnesemia) or IV methadone, because it contains chlorobutanol, which prolongs QTc intervals [49], may increase that risk [50]. Combining methadone with a CYP3A4 inhibitor such as ciprofloxin [51] potentially can increase that risk. It is recommended that a switch to methadone from another opioid be accompanied by a large (50–90 %) decrease in the calculated equipotent dose (Table 10.1) [53]. It cannot be too strongly emphasized that the dosing of methadone can be potentially lethal and must be done with knowledge and caution.

Fentanyl

Fentanyl is approximately 80 times more potent than morphine, is highly lipophilic, and binds strongly to plasma proteins. Fentanyl undergoes extensive metabolism in the liver. Fentanyl is metabolized by CYP3A4 to inactive and nontoxic metabolites [54]; however, CYP3A4 inhibitors may lead to increased fentanyl blood levels. The transdermal formulation has a onset of action lag time of 6–12 h after application and typically reaches steady state in 3–6 days. When a patch is removed, a subcutaneous reservoir remains, and drug clearance may take up to 24 h.

Conversion Tables

The usual recommendation for calculating the equipotent dose of different opioids involves calculating the 24-h dose as "morphine equivalents" (see Table 10.2). However, Hanks and Fallon [54] instead suggest relating the starting doses to 4-h doses of morphine rather than 24-h doses. For example, in patients receiving 5–20 mg oral morphine every 4 h (or the equivalent in controlled-release morphine), start with 25 mcg/h fentanyl patches every 72 h; patients on 25–35 mg oral morphine every 4 h, 50 mcg/h of fentanyl; patients on 40–50 mg oral morphine every 4 h, 75 mcg/h fentanyl; and patients on 55–65 mg oral morphine every 4 h, 100 mcg/h fentanyl. They feel that the controversies over appropriate morphine to fentanyl potency ratio calculations miss the point that fentanyl transdermally behaves differently and cannot be equated with oral routes when calculating relative potency.

Table 10.1 Oral morphine to methadone conversion

Oral morphine dose (mg)	MS: methadone ratio
30–90	4:1
90–300	8:1
300–800	12:1
800–1,000	15:1
>1,000	20:1

Ripamonti et al. [52]

Table 10.2 Opioid conversions

Drug	Initial po dose	PO:IV	PO MS:PO drug	PO drug: PO MS
Morphine	2.5–15 mg	3:1	1:1	1:1
Hydromorphone	1, 2, or 4 mg	4:1	1:0.25	1:4
Oxycodone	5 or 10 mg	N/A	1:0.66	1:1.5
Oxymorphone	2.5, 5, or 10 mg	10:1	1:0.33	1:3
Methadone	2.5 or 5 mg	2:1	a	a
TD fentanyl	25 mcg/h[b]	TD = IV/h	b	b

Modified from NHHPCO [55]

[a]See Table 10.1

[b]See section "Fentanyl"

Tramadol

A unique analgesic, tramadol, is an atypical synthetic analogue of codeine [56]. The M1 derivative (O-demethyl tramadol) produced by CYP2D6 has a higher affinity for the mu receptor than the parent compound (as much as six times). Tramadol is a racemic mixture of two enantiomers—one form is a selective mu agonist and inhibits serotonin reuptake, while the other mainly inhibits norepinephrine reuptake [57]. Maximum dose is 400 mg/day, and toxic doses cause CNS excitation and seizures. Because it requires CYP2D6 metabolism for maximal analgesic effect, coadministration of CYP2D6 inhibitors such as fluoxetine, paroxetine, and sertraline is contraindicated. In addition, because tramadol has serotonin activity, SSRIs are relatively contraindicated because of the potential of a serotonin syndrome.

Although considered a "weak" opioid, it can have significant analgesic qualities (perhaps because of its dual opioid and SNRI action). In a study of 118 patients with moderate to severe cancer pain comparing 25 mg of hydrocodone to 200 mg of tramadol, 62 % of the tramadol patients obtained relief, compared to 57 % of the hydrocodone patients [58].

Opioid Routes of Administration

Oral

Major advances in the pharmacotherapy of chronic pain have led to the development of extended-release opioid delivery systems, thereby allowing less frequent dosing than the classic short-acting formulas. It is the patterns in serum drug levels that define the difference between short-acting opioids (SAO) and long-acting opioids (LAO); with SAOs, serum opioid levels rise rapidly following administration and then decline rapidly, while LAO administration allows for less fluctuation in serum opioid levels and an extended period within the therapeutic range (Fig. 10.4) [59]. The assumption that plasma levels of opioids correspond to analgesia has led to the additional concept of minimum effective concentration (MEC), the plasma level of an opioid below which there is ineffective analgesia.

There are many proposed advantages of the long-acting opioid formulas compared to the short-acting formulas. Because of the longer duration of action, there is a lessening of the frequency and severity of end-of-dose pain [60]. Furthermore, it has been suggested that less frequent dosing leads to increased compliance and improved efficacy [61]. Sustained analgesia and uninterrupted sleep are other potential advantages of the extended-release formulation compared to the short-acting variety. However, in a recent systematic review of long-acting versus short-acting opioids, Rauck [62] noted that, while it was clear that long-acting

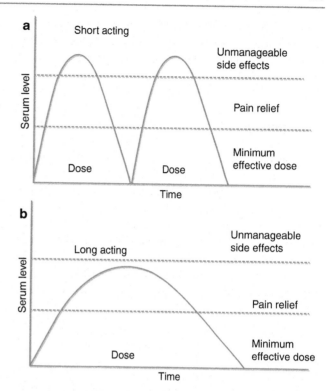

Fig. 10.4 Serum drug level following administration of (**a**) short-acting and (**b**) long-acting opioids (Modified from McCarberg and Barkin [59])

opioids achieved more stable drug levels, there was no clear evidence from appropriately designed comparative trials to make a case for the use of one type of formulation over the other on the basis of clinical efficacy.

Transmucosal

Oral transmucosal fentanyl citrate (OTFC) has become a mainstay in the treatment of breakthrough pain because it provides faster absorption of the lipophilic fentanyl than any other oral opioid formulation [63]. This "fentanyl lollipop" consists of medication on the end of a stick, which is applied to the buccal membrane. A newer formulation of fentanyl, the fentanyl buccal tablet (FBT), was designed to provide an even faster relief. Additional delivery systems for intranasal and inhaled fentanyl are being developed [64].

Intravenous

Intravenous delivery of opioids allows for rapid and reliable delivery of medicine, but veins for administration are not always available. In general, the IV dose is approximately 1/3 of the oral dose, since IV medications do not have a first-pass effect. Opioids can be delivered intermittently or continuously;

patient-controlled analgesia (PCA) is now available for outpatient use so that small doses of opioids are delivered when the patient pushes a button, with or without a continuous infusion of opioid.

Subcutaneous

Subcutaneous opioid injections can be an option for the patient unable to tolerate oral medications but without IV access. The medication is administered through a butterfly needle and can be given intermittently or continuously. Onset is slower and lower peak effect than IV, but this may be a better option for acute or escalating pain than transdermal fentanyl, which has an even slower onset and prolonged effect [65]. Subcutaneous infusions up to 10 cc/h can be usually absorbed, but patients are usually more comfortable with 2–3 cc/h.

Rectal

The rectal mucosa absorbs many medications easily, including most opioids, and the blood flow from the rectum bypasses the liver so that rectal morphine results in blood levels that are almost 90 % of the oral dose [66]. A double-blind, double-dummy, crossover study in 1995 compared oral versus rectal morphine, which was shown to be effective, easy to manage, and inexpensive, with a rapid onset of action [67].

Transdermal

The skin is the largest organ in the body, with a surface area of 1–2 m^2, which makes it appealing as a drug absorption modality. However, the skin functions as a barrier to the elements, and those same properties limit its effectiveness as a drug delivery site. Medications must have a small molecular weight with high lipid solubility to pass across the skin barrier, and fentanyl is one of the most effective opioids for transdermal delivery [68]. Although all opioids have similar side effects (see section "Opioid Side Effects"), transdermal fentanyl appears to have less constipation but did show skin reactions in 1–3 % of the 153 cancer pain patients studied [69].

Intrathecal/Epidural

Oral and parenteral opioids work by dulling the brain so that it does not recognize the pain signals as easily. Intrathecal and epidural opioids attach to opioid receptors at the spinal level, blocking pain signals from reaching the brain.

The medications are more potent in the spinal column; as an example, 300 mg of morphine by mouth is felt to be equivalent to 5 mg in the epidural space or 1 mg in the spinal fluid (intrathecal space). These dramatically lower doses result in less sedation and mental clouding. Single dose administration of intrathecal opioids has been used for acute pain, such as postoperative pain. Continuous infusions for cancer pain and chronic noncancer pain utilized implanted subcutaneous pumps connected to intrathecal catheters. However, because these systems require specialist's placement and care, they are often not considered until very late in the course of the cancer, and hematologic abnormalities such as chemotherapy-induced thrombocytopenia may severely limit the ability to safely access the spinal canal. Although intrathecal opioid pain relief can be dramatic, procedural complications remain high, including infection, pump failures, drug errors, and post-dural puncture headaches [70].

Pruritus is seen more commonly with neural axial opioids than systemic opioids, with an incidence between 30 and 100 %, and is effectively reversed by opioid antagonists. Although respiratory depression is the dreaded complication of intrathecal opioids, its incidence is low (0.09–0.4 %) [71].

Opioid Conversion

Equianalgesic tables, like the one below (Table 10.2), can guide physicians to *estimate* the new opioid optimal dose for a patient that has started to develop tolerance to their current opioid dose. These tables provide only broad guidelines for selecting the dose of an opioid because of large individual pharmacokinetic and even larger pharmacodynamic differences in opioid pharmacology. Different pain syndromes, such as osteoarticular diseases, neuropathic pain, or oncologic pain states, may demonstrate very different and unpredictable clinical responses [72]. The majority of patients need a lower dosing of the new opioid than the dose theoretically calculated with an equianalgesic table [73]. Because of an incomplete cross-tolerance, it is recommended to reduce the calculated dose by 33 % (methadone should be decreased as much as 90%) [74]. For safety reasons, the new opioid should be initiated at a low dose that, if necessary, can be gradually increased to achieve adequate analgesia [75].

Opioid in Acute Pain

Opioids have typically been used in the treatment of acute pain, such as broken bones or postsurgical pain. In the emergency department, there has been a concern that opioids would mask the physical findings for surgical problems such as acute appendicitis. Yuan and colleagues [76] prospectively evaluated 102 patients with acute appendicitis who received either morphine or normal saline IV. In the morphine group, the abdominal pain was significantly relieved, and the patient's cooperation was improved while the physical exam was unaffected, supporting the premise that morphine did not obscure the physical signs.

Unfortunately, standard doses of opioids may not work effectively for acute pain; 621 consecutive ED patients were treated with titrated boluses of IV morphine [77]. The mean total dose of morphine was 10.5 mg with a range of 2–46 mg. The authors noted that sedation could not be arbitrarily attributed to the occurrence of an adequate level of analgesia because, among patients in whom morphine titration was discontinued because of sedation, 25 % still exhibit a level of pain above 50 (0–100).

Opioids in Cancer Pain

There are many causes of cancer pain, some caused by the cancer itself, and others caused by the effects of the cancer. Recently, a large study of almost 2,000 outpatient oncology patients [78] showed that 53 % of the patients had pain only due to their cancer and/or treatment, 25.3 % had noncancer pain, and 21.7 % had both cancer and noncancer pain. However, less than 25 % received a prescription for a strong opioid, only 7 % had a coanalgesic prescribed for pain, and approximately 20 % received no analgesic prescription. This suggests that oncologists are not adequately addressing pain needs.

Noncancer Pain in Cancer Pain Patients

Although often blamed on the cancer, patients with cancer can also suffer from the same pain conditions seen in noncancer pain patients. Thus, the lung cancer patient with pain going down the arm may have tumor involvement of the brachial plexus but may also have a herniated cervical disc or suprascapular nerve entrapment. In addition, there are multiple cancer-related pain issues, such as chemotherapy-induced peripheral neuropathy or postherpetic neuralgia, that may need to be addressed with opioids.

Noncancer Pain

Although originally considered contraindicated for chronic noncancer pain, opioids are now being used much more frequently for a variety of chronic painful conditions, such as post-laminectomy syndrome, peripheral neuropathy, and postherpetic neuralgia. The American Society of Interventional Pain Physicians (ASIPP) reviewed chronic opioid use in noncancer pain [79] and concluded that opioids are commonly prescribed for chronic noncancer pain and may be effective for short-term pain relief. However, evidence of long-term effectiveness for 6 months or longer is variable, with evidence ranging from moderate for transdermal fentanyl and sustained-release morphine to limited for oxycodone and indeterminate for hydrocodone and methadone.

Opioid Tolerance Versus Hyperalgia

When opioids become less effective over time, increased pain may represent tolerance, a pharmacodynamic desensitization induced by high opioid doses [80]. One method of addressing this increase in pain is the use of adjuvant medications. The cancer patient with neuropathic pain, for instance, from tumor invasion of a nerve plexus, would not be expected to respond well to opioids but might benefit from the addition of an anticonvulsant. Another option is opioid rotation (see below), a therapeutic maneuver aiming in improving analgesic response and/or reducing adverse effects, including change to a different medication using the same administration route, maintaining the current medication but altering administration route, or both.

Decreased response to opioids may also be due to pharmacokinetic and drug delivery factors, such as poor absorption or vascular compromise. However, most concerning is the concept of opioid-induced hyperalgesia, a reduced opioid responsiveness resulting in increased pain despite (or perhaps because of) escalating doses of opioids. Opioid-induced hyperalgesia might be considered in a patient who has no evidence of disease progression, who is on clinically reasonable doses of opioids, and whose pain escalates as opioid doses are increased [81]. A reduction of opioids and the addition of a low-dose N-methyl-D-aspartate (NMDA) receptor antagonist may provide a favorable clinical outcome in those patients who have failed to benefit from opioid rotation and other adjunctive pain treatments.

Opioid Rotation

Pain patients may not respond to increasing doses of opioids because they develop adverse effects before achieving an acceptable analgesia, or the analgesic response is poor despite a rapid dose escalation. Opioid switching may significantly improve the balance between analgesia and adverse effects. According to available data, opioid switching results in clinical improvement in more than 50 % of patients with chronic pain with poor response to one opioid [82].

Addiction

We currently have no satisfactory definition or criteria for addiction in patients receiving therapeutic opioids [83]. However, the rise of prescription opioid abuse has focused attention on the need for prevention in all exposed populations. The 2006 National Survey on Drug Use and Health found that 5.2 million Americans age 12 or older misused prescription analgesics, an increase from 4.7 million in 2005 [84]. Furthermore, analgesic use was the drug category with the most new initiates. Screening patients to determine their risk for drug abuse prior to beginning opioid therapy is considered good practice. Even more vital is the monitoring of patients to ensure compliance, including urine drug monitoring and surveillance of non-sanctioned opioid use via national prescription registers, a process that was associated with a 50 % reduction in opioid abuse in 500 patients receiving controlled substances [85].

Future Directions

Opioids of lower addictive potential, such as tamper-resistant extended-release opioids, are coming on the market, in an effort to expand the use of opioids while decreasing the addiction and diversion potential. Opioid abuse screening tools (such as the Opioid Risk Tool) and fMRIs to look at brain areas associated with addiction and pain perception may also help identify those patients at risk for opioid abuse while maintaining access for those patients in whom opioids are appropriate management for their painful condition.

Conclusion

Opioids are broad-spectrum analgesics, with multiple effects and side effects. When used wisely and with appropriate caution and knowledge of metabolism and interactions, opioids can offer significant relief from soul-draining pain.

Recommended Links

American Academy of Pain Medicine code of ethics
http://www.painmed.org/pract_mngmnt/ethics.html
ASIPP opioid guidelines
http://www.asipp.org/Guidelines.htm
American Pain Foundation
http://www.painfoundation.org/

References

1. Breasted JG. Ancient records of Egypt. University of Chicago Oriental Institute Publications, vol. III. Chicago: University of Chicago Press; 1930. p. 217.
2. Schwarz S, Huxtable R. The isolation of morphine. Mol Interv. 2001;1(4):189–91.
3. The role of chemistry in history. 2010. http://itech.dickinson.edu/chemistry/?cat=107. Accessed 15 Mar 2010.
4. Jurna I. Serturner and morphine – a historical vignette. Schmerz. 2003;17(4):280–3.
5. Trescot A, Datta S, Lee M, Hansen H. Opioid pharmacology. Pain Physician. 2008;11(opioid special issue):S133–53.
6. Pert CB, Snyder SH. Opiate receptor: its demonstration in nervous tissue. Science. 1973;179:1011–4.
7. Hughes J, Smith T, Kosterlitz H, Fothergill L, Morgan B, Morris H. Identification of two related pentapeptides from the brain with potent opiate agonist activity. Nature. 1975;258:577–80.
8. Fukuda K. Intravenous opioid anesthetics. In: Miller RD, editor. Miller's anesthesia. 6th ed. Philadelphia: Elsevier; 2005.
9. Chahl LA. Opioids – mechanism of action. Aust Prescr. 1996; 19:63–5.
10. Nestler EJ. Molecular basis of long-term plasticity underlying addiction. Nat Rev Neurosci. 2001;2:119–28.
11. Fillingim RB, Kaplan L, Staud R, et al. The A118G single nucleotide polymorphism of the μ-opioid receptor gene (OPRM1) is associated with pressure pain sensitivity in humans. J Pain. 2005; 6(3):159–67.
12. Smith HS. Variations in opioid responsiveness. Pain Physician. 2008;11:237–48.
13. Klepstad P, Kaasa S, Skauge M, Borchgrevink PC. Pain intensity and side effects during titration of morphine in cancer patients using a fixed schedule dose escalation. Acta Anaesthesiol Scand. 2000;44(6):656–64.
14. Bertilsson L, Dahl ML, Ekqvist B, Jerling M, Lierena A. Genetic regulation of the disposition of psychotropic drugs. In: Meltzer HY, Nerozzi D, editors. Current practices and future developments in the pharmacotherapy of mental disorders. Amsterdam: Elsevier; 1991. p. 73–80.
15. Stamer UM, Stuber F. Genetic factors in pain and its treatment. Curr Opin Anaesthesiol. 2007;20(5):478–84.
16. Otton SV, Schadel M, Cheung SW, Kaplan HL, Busto UE, Sellers EM. CYP2D6 phenotype determines the metabolic conversion of hydrocodone to hydromorphone. Clin Pharmacol Ther. 1993;54(5):463–72.
17. Benyamin R, Trescot AM, Datta S, et al. Opioid complications and side effects. Pain Physician. 2008;11(opioid special issue):S105–20.
18. McNicol E, Horowicz-Mehler N, Fisk RA, et al. Management of opioid side effects in cancer-related and chronic noncancer pain: a systematic review. J Pain. 2003;4:231–56.
19. Swegle JM, Logemann C. Opioid-induced adverse effects. Am Fam Physician. 2006;74(8):1347–52.
20. Meuser T, Pietruck C, Radbruch L, Stute P, Lehmann KA, Grond S. Symptoms during cancer pain treatment following WHO-guidelines: a longitudinal follow-up study of symptom prevalence, severity and etiology. Pain Med. 2001;93:247–57.
21. Flake ZA, Scalley RG, Bailey AG. Practical selection of antiemetics. Am Fam Physician. 2004;69:1169–74.
22. Cherny N, Ripamonti C, Pereira J, et al. Strategies to manage the adverse effects of oral morphine: an evidence-based report. J Clin Oncol. 2001;19:2542–54.
23. Cherny NI. The management of cancer pain. CA Cancer J Clin. 2000;50:70–116.

24. Teichtahl H, Prodromidis A, Miller B, et al. Sleep-disordered breathing in stable methadone programme patients: a pilot study. Addiction. 2001;96(3):395–403.

25. Downey R, Gold PM. Obstructive sleep apnea. 2010. http://emedicine.medscape.com/article/295807-print. Accessed Apr 2010.

26. Wang D, Teichtahl H, Drummer O, et al. Central sleep apnea in stable methadone maintenance treatment patients. Chest. 2005; 128(3):1348–56.

27. Howlett TA, Rees LH. Endogenous opioid peptides and hypothalamopituitary function. Annu Rev Physiol. 1986;48:527–36.

28. Daniell HW. Opioid endocrinopathy in women consuming prescribed sustained action opioids for control of nonmalignant pain. J Pain. 2008;9:28–36.

29. Daniell HW. Hypogonadism in men consuming sustained-action oral opioids. J Pain. 2002;3:377–84.

30. Merza Z. Chronic use of opioids and the endocrine system. Horm Metab Res. 2010;42(9):621–6.

31. Roy S, Loh HH. Effects of opioids on the immune system. Neurochem Res. 1996;21(11):1375–86.

32. Zacny JP. Morphine responses in humans: a retrospective analysis of sex differences. Drug Alcohol Depend. 2001;63:23–8.

33. Zun LS, Downey LV, Gossman W, Rosenbaumdagger J, Sussman G. Gender differences in narcotic-induced emesis in the ED. Am J Emerg Med. 2002;20(3):151–4.

34. Cepeda MS, Farrar JT, Roa JH, et al. Ethnicity influences morphine pharmacokinetics and pharmacodynamics. Clin Pharmacol Ther. 2001;70(4):351–61.

35. Lotsch J, Geisslinger G. Morphine-6-glucuronide: an analgesic of the future? Clin Pharmacokinet. 2001;40:485–99.

36. Smith MT. Neuroexcitatory effects of morphine and hydromorphone: evidence implicating the 3-glucuronide metabolites. Clin Exp Pharmacol Physiol. 2000;27:524–8.

37. Wasan AD, Michna E, Janfaza D, Greenfield S, Teter CJ, Jamison RN. Interpreting urine drug tests: prevalence of morphine metabolism to hydromorphone in chronic pain patients treated with morphine. Pain Med. 2008;9:918–23.

38. MedWatch safety labeling change. 2010. www.fda.gov/medwatch/safety/2007/safety07.htm#Codeine. Accessed Jan 2010.

39. Rodriguez RF, Castillo JM, del Pilar Castillo M, et al. Codeine/acetaminophen and hydrocodone/acetaminophen combination tablets for the management of chronic cancer pain in adults: a 23-day, prospective, double-blind, randomized, parallel-group study. Clin Ther. 2007;29(4):581–7.

40. Poyhia R, Seppala T, Olkkola KT, Kalso E. The pharmacokinetics and metabolism of oxycodone after intramuscular and oral administration to healthy subjects. Br J Clin Pharmacol. 1992;33: 617–21.

41. Sloan PA, Barkin RL. Oxymorphone and oxymorphone extended release: a pharmacotherapeutic review. J Opioid Manag. 2008;4(3): 131–44.

42. Foley KM, Abernathy A. Management of cancer pain. In: Devita VT, Lawrence TS, Rosenberg SA, editors. Devita, Hellman & Rosenberg's cancer: principles & practice of oncology. 8th ed. Philadelphia: Lippincott Williams & Wilkins; 2008.

43. Murray A, Hagen NA. Hydrocodone. J Pain Symptom Manage. 2005;29:S57–66.

44. Vallner JJ, Stewart J, Kotzan JA, Kirsten EB, Honigberg IL. Pharmacokinetics and bioavailability of hydromorphone following intravenous and oral administration to human subjects. J Clin Pharmacol. 1981;214:152–6.

45. Davis MP, McPherson ML. Tabling hydromorphone: do we have it right? J Palliat Med. 2010;13(4):365–6.

46. Wright AW, Mather LE, Smith MT. Hydromorphone-3-glucuronide: a more potent neuro-excitant than its structural analogue, morphine-3-glucuronide. Life Sci. 2001;69(4):409–20.

47. Lynch ME. A review of the use of methadone for the treatment of chronic noncancer pain. Pain Res Manag. 2005;10:133–44.

48. Leavitt SB. Addiction treatment forums: methadone – drug interactions. 2009. www.atforum.com/SiteRoot/pages/rxmethadone/methadonedruginteractions.shtml. Accessed 2009.

49. Kornick CA, Kilborn MJ, Santiago-Palma J, et al. QTc interval prolongation associated with intravenous methadone. Pain. 2003; 105(3):499–506.

50. Krantz MJ, Lewkowiez L, Hays H, Woodroffe MA, Robertson AD, Mehler PS. Torsade de pointes associated with very high dose methadone. Ann Intern Med. 2002;137:501–4.

51. Herrlin K, Segerdahl M, Gustafsson LL, Kalso E. Methadone, ciprofloxacin, and adverse drug reactions. Lancet. 2000;356: 2069–70.

52. Ripamonti C, Conno FD, Groff L, et al. Equianalgesic dose/ratio between methadone and other opioid agonists in cancer pain: comparison of two clinical experiences. Ann Oncol. 1998;9(1):79–83.

53. Gazelle G, Fine PG. Methadone for the treatment of pain. J Palliat Med. 2003;6:621–2.

54. Hanks G, Cherny N, Fallon M. Opioid analgesic therapy. In: Doyle D, Hanks G, Cherny N, et al (eds) Oxford Textbook of Palliative Medicine (3rd ed). Oxford University Press, 2004; pp. 318–21.

55. New Hampshire Hospice and Palliative Care Organization. 2010. http://www.nhhpco.org/opioid.htm. Accessed Apr 2010.

56. Grond S, Sablotzki A. Clinical pharmacology of tramadol. Clin Pharmacokinet. 2004;43:879–923.

57. Raffa RB, Friderichs E, Reimann W. et al opioid and nonopioid components independently contribute to the mechanism of action of tramadol, an "atypical" opioid analgesic. J Pharmacol Exp Ther. 1992;260:275–85.

58. Rodriguez RF, Castillo JM, Castillo MP, et al. Hydrocodone/acetaminophen and tramadol chlorhydrate combination tablets for the management of chronic cancer pain: a double-blind comparative trial. Clin J Pain. 2008;24(1):1–4.

59. McCarberg B, Barkin R. Long-acting opioids for chronic pain; pharmacotherapeutic opportunities to enhance compliance, quality of life, and analgesia. Am J Ther. 2001;8:181–6.

60. Kaplan R, Parris WC, Citron ML, et al. Comparison of controlled-release and immediate-release oxycodone tablets AVINZA and chronic noncancer pain – 263 inpatients with cancer pain. J Clin Oncol. 1998;16:3230–7.

61. American Pain Society. Principles of analgesic use in the treatment of acute pain and cancer pain. Glenview: American Pain Society; 2003.

62. Rauck RL. What is the case for prescribing long-acting opioids over short-acting opioids for patients with chronic pain? A critical review. Pain Pract. 2009;9(6):468–79.

63. Coluzzi PH, Shwartzberg L, Conroy Jr JD, Charapata S, Gay M, Busch MA, et al. Breakthrough cancer pain: a randomized trial comparing oral transmucosal fentanyl citrate (OTFC®) and morphine sulfate immediate release (MSIR®). Pain. 2001;91:123–30.

64. Mercadante S, Radbruch L, Popper L, Korsholm L, Davies A. Efficacy of intranasal fentanyl spray (INFS) versus oral transmucosal fentanyl citrate (OTFC) for breakthrough cancer pain: open-label crossover trial. Eur J Pain. 2009;13:S198.

65. Ripamonti C, Fagnoni E, Campa T, et al. Is the use of transdermal fentanyl inappropriate according to the WHO guidelines and the EAPC recommendations? A study of cancer patients in Italy. Support Care Cancer. 2006;14:400–7.

66. McCaffery M, Martin L, Ferrell BR. Analgesic administration via rectum or stoma. J ET Nurs. 1992;19:114–21.

67. DeConno F, Ripamonti C, Saita L, MacEachern T, Hanson J, Bruera E. Role of rectal route in treating cancer pain: a randomized crossover clinical trial of oral versus rectal morphine administration in opioid-naive cancer patients with pain. J Clin Oncol. 1995;13(4):1004–8.

68. Jeal W, Benfield P. Transdermal fentanyl. A review of its pharmacological properties and therapeutic efficacy in pain control. Drugs. 1997;53(1):109–38.

69. Muijsers RB, Wagstaff AJ. Transdermal fentanyl: an updated review of its pharmacological properties and therapeutic efficacy in chronic cancer pain control. Drugs. 2001;61(15):2289–307.

70. Rathmell JP, Lair TR, Nauman B. The role of intrathecal drugs in the treatment of acute pain. Anesth Analg. 2005;101:S30–43.

71. Gustafsson LL, Schildt B, Jacobsen K. Adverse effects of extradural and intrathecal opiates: report of a nation-wide survey in Sweden. Br J Anaesth. 1982;54:479–86.

72. Galer BS, Coyle N, Pasternak GW, Portenoy RK. Individual variability in the response to different opioids: report of five cases. Pain. 1992;49:87–91.

73. Brant JM. Opioid equianalgesic conversion: the right dose. Clin J Oncol Nurs. 2001;5:163–5.

74. Vissers KC, Besse K, Hans G, Devulder J, Morlion B. Opioid rotation in the management of chronic pain: where is the evidence? Pain Pract. 2010;10(2):85–93.

75. Hanks GW, Conno F, Cherny N, et al. Morphine and alternative opioids in cancer pain: the EAPC recommendations. Br J Cancer. 2001;84:587–93.

76. Yuan Y, Chen JY, Guo H, et al. Relief of abdominal pain by morphine without altering physical signs in acute appendicitis. Chin Med J (Engl). 2010;123(2):142–5.

77. Lvovschi V, Aubrun F, Bonnet P, et al. Intravenous morphine titration to treat severe pain in the ED. Am J Emerg Med. 2008; 26:676–82.

78. Valeberg BT, Rustoen T, Bjordal K, Hanestad BR, Paul S, Miaskowski C. Self-reported prevalence, etiology, and characteristics of pain in oncology outpatients. Eur J Pain. 2008;12(5):582–90.

79. Trescot AM, Boswell MV, Atluri SL, et al. Opioid guidelines in the management of chronic non-cancer pain. Pain Physician. 2006; 9(1):1–39.

80. Chang G, Chen L, Mao J. Opioid tolerance and hyperalgesia. Med Clin North Am. 2007;91:199–211.

81. Vorobeychik Y, Chen L, Bush MC, Mao J. Improved opioid analgesic effect following opioid dose reduction. Pain Med. 2008; 9(6):724–7.

82. Mercadante S, Bruera E. Opioid switching: a systematic and critical review. Cancer Treat Rev. 2006;32:304–15.

83. Ballantyne J. Opioid analgesia: perspective on right use and utility. Pain Physician. 2007;10:479–91.

84. Substance Abuse and Mental Health Services Administration. Results from the 2006 national survey on drug use and health. National findings. Office of Applied Studies, NSDUH Series: H-32, DHHS Publication No. SMA 07-4293. Rockville. 2007.

85. Manchikanti L, Manchukonda R, Damron KS, Brandon D, McManus CD, Cash K. Does adherence monitoring reduce controlled substance abuse in chronic pain patients? Pain Physician. 2006;9(1):57–60.

Opioid Adverse Effects and Opioid-Induced Hypogonadism

11

Saloni Sharma and David M. Giampetro

Key Points

- Recognize that opioids are known to have potentially serious adverse effects
- Review major adverse effects including nausea and vomiting, constipation, neuroendocrine effects, immune effects, respiratory depression, central nervous system effects, and pruritis
- Consider the risks and benefits of continued opioid therapy in light of adverse effects
- Become familiar with common treatment options for opioid-related adverse effects

Nausea and Vomiting

Nausea and vomiting are well-known side effects of opioid use. When used for treatment of chronic nonmalignant pain, nausea has been reported to occur in 21–32 % of patients with vomiting reported in 10 % [1, 2]. Opioid-induced nausea and vomiting often occurs with initiation of an opioid or with recent dose escalation. The majority of patients develop a tolerance to this over several days or weeks. These effects can occur via centrally and peripherally stimulated pathways. Activation of the emesis center in the medulla is the primary mechanism for opioid-induced nausea and vomiting. The emesis center is stimulated by input from gastrointestinal

(GI) receptors, the cerebral cortex, the vestibular system, and the chemoreceptor trigger zone in the area postrema of the medulla. It also sends efferent information to the GI system (see Fig. 11.1).

Since tolerance to opioid-induced nausea and vomiting usually develops within days, prolonged treatment, if any, is usually not needed. Often, decreasing the opioid dose with a slower titration to escalating doses, changing the route of administration, or opioid rotation are sufficient strategies to manage this side effect. If possible, identifying an individual's trigger of opioid-induced nausea and/or vomiting can allow one to tailor etiology-specific treatment. If symptoms occur with movement or ambulation, the vestibular system may be involved and treatment with antihistamines or anticholinergics such as scopolamine may be of benefit. If symptoms are associated with meals, gastrointestinal causes may be triggering nausea and vomiting and the patient may benefit from multiple smaller volume meals as well as treatment with a motility agent such as metoclopramide [3].

If a clear mechanism cannot be identified, treatment is often determined based on a patient's comorbidities and other symptoms such as constipation. The potential for side effects from the treating medication must also be considered. Other potentially therapeutic drugs include prokinetic drugs, antipsychotics and related drugs, antihistamines, serotonin antagonists, anticholinergics, benzodiazepines, and steroids (see Table 11.1). Prokinetic agents such as metoclopramide improve gastric motility and decrease GI transit times and, therefore, may be beneficial to patients with nausea and constipation [4]. Antipsychotics work within the chemoreceptor trigger zone to block dopamine receptors and have been found to be effective for the treatment of opioid-associated nausea and vomiting in cancer patients [5]. Antihistamines act on the emesis center and vestibular system [3, 6]. Serotonin antagonists act by blocking serotonin release in the GI tract and the chemoreceptor trigger zone [6]. Anticholinergics act on the emesis center and GI tract [6]. Benzodiazepines act on the vestibular system and chemoreceptor trigger zone.

S. Sharma, B.A., M.D. (✉)
Rehabilitation & Pain Specialists, 107 Gamma Drive, Suite 220, Pittsburgh, PA 15238, USA
e-mail: salsharma@hotmail.com

D.M. Giampetro, M.D.
Department of Anesthesiology, Pennsylvania State University College of Medicine, 500 University Blvd, Hershey, PA 17033, USA
e-mail: dgiampetro@psu.edu

T.R. Deer et al. (eds.), *Treatment of Chronic Pain by Medical Approaches: the AMERICAN ACADEMY of PAIN MEDICINE Textbook on Patient Management*, DOI 10.1007/978-1-4939-1818-8_11,
© American Academy of Pain Medicine 2015

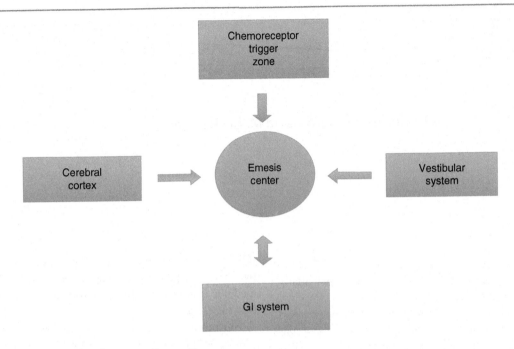

Fig. 11.1 Causes of opioid-induced nausea and/or vomiting

Table 11.1 Medications for treatment of opioid-induced nausea and/or vomiting[a] [3, 6, 7]

Motility drugs	Metoclopramide
Antipsychotics and related drugs	Haloperidol, droperidol, prochlorperazine, promethazine, chlorpromazine, methotrimeprazine
Antihistamines	Meclizine, cyclizine, hydroxyzine, diphenhydramine
Serotonin antagonists	Ondansetron, granisetron, dolasetron
Anticholinergics	Scopolamine
Benzodiazepines	Lorazepam
Steroids	Prednisone, dexamethasone
Potentially, peripherally acting mu-receptor antagonist	Methylnaltrexone, alvimopan

[a]An example(s) of each type of medication is listed and is not meant to be a comprehensive list

The mechanism of steroids in reducing nausea and vomiting is not clear [6]. Peripherally acting mu-receptor antagonists have been shown to decrease gastric transit time and diminish opioid-related nausea and vomiting [7, 8] but have not been extensively used for this purpose. Medications may be delivered in a non-oral form if nausea and vomiting impair oral intake or if oral intake is limited for other reasons. A combination of antiemetics from different classes may be needed in resistant cases. All of these medications may result in side effects of their own, and the risks and benefits of initiating these therapies as opposed to decreasing the opioid dose, changing the route of administration, changing the type of opioid, or discontinuing opioid therapy must be considered.

Additionally, some have recommended use of alternative therapies including cannabinoids and acupressure [9]. Cannabinoids have been primarily studied for the treatment of nausea and vomiting related to chemotherapy. The results of the studies in this setting have shown some efficacy in patients who have failed treatment with other antiemetics but often resulted in a high rate of therapy discontinuation secondary to adverse side effects [10]. Cannabinoids are not commonly used in the setting of opioid-induced nausea and vomiting and are not recommended for routine use in this setting. Acupuncture techniques including acupressure and electro-acutherapy treatments with use of acupuncture point Pericardium 6 have been found to be effective in the treatment of postoperative nausea and vomiting [11] as well as in a multitude of other settings including chemotherapy-induced nausea and vomiting [12]. Other alternative approaches include use of meditation and guided imagery to treat the anticipation of nausea and vomiting and have been studied in patients with cancer [13]. There is not a large amount of data

Table 11.2 Differential diagnosis nausea and vomiting[a] [14]

Gastrointestinal (GI)	*Functional* (e.g., irritable bowel syndrome, dyspepsia, gastroparesis)
	Obstruction (e.g., adhesions, malignancy, hernia, stenosis)
	Organic (e.g., appendicitis, cholecystitis, hepatitis, peptic ulcers)
Infectious	(e.g., Food-borne toxins, urinary tract infection)
Medications/toxins	(e.g., Nonsteroidal anti-inflammatories, radiation)
Metabolic	(e.g., Adrenal disorder, pregnancy, uremia)
Miscellaneous	(e.g., Nephrolithiasis, pain, psychiatric)
Central nervous system	*Increased intracranial pressure, migraine, seizure disorder, head injury, vestibular*

[a]This is a summary and is not intended to include all potential causes

supporting use of these treatments for opioid-induced nausea and vomiting, but they may be beneficial.

Most importantly, if an opioid has not recently been started or opioid dose recently escalated, or if there are other systemic signs and symptoms, other etiologies of nausea and/or vomiting must be considered (see Table 11.2).

Constipation

Constipation is a common side effect of opioid therapy. Constipation related to opioid use has been reported to occur in 15–90 % of patients [15]. Constipation as defined by the Rome III Diagnostic Criteria includes at least two of the following: less than three defecations per week, straining, lumpy or hard stools, feeling of incomplete evacuation or anorectal obstruction, and manual attempts to ease defecation [16].

There are multiple potential mechanisms for opioid-induced constipation, and it is widely known to be mediated via opioid receptors in the GI tract and central nervous system (see Table 11.3). Binding of opioid receptors, specifically mu, kappa, and delta receptors, within the enteric nervous system of the GI tract alters GI motility and contributes to constipation [17–19] as well as to nausea and vomiting. Once bound, the release of GI neurotransmitters is inhibited disrupting the appropriate intestinal contractions needed for GI motility, and mucosal secretions are decreased [15].

Constipation is thought to be dose-related, and unfortunately, tolerance to opioid-induced constipation does not typically occur [7]. Therefore, this side effect usually necessitates treatment. Lifestyle and dietary modifications including increasing physical activity, drinking more fluids, ingesting larger amounts of fiber, and creating a meal and toileting schedule may be trialed [20]. Typically, first-line treatment includes use of a stool softener such as sodium docusate and often is not effective as a sole treatment [21]. A stimulant laxative such as senna is typically added to use of stool softener. If constipation persists, addition of osmotic or bulk-forming laxatives, nonabsorbable solution, or enema may be therapeutic (see Table 11.4). Recently, peripherally acting mu-receptor antagonists have been found effective in

Table 11.3 Mechanisms of opioid-induced constipation [3, 15]

1. ↓ Peristalsis → ↓ GI motility → ↑ transit time → ↑ fluid absorption → ↓ fluid in stool
2. ↑ Segment contractions that are ineffective in propelling stool forward
3. ↑ Sphincter tone
4. ↓ Mucosal secretions

treating peripheral causes of constipation. Methylnaltrexone is approved for treatment of opioid-induced constipation in patients receiving palliative care, and alvimopan is approved for aiding GI function after bowel resection [8].

As with most opioid side effects, one may consider decreasing opioid dose, opioid rotation, changing the route of administration, or discontinuing opioid therapy. There is literature reporting diminished rates of constipation with use of buprenorphine or transdermal fentanyl, but there is also literature refuting this in regard to transdermal fentanyl [23–25]. If opioid therapy has not recently been initiated or opioid dose increased, or if there are other symptoms, one must consider other causes of constipation (see Table 11.5).

Neuroendocrine Effects Including Hypogonadism

Opioids are known to alter the functioning of the hypothalamus-pituitary-adrenal axis in both acute and chronic settings. The hypothalamus has numerous functions including controlling the secretion of gonadotropin-releasing hormone (GrH), which stimulates the pituitary gland to secrete luteinizing hormone (LH) and follicle-stimulating hormone (FSH). These hormones, then, act on the testes and ovaries to result in the secretion of testosterone and estradiol. The release of GrH, LH, and FSH are regulated by negative feedback from testosterone and estradiol (see Fig. 11.2).

Chronic opioid therapy leads to suppression of the hypothalamus and pituitary [27–30]. This results in diminished GrH secretion contributing to a decreased release of LH and FSH as well as decreased testosterone and estradiol. Studies support the finding of opioid receptors in the

Table 11.4 Medications to treat opioid-induced constipation[a] [3, 4, 15, 19, 22]

Stool softeners	Sodium docusate
Stimulants	Senna, bisacodyl
Osmotic laxatives	Sorbitol, lactulose, magnesium, polyethylene glycol
Bulk laxatives	Wheat bran, psyllium seed, polycarbophil
Lubricant	Mineral oil
Peripherally, acting mu-receptor antagonist	Methylnaltrexone, alvimopan

[a]An example(s) of each type of medication is listed and is not meant to be a comprehensive list or suggests a preferred medication

Table 11.5 Differential framework for constipation[a] [26]

Functional	Dietary reasons, motility problem
Structural	Anorectal disorders, colonic strictures, or mass lesions
Endocrine and metabolic	Diabetes mellitus, hypercalcemia, hypothyroidism
Neurogenic	Cerebrovascular events, multiple sclerosis
Smooth muscle and connective tissue disorders	Amyloidosis, scleroderma
Psychogenic	Anxiety, depression, somatization
Drugs	Narcotics, anticholinergics, antidepressants

[a]This is a summary and is not intended to include all potential causes

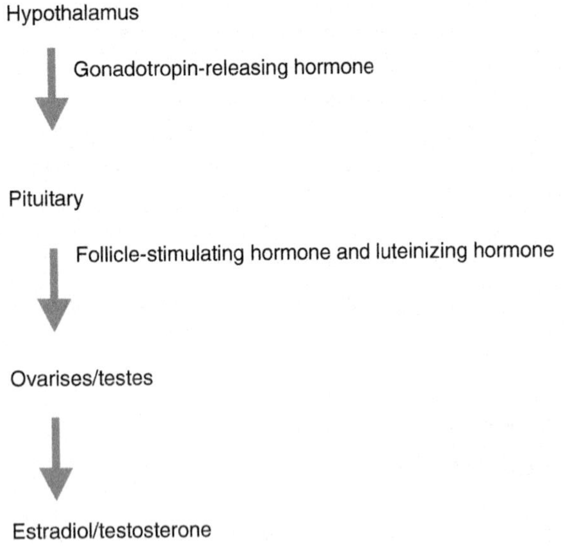

Hypothalamus

↓ Gonadotropin-releasing hormone

Pituitary

↓ Follicle-stimulating hormone and luteinizing hormone

Ovarises/testes

↓

Estradiol/testosterone

Fig. 11.2 The hypothalamus-pituitary axis

hypothalamus and pituitary as well as the gonads [27, 28, 30–33]. Therefore, opioid-induced hypogonadism is thought to be mediated via central effects on the hypothalamus and pituitary and via direct gonadal effects.

Opioids also have been shown to alter neuroendocrine function by increasing thyroid-stimulating hormone and prolactin while decreasing oxytocin [34]. Additionally, studies have shown opioids may impact the autonomic nervous system and result in altered glycemic control and insulin release [34].

Opioid suppression of the hypothalamus, pituitary, and gonads can result in hypogonadism in both males and females potentially leading to fatigue, depression, anxiety, decreased libido, infertility, decreased muscle mass, osteopenia, osteoporosis, and compression fractures in either sex (see Table 11.6) [29, 35]. In females, there may be amenorrhea and oligomenorrhea and, in males, erectile dysfunction. Daniell reported that 87% of men receiving opioids noted a decreased libido or significant erectile dysfunction after initiating use of opioids [27]. This study was followed by a study treating men with opioid-induced androgen deficiency with testosterone and revealed that testosterone treatment resulted in improved sexual function, decreased depression, and improved mood [36].

Patients receiving chronic opioid therapy with symptoms of hypogonadism should be monitored for abnormalities in sex hormones. Laboratory analysis should include free and total testosterone and estradiol in women. It has also been recommended that LH and dehydroepiandrosterone, an adrenal precursor to the primary sex hormones, be tested as well [37, 38]. If diagnosed with hypogonadism secondary to opioids, it has been suggested that the risks and benefits of continued opioid therapy be considered versus discontinuation of opioids, a trial of alternative opioid, or hormonal supplementation [37]. In current practice, sex hormones are often monitored if the patient has complaints consistent with hypogonadism as outlined above while receiving chronic opioid therapy. Hormonal supplementation may be beyond the scope of some pain management practitioners and require coordinated care through the patient's primary care physician

Table 11.6 Symptoms of hypogonadism

In females	Amenorrhea, oligomenorrhea
In males	Erectile dysfunction
In both sexes	Decreased libido, decreased fertility, decreased muscle mass, osteopenia, osteoporosis, compression fractures, fatigue, decreased ability to concentrate, depression, anxiety

Table 11.7 Differential diagnosis of hypogonadism in males[a] [35]

Pituitary tumors, pituitary insufficiency, hemochromatosis

Hyperprolactinemia

Transient hypogonadism due to serious illness or stress

Aging, metabolic syndrome

Autoimmune syndromes, acquired immunodeficiency syndrome

Fertile eunuch syndrome, mumps, orchitis

Cryptorchidism, vanishing testes syndrome, testicular trauma

Radiation treatment or chemotherapy

Sertoli cell only syndrome

Genetic syndromes:

Klinefelter's syndrome, 47 XYY syndrome, dysgenetic testes

Androgen receptor defects, testicular feminization, Reifenstein's syndrome

5 Alpha-reductase deficiency, myotonic dystrophy, Kallmann's syndrome

[a]This is a summary and is not intended to include all potential causes

or with referral to endocrinology. Nonetheless, sex hormone levels should be monitored in all symptomatic patients and potentially in all patients receiving chronic opioid therapy. In addition to monitoring of free testosterone, estradiol, and other hormones, measuring bone density may also be valuable [29]. The American Association of Clinical Endocrinologists recommends ordering bone density studies for all patients with hypogonadism [35]. Furthermore, depending on the patient's history, other causes of hypogonadism should be considered as well (see Tables 11.7 and 11.8). Many of these would likely have presented earlier in life or with additional symptoms. Detailed evaluation of these conditions may be left to an endocrinologist or other specialist.

Immune Effects

Opioids, especially morphine, are known to adversely affect the immune system. Morphine has been shown to inhibit phagocytosis as early as 1898 [41]. Numerous subsequent studies have verified this including early animal research by Kraft and Leitch in 1921 demonstrating a decreased resistance to streptococcal septicemia in animals treated with morphine [42].

This immunosuppression occurs via both central and direct cellular mechanisms. Centrally, opioids can lead to the release of corticosteroids via the hypothalamic-pituitary-adrenal axis [43], leading to suppression of immune system function with chronic use of opioids [44]. Acute exposure to morphine and related drugs is also believed to influence the immune system via activation of the sympathetic nervous system [43, 44]. The released catecholamines, including norepinephrine, bind to leukocytes to alter immune function [45]. Opioids can also directly affect immune cells via opioid receptors present on immune cells [43]. Studies suggest that opioids bind to immune cell opioid receptors resulting in a diminished ability of immune cells to produce lymphocytes and macrophage precursors [43]. Further studies reveal that immune cells possess mu-opioid receptors and are activated by morphine, which is the most immunosuppressive opioid [44].

Morphine has been the most extensively researched opioid, in both animals and humans, regarding its potentially immunosuppressive effect. In animal studies and studies of opioid abusers in which confounding factors were controlled, chronic morphine use has been shown to result in an increased risk in opportunistic infections including pneumonia, HIV, and tuberculosis [46]. In addition to morphine, fentanyl has also been studied and found to suppress immune function including natural killer cell function [47]. The immunosuppressive effects are prolonged with increased doses of fentanyl [48]. The immunomodulatory effect of other opioids has also been studied but to a lesser extent than morphine and fentanyl. Codeine has been found to suppress the immune system but to a lesser degree than morphine [49]. Both hydromorphone and oxycodone have not been found to suppress the immune system [49]. Interestingly, naloxone and naltrexone have been found to increase immune responses [49]. These findings have not been widely studied. Buprenorphine has not been found to exert a significant immunosuppressive effect when monitoring immune functioning [50, 51]. Therefore, current data suggests that morphine and fentanyl have immunosuppressive effects although the significance with short-term or long-term administration is not clear. Furthermore, buprenorphine, hydromorphone, and oxycodone have not been found to depress the immune system although there is somewhat limited data in regard to this finding.

There has been debate about the clinical significance of opioid-induced immunosuppression. Opioid-induced immune dysfunction including an increased risk for opportunistic infections may have implications for patients who already have alterations in their immune system or are already immunocompromised including cancer patients. Some practitioners suggest use of

Table 11.8 Differential diagnosis of hypogonadism in females[a] [39,40]

Reproductive organ dysfunction	Congenital, Asherman's syndrome, Turner's syndrome, premature ovarian failure including secondary to autoimmune causes, polycystic ovarian syndrome, ovarian tumors
Pituitary disorders	Tumor, hemochromatosis, sarcoidosis, traumatic brain injury
Hypothalamic dysfunction	Kallmann's syndrome, radiation
Prolactin secreting tumors	
Hypercortisolism	
Thyroid disorders	

[a]This is a summary and is not intended to include all potential causes

Table 11.9 Causes of hypoventilation resulting in respiratory acidosis[a] [60]

Pulmonary	Airway (laryngospasm)
	Parenchymal (pneumonia, chronic obstructive pulmonary disease)
Nonpulmonary	Drugs (e.g., narcotics, benzodiazepines)
	Flail chest (spinal cord injury, cardiopulmonary arrest)
	Sleep apnea
	Neuromuscular and chest wall disease (Guillain-Barre syndrome)

[a]This is a summary and is not intended to be comprehensive

opioids without immunosuppressive properties at all times [52] while others feel there is not enough clinical data to change clinical practice at this point [53]. Currently, there is no clear recommendation in regard to individualized opioid selection based on a patient's comorbidities and consideration of opioid immunosuppressive effects. A consensus statement published in 2008 generally suggests use of buprenorphine over morphine or fentanyl for chronic opioid use in light of immunosuppressive effects [54]. Beyond this, no other formal recommendations are available, and further research must be done to elucidate the clinical significance of opioid immunosuppression and develop prescribing guidelines for the application of this knowledge.

Respiratory Depression

Respiratory depression is an established and potentially life-threatening event related to opioid use. It has been defined in relation to respiratory rate as well as oxygen saturation with severe respiratory depression considered to be a respiratory rate less than 8–10 breaths/min [55]. Opioids depress brainstem respiratory centers in a dose-dependent manner. Respiratory depression typically occurs in opioid-naive patients or patients suddenly receiving doses greater than their typical doses. As the depression becomes more significant, it is often accompanied by confusion and sedation. Opioid-naive patients and patients receiving gradually increasing doses of opioids usually develop a tolerance to this side effect quickly [3, 56]. Additionally, hypoventilation results in increased levels of carbon dioxide stimulating chemoreceptors centrally to increase the respiratory rate and arterial oxygen level [57].

Naloxone is an opioid receptor antagonist that may be used to treat opioid-related respiratory depression. Such treatment should be done in an emergent or inpatient setting with appropriate monitoring. Furthermore, one must recognize, especially, with respiratory depression related to a long-acting opioid, that multiple doses of naloxone may be required as the onset of action is 1–3 min with a duration of only 45 min depending on the naloxone dose [3, 58]. Methadone, a long-acting opioid, may result in prolonged respiratory depression requiring a continuous infusion of naloxone or frequent doses secondary to its average elimination half-life being 22 h [59]. One must assess other causes of respiratory depression, especially, if opioid therapy has not recently been initiated or dose escalated or if there are other symptoms (see Table 11.9).

Central Nervous System Effects

Opioids can have various effects on the central nervous system (CNS) including sedation, psychomotor slowing, delirium, hallucinations, muscle rigidity, myoclonus, and sleep disturbances. Opioid-induced sedation and cognitive effects typically occur with the initiation of an opioid or with dose escalation [56, 61]. Cognitive effects are usually transient and last 1–2 weeks [62, 63]. If patients do not develop tolerance to the sedative effects, they may be treated with CNS stimulants such as methylphenidate or modafinil or with acetylcholinesterase inhibitors such as donepezil [3]. Studies have demonstrated that driving ability is not impaired with use of a stable and chronic dose of opioid medication [64–66].

Pruritis

Pruritis has been reported to occur in 2–10 % patients taking oral morphine [67]. It is most commonly associated with morphine use and thought to occur via histamine release [7]. The likelihood of opioid-associated pruritis is increased with epidural or intrathecal opioids [68, 69]. Antihistamines are commonly used to treat pruritis. Use of antihistamines may compound potential sedation.

Other medications including mixed opioid receptor agonist-antagonists, serotonin 5-HT$_3$ receptor antagonists, opioid antagonists, propofol, NSAIDs, and dopamine receptor antagonists have been found to reduce opioid-related pruritis [70, 71]. Specifically, methylnaltrexone, naloxone, naltrexone, and nalbuphine have demonstrated efficacy in reducing pruritis [72, 73]. Acupuncture has also been shown to be helpful in reducing morphine-related pruritis [74]. As with other side effects, opioid rotation, dose reduction, or use of non-opioid therapy may be considered.

Conclusion

Opioid-related adverse effects are well known and studied. The risks and benefits of opioid treatments must be weighed against these. The development of adverse effects requires consideration of decreasing the opioid dose, changing the route of administration, changing the type of opioid, or discontinuing opioid therapy. If medications are used to treat these adverse effects, one must also recognize that these medications may result in side effects of their own. Novel approaches and medications as well as combination medications of opioids and other drugs that minimize side effects are continually being developed.

References

1. More RA, McQuay HJ. Prevalence of opioid adverse events in chronic non-malignant pain: systematic review of randomised trials of oral opioids. Arthritis Res Ther. 2005;7(5):R1046–51.
2. Kalso E, Allan L, Dellemijn PLI, Faura CC, Ilias WK, Jensen TS, Perrot S, Plaghki LH, Zenz M. Recommendations for using opioids in chronic non-cancer pain. Eur J Pain. 2003;7(5):381–6.
3. O'Mahony S, Coyle N, Payne R. Current management of opioid related side effects. Oncology. 2001;15(1):61–74.
4. Herndon CM, Jackson 2nd KC, Hallin PA. Management of opioid-induced gastrointestinal effects in patients receiving palliative care. Pharmacotherapy. 2002;22(2):240–50.
5. Okamoto Y, Tsuneto S, Matsuda Y, et al. A retrospective chart review of the antiemetic effectiveness of risperidone in refractory opioid-induced nausea and vomiting in advanced cancer patients. J Pain Symptom Manage. 2007;34:217–22.
6. Porreca F, Ossipov MH. Nausea and vomiting side effects with opioid analgesics during treatment of chronic pain: mechanisms,

implications, and management options. Pain Med. 2009;10(4): 654–62.
7. Swegle JM, Logemann C. Management of common opioid-induced adverse effects. Am Fam Physician. 2006;74:1347–54.
8. Moss J, Rosow CE. Development of peripheral opioid antagonists' new insights into opioid effects. Mayo Clin Proc. 2008;83(10): 1116–30.
9. Harris JD. Management of expected and unexpected opioid-related side effects. Clin J Pain. 2008;24 Suppl 10:S8–13.
10. Voth EA, Schwartz RH. Medicinal applications of delta-9-tetrahydrocannabinol and marijuana. Ann Intern Med. 1997; 126(10):791–8.
11. Lee A, Fan LT. Stimulation of the wrist acupuncture point P6 for preventing postoperative nausea and vomiting. Cochrane Database Syst Rev. 2010;(2):CD003281.
12. Bao T. Use of acupuncture in the control of chemotherapy-induced nausea and vomiting. J Natl Compr Canc Netw. 2009;7(5): 606–12.
13. Mansky PJ, Wallerstedt DB. Complementary medicine in palliative care and cancer symptom management. Cancer J. 2006;12(5): 425–31.
14. Scorza K, Williams A, Phillips D, Shaw J. Evaluation of nausea and vomiting. Am Fam Physician. 2007;76(1):76–84.
15. Panchal SJ, Müller-Schwefe P, Wurzelmann JI. Opioid-induced bowel dysfunction: prevalence, pathophysiology and burden. Int J Clin Pract. 2007;61(7):1181–7.
16. Longstreth GF, Thompson WG, Chey WD, Houghton LA, Mearin F, Spiller RC. Functional bowel disorders. Gastroenterology. 2006;130:1480–91.
17. Fox-Threlkeld JE, Daniel EE, Christinck F, Hruby VJ, Cipris S, Woskowska Z. Identification of mechanisms and sites of actions of mu and delta opioid receptor activation in the canine intestine. J Pharmacol Exp Ther. 1994;268(2):689–700.
18. Holzer P. Opioids and opioid receptors in the enteric nervous system: from a problem in opioid analgesia to a possible new prokinetic therapy in humans. Neurosci Lett. 2004;361(1–3):192–5.
19. De Schepper HU, Cremonini F, Park MI, Camilleri M. Opioids and the gut: pharmacology and current clinical experience. Neurogastroenterol Motil. 2004;16(4):383–94.
20. Canty SL. Constipation as a side effect of opioids. Oncol Nurs Forum. 1994;21:739–45.
21. Michael AA, Arthur GL, Daniel C, Carla R. Principles of analgesic use in the treatment of acute pain and cancer pain. 5th ed. Glenview: American Pain Society; 2003.
22. Clemens KE, Klaschik E. Management of constipation in palliative care patients. Curr Opin Support Palliat Care. 2008;2(1):22–7.
23. Likar R. Transdermal buprenorphine in the management of persistent pain – safety aspects. Ther Clin Risk Manag. 2006;2: 115–25.
24. Bach V, Kamp-Jensen M, Jensen N-H, Eriksen J. Buprenorphine and sustained release morphine – effects and side effects in chronic use. Pain Clin. 1991;4:87–93.
25. Allan L, Hays H, Jensen NH, de Waroux BL, Bolt M, Donald R, Kalso E. Randomised crossover trial of transdermal fentanyl and sustained release oral morphine for treating chronic non-cancer pain. BMJ. 2001;322(7295):1154–8.
26. Arce DA, Ermocilla CA, Costa H. Evaluation of constipation. Am Fam Physician. 2002;65(11):2283–90.
27. Daniell HW. Hypogonadism in men consuming sustained-action opioids. J Pain. 2002;3(5):377–84.
28. Cicero TJ. Effects of exogenous and endogenous opiates on the hypothalamic–pituitary–gonadal axis in the male. Fed Proc. 1980; 39(8):2551–4.
29. Daniell HW. Opioid endocrinopathy in women consuming prescribed sustained-action opioids for control of nonmalignant pain. J Pain. 2008;9(1):28–36.

30. Genazzani AR, Genazzani AD, Volpogni C, et al. Opioid control of gonadotropin secretion in humans. Hum Reprod. 1993;8 suppl 2:151–3.

31. Jordan D, Tafani JA, Ries C, Zajac JM, Simonnet G, Martin D, Kopp N, Allard M. Evidence for multiple opioid receptors in the human posterior pituitary. J Neuroendocrinol. 1996;8(11):883–7.

32. Cicero TJ, Bell RD, Wiest WG, et al. Function of the male sex organs in heroin and methadone users. N Engl J Med. 1975;292:882–7.

33. Kaminski T. The involvement of protein kinases in signalling of opioid agonist FK 33-824 in porcine granulosa cells. Anim Reprod Sci. 2006;91:107–22.

34. Vuong C, Van Uum SH, O'Dell LE, Lutfy K, Friedman TC. The effects of opioids and opioid analogs on animal and human endocrine systems. Endocr Rev. 2010;31(1):98–132.

35. AACE Hypogonadism Task Force. American association of clinical endocrinologists medical guidelines for clinical practice for the evaluation and treatment of hypogonadism in adult male patients-2002 update. Endocr Pract. 2002;8(6):439–56.

36. Daniell HW, Lentz R, Mazer NA. Open-label pilot study of testosterone patch therapy in men with opioid induced androgen deficiency (OPIAD). J Pain. 2006;7:200–10.

37. Katz N, Mazer NA. The impact of opioids on the endocrine system. Clin J Pain. 2009;25(2):170–5.

38. Daniell HW. DHEAS deficiency during consumption of sustained-action prescribed opioids: evidence for opioid- induced inhibition of adrenal androgen production. J Pain. 2006;7:901–7.

39. Rothman MS, Wierman ME. Female hypogonadism: evaluation of the hypothalamic-pituitary-ovarian axis. Pituitary. 2008;11:163–9.

40. Makhsida N, Shah J, Yan G, Fisch H, Shabsigh R. Hypogonadism and metabolic syndrome: implications for testosterone therapy. J Urol. 2005;174(3):827–34.

41. Cantacuzene. Annales de L'Institut Pasteur. 1898; xli:273.

42. Kraft A, Leitch NM. The action of drugs in infection I. The influence of morphine in experimental septicemia. J Pharmacol Exp Ther. 1921;5:3877–84.

43. Roy S, Loh HH. Effects of opioids on the immune system. Neurochem Res. 1996;21(11):1375–86.

44. Mellon RD, Bayer BM. Evidence for central opioid receptors in the immunomodulatory effects of morphine: review of potential mechanism(s) of action. J Neuroimmunol. 1998;83(1–2):19–28.

45. Peterson PK, Molitor TW, Chao CC. Mechanisms of morphine-induced immunomodulation. Biochem Pharmacol. 1993;46:343–8.

46. Roy S, Wang J, Kelschenbach J, Koodie L, Martin J. Modulation of immune function by morphine: implications for susceptibility to infection. J Neuroimmune Pharmacol. 2006;1:77–89.

47. Shavit Y, Ben-Eliyahu S, Zeidel A, Beilin B. Effects of fentanyl on natural killer cell activity and on resistance to tumor metastasis in rats dose and timing study. Neuroimmunomodulation. 2004;11(4):255–60.

48. Beilin B, Shavit Y, Hart J, Mordashov B, Cohn S, Notti I, Bessler H. Effects of anesthesia based on large versus small doses of fentanyl on natural killer cell cytotoxicity in the perioperative period. Anesth Analg. 1996;82(3):492–7.

49. Sacerdote P, Manfredi B, Mantegazza P, Panerai AE. Antinociceptive and immunosuppressive effects of opiate drugs: a structure-related activity study. Br J Pharmacol. 1997;121(4):834–40.

50. Martucci C, Panerai AE, Sacerdote P. Chronic fentanyl or buprenorphine infusion in the mouse: similar analgesic profile but different effects on immune responses. Pain. 2004;110(1–2):385–92.

51. Sacerdote P. Opioids and the immune system. Palliat Med. 2006;20 Suppl 1:s9–15.

52. Budd K. Pain management: is opioid immunosuppression a clinical problem? Biomed Pharmacother. 2006;60(7):310–7.

53. Sacerdote P. Opioid-induced immunosuppression. Curr Opin Support Palliat Care. 2008;2(1):14–8.

54. Pergolizzi J, Böger RH, Budd K, Dahan A, Erdine S, Hans G, Kress HG, Langford R, Likar R, Raffa RB, Sacerdote P. Opioids and the management of chronic severe pain in the elderly: consensus statement of an international expert panel with focus on the six clinically most often used World Health Organization Step III opioids (buprenorphine, fentanyl, hydromorphone, methadone, morphine, oxycodone). Pain Pract. 2008;8(4):287–313.

55. Dahan A, Aarts L, Smith TW. Incidence, reversal, and prevention of opioid-induced respiratory depression. Anesthesiology. 2010;112: 226–38.

56. McNicol E, Horowicz-Mehler N, Fisk RA, Bennett K, Gialeli-Goudas M, Chew PW, Lau J, Carr D. Management of opioid side effects in cancer-related and chronic noncancer pain: a systematic review. J Pain. 2003;4(5):231–56.

57. Mueller RA, Lundberg DB, Breese GR, Hedner J, Hedner T, Jonason J. The neuropharmacy of respiratory control. Pharmacol Rev. 1982;34:255–85.

58. Olofsen E, van Dorp E, Teppema L, Aarts L, Smith TW, Dahan A, Sarton E. Naloxone reversal of morphine- and morphine-6-glucuronide-induced respiratory depression in healthy volunteers: a mechanism-based pharmacokinetic-pharmacodynamic modeling study. Anesthesiology. 2010;112(6):1417–27.

59. Eap CB, Buclin T, Baumann P. Interindividual variability of the clinical pharmacokinetics of methadone: implications for the treatment of opioid dependence. Clin Pharmacokinet. 2002;41(14): 1153–93.

60. Lerma EV, Berns JS, Nissenson AR. Current diagnosis & treatment: nephrology & hypertension. New York: The McGraw-Hill Companies; 2009. p. 58.

61. Christo PJ. Opioid effectiveness and side effects in chronic pain. Anesthesiol Clin North America. 2003;21(4):699–713.

62. Reissig JE, Rybarczyk AM. Pharmacologic treatment of opioid-induced sedation in chronic pain. Ann Pharmacother. 2005;39: 727–31.

63. Bruera E, Macmillan K, Hanson J, MacDonald RN. The cognitive effects of the administration of narcotic analgesics in patients with cancer pain. Pain. 1989;39(1):13–6.

64. Byas-Smith MG, Chapman SL, Reed B, Cotsonis G. The effect of opioids on driving and psychomotor performance in patients with chronic pain. Clin J Pain. 2005;21(4):345–52.

65. Fishbain DA, Cutler RB, Rosomoff HL, Rosomoff RS. Can patients taking opioids drive safely? A structured evidence-based review. J Pain Palliat Care Pharmacother. 2002;16(1):9–28.

66. Fishbain DA, Cutler RB, Rosomoff HL, Rosomoff RS. Are opioid-dependent/tolerant patients impaired in driving-related skills? A structured evidence-based review. J Pain Symptom Manage. 2003;25(6):559–77.

67. Cherny N, Ripamonti C, Pereira J, Davis C, Fallon M, McQuay H, Mercadante S, Pasternak G, Ventafridda V, Expert Working Group of the European Association of Palliative Care Network. Strategies to manage the adverse effects of oral morphine: an evidence-based report. J Clin Oncol. 2001;19(9):2542–54.

68. Ballantyne JC, Loach AB, Carr DB. Itching after epidural and spinal opiates. Pain. 1988;33(2):149–60.

69. Chaney MA. Side effects of intrathecal and epidural opioids. Can J Anaesth. 1995;42(10):891–903.

70. Ganesh A, Maxwell LG. Pathophysiology and management of opioid-induced pruritus. Drugs. 2007;67(16):2323–33.

71. Szarvas S, Harmon D, Murphy D. Neuraxial opioid-induced pruritus: a review. J Clin Anesth. 2003;15(3):234–9.

72. Diego L, Atayee R, Helmons P, von Gunten CF. Methylnaltrexone: a novel approach for the management of opioid-induced constipation in patients with advanced illness. Expert Rev Gastroenterol Hepatol. 2009;3(5):473–85.

73. Kjellberg F, Tramèr MR. Pharmacological control of opioid-induced pruritus: a quantitative systematic review of randomized trials. Eur J Anaesthesiol. 2001;18(6):346–57.

74. Jiang YH, Jiang W, Jiang LM, Lin GX, Yang H, Tan Y, Xiong WW. Clinical efficacy of acupuncture on the morphine-related side effects in patients undergoing spinal-epidural anesthesia and analgesia. Chin J Integr Med. 2001;16(1):71–4.

Acute Management of the Opioid-Dependent Patient

Brandi A. Bottiger, Denny Curtis Orme, and Vitaly Gordin

Key Points

- Opioid-dependent patients are at substantial risk in postoperative period for being labeled as drug seeking and therefore have their pain inadequately controlled.
- When appropriate, use of regional anesthesia and adjuvant analgesics can have a beneficial effect on postoperative pain control and decrease the total dose of opioid analgesics.
- Perioperative period is an inappropriate setting for opioid tapering.
- Adequate pain control in opioid-dependent patient will decrease the psychological and physiologic burden of poorly controlled pain. It will improve surgical outcomes, decrease hospital stay, and prevent unnecessary admission after outpatient surgery.

Introduction

Seventy million patients are afflicted by and treated for chronic pain in the United States and treated more frequently with long-term opioids, particularly morphine, oxycodone, and methadone in the treatment of non-cancer pain [1].

B.A. Bottiger, M.D. (✉)
Department of Anesthesiology, Duke University Hospital, 3094, 2301 Erwin Rd, Durham, NC 27705, USA
e-mail: brandi.bottiger@dm.duke.edu

D.C. Orme, DO, MPH
Billings Anesthesiology PC, 1155, Billings, MT 59103, USA
e-mail: dennyxorme@hotmail.com

V. Gordin
Associate Professor, Associate Vice Chair of Pain Management, Department of Anesthesiology, Pennsylvania State University, College of Medicine, Director, Pain Medicine, Milton S. Hershey Medical Center, 500 University Drive, Hershey, PA 17033, USA
e-mail: vgordin@hmc.psu.edu

Many of these patients will arrive for surgical procedures and pain management will be a major part of their hospital stay [2–4]. According to various sources, approximately 40 % of all surgical patients still experience moderate to severe pain and almost a quarter of them experience inadequate pain relief [5, 6]. Allowing patients to suffer from poorly controlled pain not only may be considered a breach of human rights [3, 7, 8] but may result in emotional and cognitive problems negatively impacting postoperative rehabilitation and quality of life.

Unfortunately, there are only a small number of reports discussing the treatment of acute pain in patients with substance abuse disorders, opioid tolerance, and physical dependence, and even less discussion on opioid-dependent patients specifically [2–4, 7, 8].

Acute pain management of opioid-dependent patients is challenging not only for the primary team but also for anesthesiologists and pain specialists. Improving perioperative pain control in these patients may result in shortening of the hospital stay [9, 10], improving patient satisfaction and rehabilitation rate, and decreasing admissions for pain control from same day surgery units. In this chapter, we will review factors responsible for opioid tolerance, physical dependence, and addiction, and provide perioperative pain management strategies.

In the perioperative period, acute surgical pain must be treated in addition to the patient's underlying chronic pain, which may or may not be adequately controlled. An opioid-tolerant patient can consume up to three times the amount of opioid analgesics than an opioid-naïve patient [11]. This can be alarming for many practitioners, and inadequate pain control may result in unnecessary suffering. Fear of the adverse effects of opioid analgesics may prevent the practitioner from adequately treating an opioid-tolerant patient. Conversely attempts to treat pain with opioid analgesics alone may put patients at increased risk for adverse events such as respiratory depression and over-sedation. The ideal focus should be on preventative pain control using a multifaceted approach, rather than controlling pain postoperatively only.

Key concepts for consideration when managing a chronic pain patient include (1) understanding the adverse consequences of acute pain; (2) exploring basic concepts as they relate to definitions of substance abuse, dependence, tolerance, and addiction; (3) differentiating opioid dependency from addiction; (4) performing preoperative and postoperative assessments; and (5) developing multifaceted, balanced pain management plan.

Consequences of Acute Pain

The consequences of pain during surgical stimulation are well known to the anesthesiologist. The intraoperative pain response can be difficult to manage and often leads to large sympathetic responses. Neuroendocrine activation along the hypothalamo-adrenal axis leads to release of not only catecholamines but also ACTH, aldosterone, angiotensin, and antidiuretic hormone (ADH) as well as cortisol and glucagon [12, 13]. This results in an overall catabolic state promoting hyperglycemia, water retention, and release of proinflammatory mediators [14].

Catecholamine release, as well as direct effects of aldosterone, cortisol, ADH, and angiotensin, has direct effect on the cardiovascular system [15]. Increased cardiac work is a direct result of increased heart rate, preload, afterload, and oxygen consumption. These changes can lead to myocardial ischemia, congestive heart failure, or lung injury in predisposed patients. Regarding the pulmonary system, increased extracellular lung water contributes to ventilation-perfusion abnormalities. Patients undergoing upper abdominal or thoracic surgery with significant pain often exhibit splinting, decreased lung compliance, and hypoventilation, resulting in atelectasis [14, 16]. In high-risk patients, there may be a reduction in functional residual capacity up to 50 %. These sequelae could have detrimental effects particularly to the patient with preexisting pulmonary disease, advanced age, or obesity [17].

Importantly, the body's response to pain and surgical stress may result in a hypercoagulable state via alteration in blood viscosity, platelet function, fibrinolysis, and coagulation pathways [18–20]. Coupling this with catecholamine release and immobilization of the patient, the risk of a thromboembolic event significantly increases. Both cellular and immune function is impaired [21–23], and with the additional problem of hyperglycemia, the patient is predisposed for wound infection and poor wound healing. Further, catecholamines may further result in increased intestinal secretions and increased smooth muscle sphincter tone in the gastrointestinal and urinary tracts, resulting in decreased bowel motility and urinary retention, respectively [24, 25]. These sequelae of the physiologic response to pain may result in prolonged hospitalization and potentially detrimental complications.

Lastly, intense painful stimuli can result in gene expression changes that influence pain perception and impulse formation in as little as 1 h, perhaps influencing the development of chronic pain [26]. The concept of preemptive and balanced analgesia becomes essential to reduce this pain response, particularly in patients who have been previously sensitized [27, 28].

Basic Concepts and Definitions

During a preoperative history and physical examination, basic concepts and terms describing substance abuse, physical and psychological dependency, and addiction should be correctly applied to describe a patient characteristic or behavior.

Substance use disorder or substance dependence has been described as a maladaptive pattern of substance use, leading to clinically significant impairment or distress, as manifested by three or more of the following described in Table 12.1. The opioid-dependent patient may be legitimately and responsibly using opioids and labeled with a substance use disorder. However, he/she may be misdiagnosed with psychological dependence or addiction (see pseudoaddiction below). Physiologic dependence must be distinguished from psychological dependence if possible and described appropriately; misdiagnosis of psychological dependence or addiction may negatively impact the patient on a personal level and inhibit future care, as well as result in undertreatment of pain. Definitions of the major terms should be reviewed in Table 12.2 and are briefly described below [6].

Psychological dependence is described as a psychological need for specific substance to obtain positive effects or to avoid negative consequences. *Addiction* refers to the aberrant use of substance, including loss of control, compulsive use, preoccupation, and continued use despite harm. Opioid abuse or addiction is more common with polydrug abuse, or dependence on other substances, such as alcohol, marijuana, or nicotine. It is important, if possible, to distinguish the chronic pain patient from the opioid-abusing patient (Table 12.3) [6]. Unfortunately, to cloud the issue, there is significant opioid addiction within the chronic pain population, approximating 3–19 % [29]. This prevalence may be underestimated because these patients have a background of emotional and psychological instability, and develop a conditioning behavior resulting from relief of increasing pain intensity experienced from opioid use [30, 31].

There is another group of patients who have well-documented chronic pain and resemble opioid abusers because of their often obsessive drug-seeking behavior. These patients may have visited many physicians but are under-medicated, seeking adequate pain relief. This phenomenon was termed *pseudoaddiction* [32]. However, unlike patients with true

Table 12.1 Criteria for substance dependence

A maladaptive pattern of substance use, leading to clinically significant impairment or distress, as manifested by three (or more) of the following, occurring at any time in the 12-month period:

1. Tolerance, as defined by either of the following:
   (a) A need for markedly increased amounts of the substance to achieve intoxication or desired effect
   (b) Markedly diminished effect with continued use of the same amount of the substance
2. Withdrawal, as manifested by either of the following:
   (a) The characteristic withdrawal syndrome for the substance (refer to criteria A and B of the criteria sets for withdrawal from the specific substances)
   (b) The same (or a closely related) substance is taken to avoid or relieve withdrawal symptoms
3. The substance is often taken in larger amounts or for a longer period than was intended
4. There is a persistent desire or unsuccessful efforts to cut down or control substance abuse
5. A great deal of time is spent in activities to obtain the substance, use the substance, or recover from its effects
6. Important social, occupational, or recreational activities are given up or reduced because of substance use
7. The substance use is continued despite knowledge of having a persistent or recurrent physical or psychological problems that is likely to have been caused or exacerbated by the substance

With physiologic dependence: evidence of tolerance or withdrawal (i.e., either item 1 or item 2 is present)

Without physiologic dependence: no evidence of tolerance or withdrawal (i.e., neither item 1 nor item 2 is present)

Criteria for opioid withdrawal

(A) Either of the following:
   1. Cessation of (or reduction in) opioid use that has been heavy and prolonged (several weeks or longer)
   2. Administration of an opioid antagonist after a period of opioid use
(B) Three (or more) of the following, developing within minutes to several days after criterion A:
   1. Dysphoric mood
   2. Nausea or vomiting
   3. Muscle aches
   4. Lacrimation or rhinorrhea
   5. Pupillary dilation, piloerection, or sweating
   6. Diarrhea
   7. Yawning
   8. Fever
   9. Insomnia

Reproduced with permission from Mitra and Sinatra [6]

addiction, the pseudoaddicted patient will obtain pain relief if the dose of opioid is increased and the behavior will be eliminated.

Physiologic dependence is described as an alteration in physiologic response to a drug resulting from opioid binding to receptors, leading to withdrawal syndrome if drug is stopped. This can be seen both in patients in whom opioids are legitimately prescribed and in those abusing opioids. In general, the higher the daily dose is, the greater the degree of physiologic dependence and tolerance [33–35].

The opioid *withdrawal* syndrome is described as increased sympathetic and parasympathetic responses mediated via the myenteric plexus, brainstem vagal, and hypothalamic nuclei. These responses include hypertension, tachycardia, diaphoresis, abdominal cramping, and diarrhea. Quitting "cold turkey" is related to the abrupt withdrawal of opioids causing piloerection of the skin. Behavioral responses such as shaking, yawning, and leg jerking occur as well [33, 36, 37]. Rarely life threatening, these symptoms are extremely unpleasant and may be missed in the perioperative period [37].

The time course of withdrawal varies depending on the opioid being used; however, that for intermediate acting agents (e.g., morphine, heroine), it is listed in Table 12.4 [33, 38]. Abrupt halt of short-acting agents such as fentanyl or meperidine may result in withdrawal as early as 2–6 h after stopping the drug and have symptoms lasting only 4–5 days. In contrast, withdrawal from long-acting agents like methadone occurs 24–48 h after use and may last up to 6–7 weeks.

Opioid tolerance is a pharmacologic adaptation occurring when patients require increasing amounts of drug for same effect, shifting the dose-response curve to the right. Tolerance develops to the analgesic, euphoric, sedative, respiratory depression, and nauseating effects but not to miosis and constipation [33, 36, 37]. Duration of exposure, daily dose requirement, and receptor association/disassociation kinetics are predictive of the degree of opioid tolerance. Opioid agonists binding to the same receptor show asymmetric cross-tolerance depending on their intrinsic efficacy [33]. The number of receptors that need to be occupied to create an analgesic effect is inversely proportional to the intrinsic efficacy.

Table 12.2 Commonly used terms in substance dependence

Addiction	Commonly used term meaning the aberrant use of a specific psychoactive substance in a manner characterized by loss of control, compulsive use, preoccupation, and continued use despite harm; pejorative term, replaced in the "DSM-IV" in a nonpejorative way by the term *substance use disorder* (SUD) with psychological and physical dependence
Dependence	1 Psychological dependence: need for a specific psychoactive substance either for its positive effects or to avoid negative psychological or physical effects associated with its withdrawal 2. Physical dependence: a physiologic state of adaptation to a specific psychoactive substance characterized by the emergence of a withdrawal syndrome during abstinence, which may be relieved in total or in part by re-administration of the substance 3. One category of psychoactive substance use disorder
Chemical dependence	A generic term relating to psychological and/or physical dependence on one or more psychoactive substances
Substance use disorders	Term of DSM-IV comprising two main groups: 1. Substance dependence disorder and substance abuse disorder 2. Substance-induced disorders (e.g., intoxication, withdrawal, delirium, psychotic disorders)
Tolerance	A state in which an increased dosage of psychoactive substance is needed to produce a desired effect; cross-tolerance: induced by repeated administration of one psychoactive substance that is manifested toward another substance to which the individual has not been recently exposed
Withdrawal syndrome	The onset of a predictable constellation of signs and symptoms after the abrupt discontinuation of or a rapid decrease in dosage of a psychoactive substance
Polydrug dependence	Concomitant use of two or more psychoactive substances in quantities and frequencies that cause individually significant physiologic, psychological, and/or sociological distress or impairment (polysubstance abuser)
Recovery	A process of overcoming both physical and psychological dependence on a psychoactive substance with a commitment to sobriety
Abstinence	Non-use of any psychoactive substance
Maintenance	Prevention of craving behavior and withdrawal symptoms of opioids by long-acting opioids (e.g., methadone, buprenorphine)
Substance abuse	Use of a psychoactive substance in a manner outside of sociocultural conventions

Reproduced with permission from Mitra and Sinatra [6]

Table 12.3 Distinguishing the chronic pain patient from the opioid-abusing patient

Chronic pain patient	Opioid-abusing patient
Using opioids as prescribed, follows treatment plan	Out of control with opioid use, does not follow treatment plan
Use of opioid improves quality of life	Opioids impair quality of life
Aware and concerned about side effects	Unconcerned about side effects
Will save previous medications, prescriptions	"Loses" prescriptions, runs out of medication early, makes excuses

In other words, a potent agonist with high efficacy binds to a small number of receptors to achieve analgesia (e.g., sufentanil). The patient treated with this agent will develop tolerance more slowly than a patient treated with opioids having low intrinsic efficacy binding to a large number of receptors (e.g., morphine) [34, 39–42]. Briefly, acquired opioid tolerance can be classified into pharmacokinetic tolerance, learned tolerance, and pharmacodynamic tolerance. The pharmacokinetic tolerance refers to enzyme induction and subsequent acceleration of opioid metabolism [43, 44]. Learned tolerance refers to decreased drug affect due to learned compensatory mechanisms (i.e., can walk a straight line while intoxicated) [45, 46]. Pharmacodynamic tolerance refers to neuroadaptive changes that take place after long-term exposure to the drug [6]. The molecular mechanisms of these adaptations are complex and result in long-term persistent neural adaptations, involving increased levels of cAMP, spinal dynorphin, glutamine, and activation of NMDA receptors [47–50]. These changes ultimately result in receptor desensitization, decreased receptor density, and alterations in receptor coupling to G proteins and signal transduction pathways [33, 46, 48, 51, 67].

Table 12.4 Typical withdrawal symptoms associated of opioid withdrawal, by stage

Stage 1 (1–36 h)
Anxiety
Craving for drug
Lacrimation
Rhinorrhea
Yawning
Stage II (12–72 h)
Diaphoresis
Piloerection
Anorexia
Mydriasis
Irritability
Mild-moderate sleep disturbance
Tremor
Stage III (24–72 h)
Abdominal pain
Muscle spasms
Nausea, vomiting, diarrhea
Severe insomnia
Violent yawning

Vignette #1

An example of a particularly difficult patient is the patient with history of opioid addiction presenting for an elective ventral abdominal hernia repair. In this example, the patient is taking an antidepressant for depression, oxyContin for chronic abdominal pain, and gabapentin for neuropathic symptoms. The preoperative appointment should be utilized to discuss clarify expectations and create a management strategy for post operative pain.

Issues relative to undergoing the procedure include the necessity to continue her current medications and then plan for treatment of acute surgical pain from tissue trauma. A prudent approach for this patient should start with preoperative assessment and discussion with the surgeon, anesthesiologist, psychiatrist, and social work to clarify expectations. Placement of an epidural, if feasible, would be useful in perioperative pain control. In addition to general anesthesia, adjuncts may include intravenous infusions of dexmedetomidine or other alpha 2 agonist to reduce sympathetic outflow and an NMDA antagonist. In the acute postoperative period, adequate dosing of the epidural would provide analgesia with breakthrough intravenous opioids, perhaps via patient-controlled analgesia (PCA). This may avoid acute withdrawal and treat breakthrough pain. As early as possible, the home dose of opioids should be reinstated with adequate short-acting breakthrough pain medication to cover surgical pain. This is one possible regimen to obtain pain control and subsequent early discharge.

Types and Mechanisms of Pain

Although chronic back pain is by far the most common cause of chronic pain, peripheral neuropathy, cancer, abdominal disorders, or musculoskeletal disorders such as rheumatoid arthritis and fibromyalgia are common. Many patients are afflicted with multiple disorders, which can cause different types of pain, e.g., somatic and/or neuropathic, and may benefit from targeted non-opioid modalities or a multimodal approach.

Pain begins with the stimulation of specialized nerve endings called nociceptors, which exist throughout the body on sensory nerves. Nociceptive pain accounts for both visceral (related to internal organs) and somatic (related to bones, joints, muscles) pains involved with surgery. Nociceptors respond to direct stimulation as well as to mediators such as prostaglandins, bradykinins, histamine, and serotonin, which are released at the site of tissue injury [26, 52, 53]. These act via nerve endings to cause pain impulse formation as well as amplifying further signals caused by direct stimulation [54].

Slow conduction takes place in the visceral unmyelinated C fibers which join somatic nerves and are responsible for referred pain. After entry into the dorsal horn, pain and temperature fibers cross the midline and ascend via the lateral spinothalamic tract. At this level, substance P is the primary mediator. Ascending fibers terminate primarily in the brainstem and thalamus, which then relay the information to the cerebral cortex. Here, the impulse is perceived and localized, and further signals to the limbic system are responsible for the emotional response to pain.

Descending pain fibers from the cerebral cortex and midbrain modulate the afferent nerve stimuli that transmit pain signals to the central nervous system. Enkephalin, norepinephrine, serotonin, and gamma aminobutyric acid (GABA) have been shown to modulate and inhibit the frequency and intensity of nociceptive impulses, thereby attenuating the pain response [28]. Endogenous opioids and endorphins are released from the central nervous system, bind to mu, delta, and kappa opioid receptors, and prevent presynaptic release of neurotransmitters, including substance P. They aslo inhibit the perception and response to painful stimuli.

Both ascending and descending pain pathways can be summarized in Fig. 12.1. Inflammatory pain acts via upregulation of nociceptors and recruiting nonstimulated or dormant receptors [52, 55–57]. Proinflammatory mediators such as IL-1, IL-6, and TNF alpha interferons decrease the threshold for impulse generation and raise the intensity of the impulse as well as the rate of impulse discharge. Further, inflammation perpetuates itself by neurogenic inflammation in which substance P is released and acts peripherally to induce more inflammation, vascular permeability, and ongoing tissue injury [26, 53].

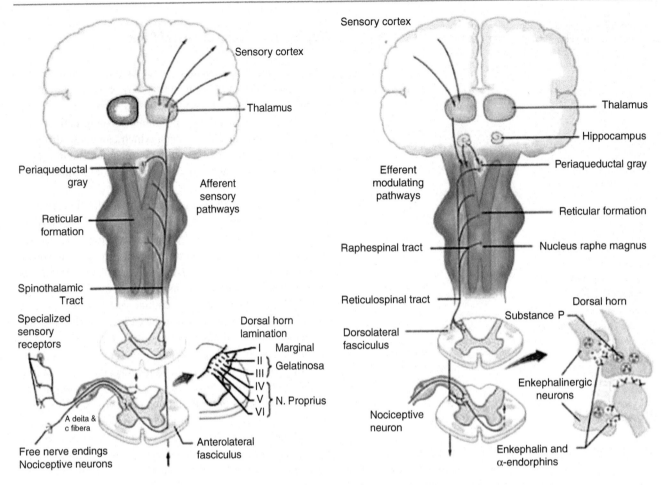

Fig. 12.1 Ascending and descending pathways of nociception (Reproduced with permission from Macres et al. [55])

Neuropathic pain occurs secondary to direct injury of peripheral or central nervous structures, or as a result of compression or tumor invasion. Opioid receptors (mu, kappa, and sigma) exist in the periphery, spinal cord, and central nervous system, as well as inflammatory and immunologic cells [59]. Most receptors are concentrated in the central nervous system, with the highest concentration in the dorsal horn of the spinal cord, periaqueductal gray matter, and rostral ventromedial medulla of the brainstem. Opioids are a mainstay for postoperative and intraoperative analgesia because of their potency. They act by binding to presynaptic receptors and preventing the release of substance P and impulse transmission. The mu receptor is responsible for spinal and supraspinal analgesia as well as having the undesirable side effects of respiratory depression, bowel dysmotility, urinary retention, and pruritis. Kappa, while providing supraspinal and spinal analgesia, also mediates miosis, sedation, and dysphagia. Lastly, the delta receptor mediates spinal and supraspinal analgesia only. A majority of opioids utilized in the perioperative period are mu agonists, having different degree of affinity for mu subtypes.

Thus, a "new" opioid may have a different selectivity for the individual mu receptor subtype, explaining "incomplete cross-tolerance" [42]. As a class, opioids do not have a ceiling effect and escalating doses will stop pain once enough opioid is given [54]. The characteristics, pharmacokinetics, and pharmacodynamics of each drug are discussed in other chapters.

Opioid-Induced Hyperalgesia

The chronic pain patient may present perioperatively with an amplified pain response or hyperesthesia. They may also present with allodynia, or pain elicited by a normally non-painful stimulus. Compared to narcotic-naïve patients, opioid-dependent patients have relative pain intolerance and significantly increased sensitivity during cold, pressor, and thermal testing [58, 59]. This is referred to as drug-induced hyperalgesia and is thought to result after continuous opioid receptor occupation. This occurs regardless of route of administration, dosing, and administration schedules [60, 61].

Both central and peripheral neural processes are influenced by the neuronal and humoral inputs caused by nociception [35, 62]. Generally, both types of hyperalgesia share underlying mechanisms mediated by glutamate via the *N*-methyl-D-aspartate (NMDA) receptor [63, 64]. Because of their amplified pain response, these patients might have extreme difficulty coping with sudden acute pain [11, 58, 65].

Treatment of the Chronic Pain Patient in the Perioperative Period

There are few controlled studies to guide the anesthesiologist in optimizing anesthetic and analgesic care in these patients although the prevalence of opioid dependency continues to increase [2–4, 11, 66]. Scientific literature in this area is mostly case reports and expert opinion. Although these have not been tested specifically, below are guidelines that may serve to improve analgesia and patient satisfaction based on the information we have.

The patient should take their daily maintenance opioid dose before induction of any anesthetic if possible. Most sustained release opioids provide 12 h or more of analgesic effect and should maintain baseline requirements during the preoperative and intraoperative period, particularly for an ambulatory surgery. If the patient forgets or is instructed not to take his or her baseline medication, they should be loaded with an equivalent loading dose of intravenous narcotic at induction or during the procedure. Transdermal fentanyl patches should be maintained. The patient may safely change the patch on their scheduled date if it happens to be the scheduled surgery date without the need for intravenous fentanyl. However, if removed >6–12 h prior this, it can be replaced with an equivalent intravenous maintenance rate. Replacing the patch may take 6–12 h to take full effect and intravenous fentanyl may be weaned after that time [67, 68]. Implanted intrathecal or epidural narcotic infusions are generally continued. If the baseline narcotic requirement is not maintained, withdrawal symptoms may be experienced, as demonstrated by some case reports [34]. While there are many computerized programs and online calculators available to convert various types of oral narcotic dosages to different available types of narcotics via intravenous and intramuscular routes, a narcotic conversion chart may be a useful place to start when calculating baseline opioid requirements (Table 12.5).

Some intravenous or intramuscular doses of morphine or hydromorphone may be titrated down from oral doses because parenteral administration bypasses first pass metabolism, having 2–3 times the bioavailability of oral dosing [70–72]. However, newer formulations such as oxycodone and oxymorphone have high oral bioavailability, approaching 83 % [70, 73, 74].

When providing these doses, close monitoring of patient the baseline oral dose can be approximated by nearly similar doses of intravenous awareness, oxygenation, heart rate, respiratory rate, and pupil diameter should be undertaken to avoid both under- and overmedication.

In an ambulatory surgery setting, patients may benefit from intraoperative boluses of fentanyl and sufentanil. After stabilization in the recovery area, they should be started on early oral opioids and might require doses higher than baseline, depending on the invasiveness of the procedure [75, 76]. Doses may need to be increased 30–100 % in comparison to opioid-naïve patients [3, 8, 76]. In a nonambulatory surgery setting, where a patient may be unable to take oral medications postoperatively, judicious doses of morphine, hydromorphone, or fentanyl can be provided to cover both baseline and postsurgical pain. Some anesthesiologists may prefer to titrate opioids preoperatively or "preemptively" while maintaining active communication with the patient and monitoring vital signs. Others prefer to give half the estimated dose before the induction of anesthesia and the remainder as the case progresses [76].

Patient-Controlled Analgesia (PCA)

Lastly, use of an intravenous patient-controlled analgesia (PCA) to control postoperative pain has been shown to be useful in this population. These can be set to fulfill a patient's basal pain requirements as well as add a patient-controlled dose to provide acute pain relief [77, 78]. Due to receptor downregulation and opioid tolerance, higher than normal doses of morphine or hydromorphone may be required. Basal requirements can be met by converting the oral or transdermal daily dose to intravenous equivalent and starting a basal infusion *or* adding 1–2 boluses per hour to maintain baseline opioid requirements [77]. Although some studies first were concerned that individuals may self-administer excessive amounts of opioid [4, 75, 76], it is now widely accepted that PCA can be offered to selected patients provided that pain intensity, opioid consumption, and side effects are monitored [79].

Methadone has also been advocated for use in patients who have inadequate pain control despite treatment with high doses of morphine [80]. Methadone may have the ability of activating a different mu receptor subtype to which morphine tolerance has not developed as well as having the added benefits of alpha 2 agonist properties and NMDA receptor antagonism [59, 81, 82]. However, initial dosing of methadone should be started cautiously due to the prolonged half-life in some patients and potentially unclear dose conversion when compared to higher total dosages of morphine equivalents.

Table 12.5 Equianalgesic dosing of opioids for pain management

Drug[a]	Equianalgesic doses (mg)		Approximate equianalgesic 24-h dose (assumes around-the-clock dosing)[b]		Usual starting dose (adults) (doses not equianalgesic)	
	Parenteral	Oral	Parenteral	Oral/other	Parenteral	Oral/other
Morphine (immediate-release tablets, oral solution)	10	30	3–4 mg q 4 h	10 mg q 4 h	2–5 mg q 3–4 h	5–15 mg q 3–4 h
Controlled-release morphine (e.g., MS Contin, Kadian)	NA	30	NA	30 mg q 12 h (Kadian may be given as 60 mg q 24 h)	NA	15 mg q 8–12 h (Kadian may be started at 10–20 mg q 24 h)[g]
Extended-release morphine (Avinza [USA], Embeda [with naltrexone USA])	NA	30	NA	60 mg q 24 h	NA	Avinza: 30 mg q 24 h / Embeda: 20 mg q 24 h
Hydromorphone (Dilaudid)	1.5–2	7.5–8	0.5–0.8 mg q 4 h	2–4 mg q 4 h	See footnotes c,d	See footnote c
Extended-release hydromorphone (Exalgo, Jurnista [Canada])	NA	See footnote e	NA	See footnote e	NA	See footnotes f,g
Oxycodone (e.g., Roxicodone [USA], OxyIR [Canada], also in Percocet, others)	NA	20–30	NA	5–10 mg q 4 h	NA	5 mg q 3–4 h
Controlled-release oxycodone (OxyContin)	NA	20–30	NA	20–30 mg q 12 h	NA	10 mg q 12 h
Oxymorphone (Opana [USA])	1	10	0.3–0.4 mg q 4 h	5 mg q 6 h	0.5 mg q 4–6 h	10 mg q 4–6 h
Extended-release oxymorphone (Opana ER [USA])[b]	NA	10	NA	10 mg q 12 h	NA	5 mg q 12 h
Hydrocodone (in Lortab [USA], Vicodin [USA], others)	NA	30–45	NA	10–15 mg q 4 h	NA	2.5–10 mg q 3–6 h
Codeine	100–130	200	30–50 mg q 4 h	60 mg q 4 h	10 mg q 3–4 h	15–30 mg q 3–4 h
Methadone (Dolophine [USA], Metadol [Canada])	Variable	Variable	The conversion ratio of methadone is highly variable depending on factors such as patient tolerance, morphine dose, and length of dosing (short term versus chronic dosing). Because the analgesic duration of action is shorter than the half-life, toxicity due to drug accumulation can occur within 3–5 days (see our detail document "Opioid Dosing")			
Fentanyl	0.1	NA	All non-injectable fentanyl products are for opioid-tolerant patients only. Do not convert mcg for mcg among fentanyl products (i.e., patch, transmucosal [Actiq (USA)], buccal [Fentora (USA)], buccal soluble film [Onsolis]). See specific product labeling for dosing			
Meperidine (Demerol)	75	300	Should be used for acute dosing only (short duration of action (2.5–3.5 h) and neurotoxic metabolite, normeperidine [1]. Avoid in renal insufficiency and use caution in hepatic impairment and in the elderly (potential for toxicity due to accumulation of normeperidine). Seizures, myoclonus, tremor, confusion, and delirium may occur			

An equianalgesic dose calculator is available at http://www.hopweb.org

From Therapeutic Research Center [69]

Project leaders in preparation of this detail document: Melanie Cupp, Pharm.D., BCPS (May 2010 update) Jennifer Obenrader, Pharm.D (original author 2004)

NA not available

Equianalgesic doses contained in this chart are approximate and should be used only as a guideline. Dosing must be titrated to individual response. There is often incomplete cross-tolerance among these drugs. It is, therefore, typically necessary to begin with a dose lower (e.g., 25–50 % lower) than the equianalgesic dose when changing drugs and then titrate to an effective response. Dosing adjustments for renal or hepatic insufficiency and other conditions that affect drug metabolism and kinetics may also be necessary. Most of the above opioids are available as generics. Exceptions (with example cost from drugstore.com) include Kadian ($4.81/30 mg cap), Avinza ($4.47/30 mg cap), Opana, Opana ER ($4.40/10 mg tab), Embeda ($4.60/20 mg cap), and Exalgo ($10/8 mg [AWP]). As a comparison, generic morphine controlled release = $1.63/30 mg tab

[a] Tramadol (e.g., Ultram [USA], Ralivia [Canada], potency is about one-tenth that of morphine, similar to codeine. The maximum daily dose of tramadol is 300–400 mg, depending on the product. Also check product information regarding appropriate dosing in elderly or in renal or hepatic dysfunction

[b] Examples of doses seen in clinical practice, taking into account available dosage strengths

[c] Product labeling for hydromorphone recommends a starting dose of 1 mg to 2 mg IV every 4–6 h or 2–4 mg orally every 4–6 h. Some institutions use even lower doses of hydromorphone (e.g., 0.2–0.5 mg every 2 h as needed). One regimen starts opioid-naïve patients at 0.2 mg IV every 2 h as needed for mild or moderate pain, with the option in moderate pain to give an extra 0.2 mg after 15 min if relief is inadequate after the first 0.2-mg dose. For severe pain, 0.5 mg IV every 2 h as needed is used initially. In adults <65 years of age, the 0.5-mg dose can be repeated in 15 min if relief is inadequate, for a maximum of 1 mg in 2 h

[d] Dilaudid Canadian monograph recommends parenteral starting dose of 2 mg. See footnote "c" for additional information and precautions

[e] Per the product labeling, convert to Exalgo 12 mg from oral codeine 200 mg, hydrocodone 30 mg, morphine 60 mg, oxycodone 30 mg, and oxymorphone 20 mg. The Jurnista product monograph recommends a 5:1 oral morphine to oral hydromorphone conversion ratio

[f] No initial dose for Exalgo. For opioid-tolerant patients only. Initial Jurnista dose (opioid naïve or <40 mg daily oral morphine equivalents) is 4–8 mg q 24 h

[g] Labeling for some products (MS Contin [USA], Kadian, Jurnista) suggests beginning treatment with an immediate-release formulation

[h] Per the product labeling, oral oxymorphone 10 mg ER is approximately equivalent to hydrocodone 20 mg or oxycodone 20 mg

Postoperative Oral Narcotic Regimens

When a postoperative oral narcotic regimen is chosen, baseline requirements should be supplemented with additional 20–50 % above baseline to accommodate pain associated with surgical injury [76]. These should be slowly titrated down over 5–7 days to presurgical amounts, thereby reducing the risk of withdrawal. If the procedure reduces chronic pain (e.g., cordotomy, spine surgery, neurolysis) then the baseline dose may be reduced by 25–50 % the first postoperative day and then tapered 25 % every 24–48 h, as tolerated. Of course, during this time, the signs and symptoms of withdrawal should be closely monitored. Weaning of opioids and the prevention of withdrawal reaction can be facilitated by adding an alpha 2 agonist such as clonidine.

Use of Mixed Agonists/Antagonists

Buprenorphine is a mixed partial opioid agonist/antagonist approximately 30 times more potent than morphine, with less respiratory depression than pure mu agonists [83]. Buprenorphine may be delivered via oral, intravenous, intramuscular, sublingual, or epidural routes. Although it may be used in the management of acute pain, it may be encountered in the patient receiving chronic treatment for past narcotic addiction. Like other chronic opioid use, long-term use of buprenorphine will result in physical dependence, but withdrawal symptoms will be less severe when compared with full mu agonists. Side effects to be wary of include constipation, headache, nausea, vomiting, sweating, dizziness, as well as respiratory depression, and changes in blood pressure and heart rate [84–87].

One approach to the patient taking chronic buprenorphine [88] is described below. Firstly, the prescribing physician should be contacted and be made aware of the surgery. If buprenorphine is being taken, the patient should continue as long as pain is controlled, and non-narcotic adjuncts should be provided for home use. If pain is uncontrolled preoperatively and surgery is elective, consider delaying the surgery until the prescribing physician can transition to short-acting opioids for 5 days. If surgery is emergent and pain is uncontrolled, buprenorphine should be discontinued and a PCA should be started if possible, realizing that patient requirements will be high due to opioid tolerance. Non-narcotic adjuncts with regional or neuraxial anesthesia should be considered. If they have been off buprenorphine for more than 5 days and pain is uncontrolled, the patient should be treated with pure opioid receptor agonists such as morphine, and the physician prescribing buprenorphine should be made aware of the switch. Buprenorphine can then be restarted by that physician after postoperative pain returns to baseline.

Use of Adjuvant Analgesics

Non-narcotic adjuvants are valuable resources in the treatment of acute pain. Each adjuvant works via a different mechanism to provide analgesia and diminished sensation of pain. All come with varying side effect profiles and efficacies. It is important to recognize these available options, and if begun preemptively, these medications can have opioid-sparing effect in the perioperative period. Effective perioperative analgesia with a combination of agents results in reducing perioperative morbidity, shortens hospital stays, and improves patient satisfaction [89–92].

Firstly, anxiolytics in the preoperative period may help the patient cooperate without fear or anxiety as well as reduce intraoperative anesthesia and postoperative analgesia requirements. The use of anxiolytic pretreatment may further lead to decrease in postoperative pain scores and postoperative anxiety [93, 94].

Local anesthetics bind to receptors in the sodium channel and block sodium influx, arresting depolarization, thereby interrupting afferent nerve conduction. Local anesthesia or peripheral nerve blockade is useful to provide incisional pain relief in the immediate perioperative period [95]. Although lidocaine patches have only been FDA approved for use in postherpetic neuralgia [94], they can also be used to decrease the incisional pain. The patches can be cut according to the size of a painful area; the manufacturer recommends leaving the patch on for 12 h and then off for 12 h. Some texts discuss the use of lidocaine patches 2–3 in. from the incision to help with incisional pain [14]. This allows lidocaine to diffuse into the dermis and epidermis, producing analgesia without numbness of the skin, with minimal systemic absorption [94]. Other medications such as tramadol, morphine, and ketorolac injected subcutaneously at the incision site have been used to decrease oral analgesic consumption [96, 97].

The use of non-opioid analgesic adjuvants may also reduce the amount of narcotic required. Acetaminophen is a commonly used agent that can be clinically useful in reducing postoperative opioid consumption and reduces inflammation via COX-2 and COX-3 inhibition. Doses less than 3 g over 24 h make hepatotoxicity unlikely in the patient without hepatic dysfunction, and it has an excellent safety profile. Intraoperative and postoperative opioid consumption is reduced via the use of nonsteroidal anti-inflammatory drugs (NSAIDs) as well. Postoperative opioid consumption may be reduced up to 50 % [98–101] and is particularly useful in same day surgeries [102]. These include the salicylates, propionic acids, acetic acids, oxylates, and fenamates. Although most NSAIDs are orally delivered, ketorolac is unique in that it can be delivered intramuscularly or intravenously in the perioperative period.

In general, NSAIDs inhibit the conversion of arachidonic acid to prostaglandins, bradykinins, and phospholipids via the cyclooxygenase enzyme. Cyclooxygenase (COX) inhibition increases leukotriene production, leading to rare asthmatic and anaphylactic reactions [103, 104]. COX-1 specifically influences platelet function, gastric mucosal protection, and hemostasis, while COX-2 affects inflammatory cascade and pain specifically [104]. The inhibition of COX-1 enzyme can thereby result in platelet inhibition, increased risk of gastric ulcers and gastrointestinal bleeding, as well as renal dysfunction. Initial enthusiasm regarding selective cyclooxygenase COX-2 inhibition has been quenched in recent years, as these have been associated with adverse cardiovascular events such as myocardial infarction and cerebrovascular accident [89, 105–110]. Despite this controversy, some authors still recommend its use in the acute setting as these agents are readily available, easy to administer, and effective [94].

Use of ketamine intraoperatively as an induction agent (1–2 mg/kg IV) or low-dose ketamine (0.5 mg/kg IV) postoperatively has been shown to reduce opioid dose requirements and provide analgesia via direct interaction with kappa opioid receptors [111] but more importantly via NMDA antagonism, inhibiting monoaminergic pain pathways [112, 113]. It also has mild local anesthetic properties, interacting with voltage-gated sodium channels. Ketamine is unique in that it does not cause respiratory depression while providing anesthesia and analgesia; however, it may be associated with increased salivation, emergence delerium, sympathetic stimulation, tachycardia, and hypertension at induction doses.

Clonidine and dexmedetomidine have also been shown to reduce total opioid requirements without respiratory depression via alpha 2 agonism and reduction of sympathetic outflow [46]. Clonidine is typically applied in a 0.1–0.2-mg/h transdermal patch or via oral routes. Dexmedetomidine is an alpha 2 receptor agonist, with less effect on alpha 1 receptors than clonidine, and may be used in the perioperative period in doses approximating 0.5 mg/kg/h via intravenous route. However, both may have side effects including sedation, dry mouth, hypotension, and bradycardia; abrupt discontinuation of clonidine may result in reflex hypertension and tachycardia.

Although it has not been studied in the chronic pain patient in the perioperative period, gabapentin has been shown to be particularly useful in patients with neuropathic pain. It has been shown to reduce postoperative morphine requirements in patients undergoing radical mastectomy and enhances morphine analgesia in healthy volunteers [114, 115]. It is renally excreted and has a few known drug interactions and can cause sedation. Although pregabalin works via a similar mechanism, this has not been studied as extensively. Both agents have been found to be effective in reducing nociception-induced hyperalgesia [35] and should be considered in a preemptive multimodal pain management plan. Ongoing study is necessary in the area of the opioid-tolerant patient.

Patients may also be chronically on antidepressants for chronic pain management, such as serotonin, norepinephrine reuptake inhibitors (SNRIs), and tricyclic antidepressants or (TCAs). These should be continued during the perioperative period, although the anesthesiologist should be aware of the profound response to pressor administration, particularly indirect agents such as ephedrine. TCAs also have anticholinergic effects and may cause somnolence.

Magnesium is thought to work as an NMDA antagonist and may be an adjuvant to consider in a comprehensive pain strategy. Its use is still an area of controversy and research. Some studies have shown a reduction of total intraoperative opioid requirements after an intravenous dose of 50 mg/kg [116, 117], while others showed reduction in postoperative opioid consumption after spinal anesthetics [118]. Evidence provided by a recent systematic review [119] demonstrated that magnesium is an inexpensive, available treatment for hypomagnesemia and shivering, and may or may not reduce postoperative opioid requirements. There are little to no recommendations from this review provided specifically to the chronic pain population.

Lastly, dextromethorphan, a commonly used antitussive, is also a low-affinity NMDA antagonist and may be used as an adjunct. More therapies are being actively developed to reduce opioid tolerance via NMDA receptors and production of nitric oxide synthase [114]. Recent studies have shown increasing levels of nitric oxide via transdermal nitroglycerin decreases the postoperative opioid requirements in cancer patients [120]. There may be some role for M5 muscarinic acetycholine receptors in mediating reward and withdrawal symptoms related to opioid use [121].

Neuraxial Analgesia for Postoperative Pain

Administration of opioids via the neuraxial rouge may be more efficacious than parenteral or oral opioids [40, 122]. Intrathecal and epidural doses are approximately 100 and 10 times more efficacious peroperatively than parenteral administration [24]. This increased efficacy may be due to downregulation of spinal opioid receptors. There have only been a few studies in opioid-dependent patients, on this route of administration and should be further explored.

Continuous epidural catheters are most appropriate in orthopedic, abdominal, pelvic, and thoracic procedures and in the treatment of blunt chest injury. When placed prior to induction of anesthesia, intraoperative and postoperative anesthetic requirements are reduced [123–127]. Ileus as well as postoperative nausea and vomiting, postoperative pulmonary complications, myocardial infarction, and thromboembolism are all reduced with epidural anesthesia [128].

If epidural anesthesia is chosen, serious complications can occur including inadvertent intravascular or intrathecal injection, epidural abscess, and epidural hematoma [129]. These risks should be assessed preoperatively and discussed with the patient.

Peripheral Nerve Blockade for Postoperative Pain

If possible and applicable for a given surgery, peripheral nerve blockade (PNB) should be considered in developing a comprehensive pain management plan for a chronic pain patient, particularly in extremity surgery. Advantages include reduction in parenteral and oral opioid requirements both intraoperative and several hours postoperatively with a "single-shot" technique, and some centers have trialed discharging patients home with an indwelling catheter for up to 48 h via disposable pumps. The goal is to minimize pain perception while reducing the need for oral or parental opioids beyond baseline requirements [4, 76].

Conclusions

In the opioid-dependent patient, preventing not only the withdrawal symptoms but also the adverse physiologic, emotional, and long-term effects of surgical pain are vital in humane perioperative pain treatment. There is a significant risk of both overdosing and underdosing narcotics in this patient population. Patients must be assessed preoperatively to determine the most appropriate plan of action for pain control. In developing a balanced analgesic plan, pain must be treated with the least amount of the most specific drug with a goal of treating stimulation, modulation, inflammation, and psychology of pain. Using a multimodal approach appropriately may reduce the amount of opioid consumed and thereby reduce the number of dose related side effects.

Vignette #2

A 33-year-old male presents for operative treatment of an ankle fracture 1 month after a severe motorcycle injury where he suffered injuries to both lower extremities. Since the accident, he has undergone multiple procedures including exploratory laparotomy, pelvic reconstruction, and femur and tibia surgeries. In the last month, he has become severely opioid tolerant and feels his pain has been vastly undertreated. This patient presents a significant challenge in the attempt to provide adequate pain control perioperatively. Even though he was in excellent health prior to his injury, over the last month, his increasing narcotic requirement and psychological impairment have led to uncontrolled pain.

The need for thorough counseling and discussion of expectations are highly important. In this patient, a balanced approach with preemptive analgesia will lead to a higher satisfaction rate and less risk of narcotic overdose and side effects of medications. The preoperative placement of popliteal and saphenous peripheral nerve blockade with local anesthesia and clonidine provides complete blockade of ongoing pain from the operative extremity. Intraoperatively, intermittent ketamine and intravenous narcotics with the peripheral nerve blockade provide analgesia. Intravenous magnesium could be considered intraoperatively. Upon emergence, patient-controlled analgesia with a basal rate to compensate for his preoperative requirements could be instated as well. Oral home medications reinstituted as soon as possible to allow for an easy transition to discharge.

References

1. Bell JR. Australian trends in opioid prescribing for chronic non-cancer pain, 1986–1996. Med J Aust. 1997;167:26–9.
2. Jage J, Bey T. Postoperative analgesia in patients with substance use disorders. Acute Pain. 2000;3:140–55.
3. May JA, White HC, Leonard-White A, Warltier DC, Pagel PS. The patient recovering from alcohol or drug addiction: special issues for the anesthesiologist. Anesth Analg. 2001;92:160–1.
4. Hord AH, Sinatra RS. Postoperative analgesia in the opioid dependent patient. In: Hord AH, Ginsberg B, Preble LM, editors. Acute pain: mechanisms and management. St Louis: Mosby Yearbook; 1992. p. 390–8.
5. Dolin SJ, Cashman JN, Bland JM. Effectiveness of acute postoperative pain management: evidence from published data. Br J Anaesth. 2002;89:409–23.
6. Mitra S, Sinatra RS. Perioperative management of acute pain in the opioid dependent patient. Anesthesiology. 2004;101:212–27.
7. Streitzer J. Pain management in the opioid dependent patient. Curr Psychiatr Rep. 2001;3:489–96.
8. Collett BJ. Chronic opioid therapy for non cancer pain. Br J Anaesth. 2001;87:133–43.
9. Miaskowski C, Crews J, Ready LB, et al. Anesthesia-based pain services improve the quality of postoperative pain management. Pain. 1999;80:23–9.
10. Finlay RJ, Keeri-Szanto M, Boyd D. New analgesic agents and techniques shorten port-operative hospital stay. Pain. 1984;19:S397.
11. Rapp SE, Ready LB, Nessly ML. Acute pain management in patients with prior opioid consumption: a case-controlled retrospective review. Pain. 1995;61:195–201.
12. Weissman C. The metabolic response to stress: an overview and update. Anesthesiology. 1990;73:308.
13. Hagen C, Brandt MR, Kehlet H. Prolactin, LH, FSH, GH, and cortisol response to surgery and the effect of epidural analgesia. Acta Endocrinol Copenh. 1980;94:151.
14. Lubenow T, Ivankovich A, Barkin R. Management of acute postoperative pain. In: Barash P, Cullen B, Stoelting R, editors. Clinical anesthesia. 5th ed. Philadelphia: Lippincott, Williams & Wilkins; 2006. p. 1413.
15. Lee D, Kimura S, DeQuattro V. Noradrenergic activity and silent ischemia in hypertensive patients with stable angina: effect of metoprolol. Lancet. 1989;1:403.
16. Rademaker BM, Ringers J, Oddom JA, et al. Pulmonary function and stress response after laparoscopic cholecystectomy: comparison with subcostal incision and influence of thoracic epidural anesthesia. Anesth Analg. 1992;75:381.

17. Rawal N, Sjostrand U, Christoffersson E, et al. Comparison of intramuscular and epidural morphine for postoperative analgesia in the grossly obese; influence on postoperative ambulation and pulmonary function. Anesth Analg. 1984;63:583.

18. Tuman K, McCarthy R, March R, et al. Effects of epidural anesthesia and analgesia on coagulation and outcome after major vascular surgery. Anesth Analg. 1991;73:696.

19. Rosenfeld B, Beattie C, Christopherson R, et al. The effects of different anesthetic regimens on fibrinolysis and the development of postoperative anesthetic regimens on fibrinolysis and the development of postoperative arterial thrombosis. Anesthesiology. 1993; 79:435.

20. Breslow MJ, Parker S, Frank S, et al. Determinants of catecholamine and cortisol responses to lower-extremity revascularization. Anesthesiology. 1993;79:1202.

21. Saol M. Effects of anesthesia and surgery on the immune response. Acta Anaesthesiol Scand. 1992;36:201.

22. Toft P, Svendsen P, Tonnesen E. Redistribution of lymphocytes after major surgical stress. Acta Anaesthesiol Scand. 1993;37:245.

23. Davis JM, Albert JD, Tracy KJ. Increased neutrophil mobilization and decreased chemotaxis during cortisol and epinephrine infusions. J Trauma. 1991;31:725.

24. Cousins M. Acute and postoperative pain. In: Wall P, Melzack R, editors. Textbook of pain. New York: Churchill Livingstone; 1999. p. 357–85.

25. Nimmo WS. Effect of anaesthesia on gastric motility and emptying. Br J Anaesth. 1984;56:29–36.

26. Carr DB, Goudas LC. Acute pain. Lancet. 1999;353:2051–8.

27. Wu CL, et al. Gene therapy for the management of pain: part I: methods and strategies. Anesthesiology. 2001;94:1119–32.

28. Wallace KG. The pathophysiology of pain. Crit Care Nurs Q. 1992;15:1–13.

29. Fishbain DA, Rosomoff HL, Rosomoff RS. Drug abuse, dependence, and addiction in chronic pain patients. Clin J Pain. 1992;8:77–85.

30. Savage SR. Addiction in the treatment of pain: significance, recognition and treatment. J Pain Symptom Manage. 1993;8:265–78.

31. Strain EC. Assessment and treatment of comorbid psychiatric disorders in opioid-dependent patients. Clin J Pain. 2002;18(suppl): S14–27.

32. Weissman DE, Haddox JD. Opioid pseudoaddiction: an iatrogenic syndrome. Pain. 1989;36:363–6.

33. Gustin HB, Akil H. Opioid analgesics. In: Hardman JG, Limbird LE, editors. Goodman and Gilman's the pharmacological basis of therapeutics. New York: McGraw-Hill; 2001. p. 569–619.

34. de Leon-Casasola OA, Lema MJ. Epidural sufentanil for acute pain control in a patient with extreme opioid dependency. Anesthesiology. 1992;76:853–6.

35. Wilder-Smith OH, Arendt-Nielsen L. Postoperative hyperalgesia: its clinical importance and relevance. Anesthesiology. 2006;104: 601–7.

36. Stoelting RK, Hillier SC. Chapter 6: nonbarbiturate intravenous anesthetic drugs. In: Pharmacology & physiology in anesthetic practice. Philadelphia: Lippincott Williams & Wilkins; 2006. p. 167–75.

37. Stoelting RK, Miller RD. Opioids. Basics of anesthesia. 5th ed. Philadelphia: Churchill -Livingstone Elsevier; 2007. p. 113–21.

38. Kosten T, O'Connor PG. Management of drug and alcohol withdrawal. N Engl J Med. 2003;348:1786.

39. Sosnowski M, Yaksh TL. Differential cross-tolerance between intrathecal morphine and sufentanil in the rat. Anesthesiology. 1990;73:1141–7.

40. de Leon-Casasola OA, Lema MJ. Epidural bupivacaine/sufentanil therapy for postoperative pain control in patients tolerant to opioid and unresponsive to epidural bupivacaine/morphine. Anesthesiology. 1994;80:303–9.

41. Saeki S, Yaksh TL. Suppression of nociceptive responses by spinal mu opioid agonists: effects of stimulus intensity and agonist efficacy. Anesth Analg. 1993;77:265–74.

42. Dupen A, Shen D, Ersek M. Mechanisms of opioid induced tolerance and hyperalgesia. Pain Manag Nurs. 2007;8:113–21.

43. Howard LA, Sellers EM, Tyndale RF. The role of pharmacogenetically variable cytochrome P450 enzymes in drug abuse and dependence. Pharmacogenomics. 2002;3:85–99.

44. Liu J-G, Anand KJS. Protein kinases modulate the cellular adaptations associated with opioid tolerance and dependence. Brain Res Rev. 2001;38:1–19.

45. Liu S, Wu C. The effect of analgesic technique on postoperative patient-reported outcomes including analgesia: a systematic review. Pain Med. 2007;105:789–807.

46. O'Brien CP. Drug addiction and drug abuse. In: Hardman JG, Limbird LE, editors. Goodman and Gilman's the pharmacological basis of therapeutics. New York: McGraw-Hill; 2001. p. 621–42.

47. Nestler EJ, Aghajanian GK. Molecular and cellular basis of addiction. Science. 1997;278:58–63.

48. Nestler EJ. Molecular basis of long-term plasticity underlying addiction. Nat Rev Neurosci. 2001;2:119–28.

49. Nestler EJ. Molecular neurobiology of addiction. Am J Addict. 2001;10:201–17.

50. Mao J. Opioid-induced abnormal pain sensitivity: implications in clinical opioid therapy. Pain. 2002;100:213–7.

51. Kieffer BL, Evans CJ. Opioid tolerance: in search of the holy grail. Cell. 2002;108:587–90.

52. Caterina MJ, Julius D. The vanilloid receptor: a molecular gateway to the pain pathway. Annu Rev Neurosci. 2001;24:487–517.

53. Desborough JP. The stress response to trauma and surgery. Br J Anaesth. 2000;85:109–17.

54. Cohen M, Schecter WP. Perioperative pain control: a strategy for management. Surg Clin North Am. 2005;85:1243–57.

55. Macres S, Moore P, Fishman S. Acute pain management. In: Barash P, Cullen B, Stoelting R, Calahan M, Stock C, editors. Clinical anesthesiology. 6th ed. Philadelphia: Lippincott, Williams & Wilkins; 2009. p. 1474.

56. Schaible HG, Richter F. Pathophysiology of pain. Langenbecks Arch Surg. 2004;389:237–43.

57. Winkelstein BA. Mechanisms of central sensitization, neuroimmunology & injury biomechanics in persistent pain: implications for musculoskeletal disorders. J Electromyogr Kinesiol. 2004;14:87–93.

58. Compton MA. Cold-pressor pain tolerance in opiate and cocaine abusers: correlates of drug type and use status. J Pain Symptom Manage. 1994;9:462–73.

59. Doverty M, Somogyi AA, White JM, Bochner F, Ali R, Ling W. Hyperalgesic responses in methadone maintenance patients. Pain. 2001;90:91–6.

60. Angst MS, Clark JD. Opioid-induced hyperalgesia: a qualitative systematic review. Anesthesiology. 2006;104:570–87.

61. Ossipov MH, Lai J, King T, Vanderah TW, Porreca F. Underlying mechanisms of pronociceptive consequences of prolonged morphine exposure. Biopolymers. 2005;80:319–24.

62. Wilder-Smith OH, Tassonyi E, Crul BJ, Arendt-Nielsen L. Quantitative sensory testing and human surgery: effects of analgesic management on postoperative neuroplasticity. Anesthesiology. 2003;98:1214–22.

63. Koppert W, Sittl R, Scheuber K, Alsheimer M, Schmelz M, Schuttler J. Differential modulation of remifentanil-induced analgesia and postinfusion hyperalgesia by S-ketamine and clonidine in humans. Anesthesiology. 2003;99:152–9.

64. Simonnet G, Rivat C. Opioid-induced hyperalgesia: abnormal or normal pain? Neuroreport. 2003;14:1–7.

65. Laulin JP, Celerier E, Larcher A, LeMoal M, Simmonet G. Opiate tolerance to daily heroin administration: an apparent phenomenon associated with enhanced pain sensitivity. Neuroscience. 1999; 89:631–6.

66. Compton P, Charuvastra VC, Kintaudi K, Ling W. Pain responses in methadone-maintained opioid abusers. J Pain Symptom Manage. 2000;20:237–45.

67. Caplan RA, Ready B, Oden RV, Matsen FA, Nessly ML, Olsson GL. Transdermal fentanyl for postoperative pain management. JAMA. 1989;261:1036–9.

68. Sevarino FB, Ning T, Sinatra RS, Hord AH, Ginsberg B, Preble LM. Transdermal fentanyl for acute pain management. In: Acute pain: mechanisms and management. St. Louis: Mosby Yearbook; 1992. p. 364–9.

69. Melanie C, Jennifer O. Therapeutic Research Center. Equianalgesic dosing of opioids for pain management. Canadian Pharm Lett. 2010;26(7):260712.

70. Foley RM. Opioids II: opioid analgesics in clinical pain management. In: Herz AAH, Simon EJ, editors. Handbook of experimental pharmacology. New York: Springer-Verlag; 1993. p. 697–743.

71. Pereira J, Lawlor P, Vigano A, Dorgan M, Bruera E. Equianalgesic dose ratios for opioids: a critical review and proposals for long-term dosing. J Pain Symptom Manage. 2001;22:672–87.

72. Steindler EM. ASAM addiction terminology. In: Graham AW, Schultz TK, editors. Principles of addiction medicine. 2nd ed. Chevy Chase: American Society of Addiction Medicine; 1998. p. 1301–4.

73. Ginsberg B, Sinatra RS, Adler LJ, Crews JC, Hord AH, Laurito CE, Ashburn MA. Conversion to oral controlled-release oxycodone from intravenous opioid analgesic in the postoperative setting. Pain Med. 2003;4:31–8.

74. Poyhia R, Vainio A, Kaiko E. A review of oxycodone's clinical pharmacokinetics and pharmacodynamics. J Pain Symptom Manage. 1993;8:63–7.

75. Pasero CL, Compton P. Pain management in addicted patients. Am J Nurs. 1997;4:17–9.

76. Saberski L. Postoperative pain management for the patient with chronic pain. In: Sinatra RS Hord AH, Ginsberg B, Preble LM, editors. Acute pain: mechanisms and management. St. Louis: Mosby Yearbook; 1992. p. 422–31.

77. Parker RK, Holtman B, White PF. Patient-controlled analgesia: does a concurrent opioid infusion improve pain management after surgery? JAMA. 1992;266:1947–52.

78. Macintyre PE. Safety and efficacy of patient-controlled analgesia. Br J Anaesth. 2001;87:36–46.

79. Hudcova J. Patient controlled opioid analgesia versus conventional opioid analgesia for postoperative pain. Cochrane Database Syst Rev. 2006;4:CD003348.

80. Sartain JB, Mitchell SJ. Successful use of oral methadone after failure of intravenous morphine and ketamine. Anaesth Intensive Care. 2002;30:487–9.

81. Morley JS, Makin MK. The use of methadone in cancer pain poorly responsive to other opioids. Pain Rev. 1998;5:51–8.

82. Davis AM, Inturrisi CE. d-Methadone blocks morphine tolerance and nmethyl-D-aspartate-induced hyperalgesia. J Pharmacol Exp Ther. 1999;289:1048–53.

83. Johnson RE, Jaffe JH, Fudala PJ. A controlled trial of buprenorphine treatment for opioid dependence. JAMA. 1992;287:2750–5.

84. Pickworth WB, Johnson RE, Holicky BA, Cone EJ. Subjective and physiologic effects of intravenous buprenorphine in humans. Clin Pharmacol Ther. 1993;53:570–6.

85. Lange WR, Fudala PJ, Dax EM, Johnson RE. Safety and side-effects of buprenorphine in the clinical management of heroin addiction. Drug Alcohol Depend. 1990;26:19–28.

86. Ling W, Wesson DR, Charuvastra C, Klett CJ. A controlled trial comparing buprenorphine and methadone maintenance in opioid dependence. Arch Gen Psychiatry. 1996;53:401–7.

87. Ling W, Charuvastra C, Collins JF, et al. Buprenorphine maintenance treatment of opiate dependence: a multicenter, randomized clinical trial. Addiction. 1998;93:475–86.

88. Brummett C. Perioperative management of buprenorphine. Department of Anesthesiology, Division of Pain Medicine, University of Michigan, 2008.

89. Barratt SM, et al. Multimodal analgesia and intravenous nutrition preserves total body protein following major upper gastrointestinal surgery. Reg Anesth Pain Med. 2002;27:15–22.

90. Basse L, et al. Accelerated postoperative recovery programme after colonic resection improves physical performance, pulmonary function and body composition. Br J Surg. 2002;89:446–53.

91. Brodner G, et al. Acute pain management: analysis, implications and consequences after prospective experience with 6349 surgical patients. Eur J Anaesthesiol. 2000;17:566–75.

92. Brodner G, et al. Multimodal perioperative management combining thoracic epidural analgesia, forced mobilization, and oral nutrition reduces hormonal and metabolic stress and improves convalescence after major urologic surgery. Anesth Analg. 2001;92:1594–600.

93. Kain ZN, Sevarino F, Pincus S, et al. Attenuation of the preoperative stress response with midazolam: effects on postoperative outcomes. Anesthesiology. 2000;93:141–7.

94. Olorunto WA, Galandiuk S. Managing the spectrum of surgical pain: acute management of the chronic pain patient. J Am Coll Surg. 2006;202:169–75.

95. Morrison JEJ, Jacobs VR. Reduction or elimination of postoperative pain medication after mastectomy through use of a temporarily placed local anesthetic pump vs control group. Zentralbl Gynakol. 2003;125:17–22.

96. Altunkaya H, Ozer Y, Kargi E, et al. The postoperative analgesic effect of tramadol when used as subcutaneous local anesthetic. Anesth Analg. 2004;99:1461–4.

97. Connelly NR, Reuben SS, Albert M, Page D. Use of preincisional ketorolac in hernia patients: intravenous versus surgical site. Reg Anesth. 1997;22:229–32.

98. Souter AJ, Fredman B, White PF. Controversies in the perioperative use of nonsterodial antiinflammatory drugs. Anesth Analg. 1994;79:1178–90.

99. Reuben SS, Connelly NR. Postoperative analgesic effects of celecoxib or rofecoxib after spinal fusion surgery. Anesth Analg. 2000;91:1221–5.

100. Katz WA. Cyclooxygenase-2-selective inhibitors in the management of acute and perioperative pain. Cleve Clin J Med. 2002;69:SI65–75.

101. Mercadante S, Sapio M, Caligara M, Serrata R, Dardanoni G, Barresi L. Opioid-sparing effect of diclofenac in cancer pain. J Pain Symptom Manage. 1997;14:15–20.

102. Rawal N. Analgesia for day-case surgery. Br J Anaesth. 2001; 87:73–87.

103. Schecter WP, et al. Pain control in outpatient surgery. J Am Coll Surg. 2002;195:95–104.

104. Zuckerman LF. Nonopioid and opioid analgesics. In: Ashburn MRL, editor. The management of pain. New York: Churchill Livingstone; 1998. p. 111–40.

105. Lefkowith JB. Cyclooxygenase-2 specificity and its clinical implications. Am J Med. 1999;106:43S–50.

106. Bresalier RS, et al. Cardiovascular events associated with rofecoxib in a colorectal adenoma chemoprevention trial. N Engl J Med. 2005;352:1092–102.

107. Drazen JM. COX-2 inhibitors: a lesson in unexpected problems. N Engl J Med. 2005;352:1131–2.

108. Nussmeier NA, et al. Complications of the COX-2 inhibitors parecoxib and valdecoxib after cardiac surgery. N Engl J Med. 2005;352:1081–91.

109. Seibert K, et al. COX-2 inhibitors is there cause for concern? Nat Med. 1999;5:621–2.

110. Solomon DH, et al. Relationship between selective cyclooxygenase-2 inhibitors and acute myocardial infarction in older adults. Circulation. 2004;109:2068–73.

111. Hurstveit O, Maurset A, Oye I. Interaction of the chiral forms of ketamine with opioid, phencyclidine, and muscarinic receptors. Pharmacol Toxicol. 1995;77:355–9.

112. Connor DFJ, Muir A. Balanced analgesia for the management of pain associated with multiple fractured ribs in an opioid addict. Anaesth Intensive Care. 1998;26:459–60.

113. Clark JL, Kalan GE. Effective treatment of severe cancer pain of the head using low-dose ketamine in an opioid-tolerant patient. J Pain Symptom Manag. 1995;10:310–4.

114. Barton SF, Langeland FF, Snabes MC, LeComte D, Kuss ME, Dhadda SS, Hubbard RC. Efficacy and safety of intravenous parecoxib sodium in relieving acute postoperative pain following gynecologic laparotomy surgery. Anesthesiology. 2002;97: 306–14.

115. Eckhardt K, Ammon S, Hofmann U, Riebe A, Gugeler N, Mikus G. Gabapentin enhances the analgesic effect of morphine in healthy volunteers. Anesth Analg. 2000;91:185–91.

116. Koinig H, Wallner T, Marhofer P, Andel KH, Mayer N. Magnesium sulfate reduces intra- and postoperative analgesic requirements. Anesth Analg. 1998;87:206–10.

117. Ryu JH, Kang MH, Park KS, Do SH. Effects of magnesium sulphate on intraoperative anaesthetic requirements and postoperative analgesia in gynaecology patients receiving total intravenous anaesthesia. Br J Anaesth. 2008;100:397–403.

118. Hwang JY, Na HS, Jeon YT, Ro YJ, Kim CS, Do SH. IV infusion of magnesium sulphate during spinal anaesthesia improves postoperative analgesia. Br J Anaesth. 2010;104:89–93.

119. Lysakowsky C, Dumont L, Czarnetzki C, Tramer MR. Magnesium as an adjuvant to postoperative analgesia: a systematic review of randomized trials. Anesth Analg. 2007;104:1532–9.

120. Lauretti GR, Perez MV, Reis MP, Pereira NL. Double-blind evaluation of transdermal nitroglycerine as adjuvant to oral morphine for cancer pain management. J Clin Anesth. 2002;14:83–6.

121. Basile AS, Fedorova I, Zapata A, Liu X, Shippenberg T, Duttaroy A, Yamada M, Wess J. Deletion of the M5 muscarinic acetylcholine receptor attenuates morphine reinforcement and withdrawal but not morphine analgesia. Proc Natl Acad Sci U S A. 2002; 99:11452–7.

122. Harrison DH, Sinatra RS, Morgese L, Chung JH. Epidural narcotic and patient-controlled analgesia for post-cesarean section pain relief. Anesthesiology. 1988;68:454–7.

123. Fernandez MI, et al. Does a thoracic epidural confer any additional benefit following videoassisted thoracoscopic pleurectomy for primary spontaneous pneumothorax? Eur J Cardiothorac Surg. 2005;27:671–4.

124. Holte K, Kehlet H. Epidural analgesia and risk of anastomotic leakage. Reg Anesth Pain Med. 2001;26:111–7.

125. Holte K, Kehlet H. Effect of postoperative epidural analgesia on surgical outcome. Minerva Anestesiol. 2002;68:157–61.

126. Subramaniam B, Pawar DK, Kashyap L. Pre-emptive analgesia with epidural morphine or morphine and bupivacaine. Anaesth Intensive Care. 2000;28:392–8.

127. Wu CT, et al. Pre-incisional epidural ketamine, morphine and bupivacaine combined with epidural and general anaesthesia provides pre-emptive analgesia for upper abdominal surgery. Acta Anaesthesiol Scand. 2000;44:63–8.

128. Carli F, Mayo N, Klubien K, et al. Epidural analgesia enhances functional exercise capacity and health-related quality of life after colonic surgery: results of a randomized trial. Anesthesiology. 2002;97:540–9.

129. Cullen DJ, Bogdanov E, Htut N. Spinal epidural hematoma occurrence in the absence of known risk factors: a case series. J Clin Anesth. 2004;16:376–81.

Opioids and the Law

13

Selina Read and Jill Eckert

Key Points

- Opioids have been used for medicinal purposes since as early as 3000 B.C.; problems such as abuse and addiction have also been reported alongside.
- Understanding the definitions, incidence, and cost of chronic pain is important for anyone who will be prescribing these medications.
- The clinician must become familiar with both state and federal laws pertaining to opioid prescribing. Not adhering to both state and federal laws can put the prescriber at risk.
- Clinicians who prescribe opioids must be well versed in detecting abuse and be able to find avenues for treatment of both the abuse alongside with the chronic pain issue.
- Prescription monitoring programs have become a valuable tool in preventing diversion of controlled substances.

Introduction

As physicians, one of the most important aspects of our job is the alleviation of pain, both acute and chronic. Opioids have been an integral part of easing pain for thousands of

years and continue to play an important role in the medical landscape today. The downside of these often powerful medications is the possibility of those taking them to become addicted and divert them away from the intended use.

History of Opioids and the Law

The earliest use of opioids dates back several thousand years, where in 3000 B.C. residents of Sumer, what is modern-day Iraq, used opium for both its medicinal and recreational characteristics. Hippocrates, one of the most important Greek physicians of his time, used opium to cure several ailments ranging from headache to depression. Other ancient Greeks and Romans used opium to relieve aches and pains. They also used opium for entertainment, enjoying the euphoric effects. Opium made its way to Europe and China sometime in the tenth century when Arab traders brought it from the Middle East. This efflux into Europe brought with it many of the problems we face today, namely, addiction. As early as the sixteenth century, manuscripts can be found discussing addiction and tolerance. It may be China that experienced the most problems with abuse in the seventeenth century when tobacco was outlawed, and the population began smoking opium as an alternative. There are no records of any of these ancient civilizations trying to pass laws to decrease or ban the use of opioids; however, many records indicate that abuse was prevalent and caused problems in society.

It wasn't until the nineteenth century when chemist Friedrich Sertürner isolated the active ingredient in opium that this plant found its birth in modern medicine. Sertürner named this isolated chemical morphine, after the Greek god of dreams, Morpheus. The safety of morphine was marginal as evidenced by untreatable respiratory depression which caused several deaths. Many companies began the search for a "safer, nonaddictive" opioid. Chemical modification of morphine began at the end of the nineteenth century when

S. Read, M.D. (✉)
Department of Anesthesiology, Penn State College of Medicine, Penn State Milton S. Hershey Medical Center, 500 University Drive, H187, Hershey, PA 17033, USA
e-mail: sread@hmc.psu.edu

J. Eckert, DO
Pennsylvania State University College of Medicine, Hershey, PA, USA

Department of Anesthesiology, Pennsylvania State Milton S. Hershey Medical Center, 850, Hershey, PA 17033, USA
e-mail: jeckert@psu.edu

T.R. Deer et al. (eds.), *Treatment of Chronic Pain by Medical Approaches: the AMERICAN ACADEMY of PAIN MEDICINE Textbook on Patient Management*, DOI 10.1007/978-1-4939-1818-8_13,
© American Academy of Pain Medicine 2015

German chemists added two acetyl groups to the drug, forming heroin. This modification allowed the opioid to dissolve faster through the blood-brain barrier, making it twice as potent. Interestingly, this German company, known as Bayer, marketed heroin as a cough suppressant. Unfortunately, heroin had the same addictive properties and dangers as morphine, and the search continued into the twentieth century where meperidine and methadone were added to the physician's arsenal. An important discovery by Wejilard and Erikson in the middle of the twentieth century was nalorphine, the first opioid antagonist, providing clinicians the ability to reverse the dangerous effects of opioids [1].

As opioid use became more widespread, the United States government started placing heavy taxes on the medications, in an attempt to prevent unintended usage. The International Opium Convention of 1912 committed governments to restrict trade of these substances to medical and scientific purposes only. In 1924, the US banned all nonmedical use of opioids along with creating the Permanent Central Opium Board, which became the agency in charge of determining whether there was too much or too little opioid production around the world. The US government passed the federal Controlled Substance Act in 1970 which scheduled opioids according to their abuse potential. This act prohibited the use of opioids by any individuals not under a physician's care and assured the safety of the medications being prescribed. Then, in 1990, the International Narcotics Control Board, which was initially formed in 1961 to unite all the international agencies under one umbrella, determined that opioids are not sufficiently available for legitimate medical purposes and called for governments to take corrective actions to repair the problem [2].

Important Definitions

When discussing opioids, certain terminology must be understood to apply the prescribing laws, treating pain in patients with addiction/dependence and understanding a clinician's practice. Furthermore, not understanding or mislabeling definitions may actually hinder effective pain treatment, leading to unnecessary suffering.

In 1999, the American Academy of Pain Medicine, the American Pain Society, and the American Society of Addiction Medicine formed the Liaison Committee on Pain and Addiction (LCPA), allowing collaboration between these groups to develop consensus definitions regarding terminology. Prior to this, most clinicians would use the World Health Organization's definitions along with the DSM and ICD-10 classifications; however, consensus was needed because practitioners need a way to communicate in the same language, along with easily understood definitions to implement into their practice [3].

Addiction is defined as a primary, chronic, neurobiologic disease with genetic, psychosocial, and environmental factors influencing its development and manifestations. It is characterized by behaviors that include one or more of the following: impaired control over drug use, compulsive use, or continued use despite harm and craving.

Physical dependence is defined as a state of adaptation that is manifested by a drug class that causes specific withdrawal syndrome that can be produced by abrupt cessation, rapid dose reduction, decreasing blood level of the drug, and/or administration of antagonist.

Tolerance is defined as a state of adaptation in which exposure to a drug induces change that results in a diminution of one or more of the drug's effects over time.

Clearly, both addiction and physical dependence can occur in the same patient; however, it is important to realize that physical dependence does not equal addiction. It is essential to understand that even though these are universally understood definitions, often state and federal governments have their own defined terminology. Whenever prescribing opioids, the prescriber should review not only the above definitions but also those set forth by their respective governing agencies they are prescribing under.

Incidence of Pain and Its Cost

It is expected that a patient will have pain following acute injury such as trauma or surgery; this pain is generally easily treated with current therapies, including opioids for short periods of time. Chronic pain presents a different set of problems due to the length of time needed for treatment, and the increasing dosage of medications that occurs with tolerance.

Chronic pain is defined as pain that persists beyond the usual course of an acute disease or pain that is not amenable to routine pain control methods. The prevalence of chronic pain ranges from 2 to 40 % in the adult population [4]. A survey in 1999 found that almost half of American households had at least one family member who suffers from chronic pain. The same survey found that one third of chronic pain sufferers did not feel they could function in society due to their pain; a majority of them felt that the pain was so horrible that they sometimes wanted to die [5]. More recently, a study from 2011 found that at least 116 million American adults suffer from pain, more than those affected by heart disease, cancer, and diabetes combined [6].

All of this adds up to billions of dollars in costs each year, $635 billion to be exact [6]. It is projected that the healthcare costs of patients with chronic pain may exceed the cost for treating patients with coronary artery disease, cancer, and AIDS combined [4].

How Common Is Abuse?

The statistics regarding abuse of prescription drugs is startling. In 2004, an estimated 19 million Americans, or 8 % of the population, admitted to abusing illicit drugs in the past year, and more than half of the public has tried an illicit drug during their lifetime [4]. The National Co-morbidity Study suggests that up to 14 % of Americans will develop alcohol addiction, and up to 7.5 % will develop addiction to illicit drugs over their lifetime [3]. According to the DEA, more than 6 million Americans are abusing prescription drugs – more than the number abusing cocaine, heroin, hallucinogens, and inhalants, combined. In the past 20 years, more people began abusing prescription pain medications (2.4 million) compared with marijuana (2.1 million) or cocaine (1.0 million) [4].

There are many types of prescription drugs abused, including opioid analgesics, tranquilizers, stimulants, and sedatives. About 75 % of the abuse is in the opioid analgesic class, with OxyContin, hydrocodone, Vicodin, morphine, and Dilaudid being the most commonly abused [4].

Although the true extent of prescription drug abuse is unknown, 10 % of patients receiving treatment for illicit drugs abuse prescription drugs only. The number abusing prescription medications is staggering, and the figures are climbing each year. Between 1992 and 2003, the United States population increased by 14 %; however, prescription drug abuse increased 94 %. During this time, the abuse rate for 12–17-year-olds increased 212 %, and it is known that those teens who abuse prescription drugs are more likely to abuse other illicit drugs such as alcohol, marijuana, cocaine, and heroin [4].

Demographics regarding abuse are varied, with the two extremes of age appearing to be the most susceptible. In 2004, the number of adolescents abusing tobacco, alcohol, marijuana, cocaine, and heroin appeared to be decreasing; however; this may be linked to an increase in the rate of prescription drug use. Monitoring the future, which is an epidemiological and etiological research project based at the University of Michigan, reported that OxyContin use among 12th graders increased almost 40 % over the previous 3 years. At the other extreme of age is the elderly who often are taking multiple prescriptions, which may lead to abuse or unintentional misuse [4].

Abuse is frequent in patients being treated for a chronic pain conditions, 15 % are concomitantly abusing prescription drugs, while 35 % are abusing illicit drugs. The direct cost of medical care is staggering in a pain clinic for those who abuse opioids, costing approximately $15,000 a year, compared with $1,800 for those on opioid therapy not abusing the prescriptions [4].

Possible Causes for Increased Abuse

It's not completely clear why there is such a significant rise in abuse rates. Some postulate it's due to increased supply, rising street values, and perceived safety of prescription medications in the general public [4].

Increased supply and demand can certainly play a large role in the ability of abusers to obtain controlled substances due to the simple fact that more medications being prescribed lend to more being available. The estimated number of prescriptions filled for controlled substances has been increasing dramatically since the early 1990s. Approximately 222 million controlled substance prescriptions were filled in 1994, compared with 354 million in 2003. This represents a 154 % increase in prescription filled for controlled substances contrasted with only a 57 % increase in all other prescription medications [4].

The street value for controlled substances is staggering; these medications sell for much more than most illicit drugs. Just a few examples will help the reader understand. The cost of 100 OxyContin 80-mg tablets to insurance is $1,081; the estimated street value for this same amount is $8,000. The pharmacy cost for 100 4-mg Dilaudid tablets is $88 where the street value is $10,000 [4]. Drug dealers will do almost anything to obtain prescriptions for these controlled substances because there is a large profit margin to be made.

The public may believe that prescribed medications are safer than the similar illicit drugs that may be found on the street. Most feel that if a doctor prescribes the medication, it must be safe. Furthermore, the acquisition of licit drugs poses much less of a threat, compared with purchasing a similar drug on the street.

Sequelae of Abuse

The increased incidence of prescription drug abuse has led to many socioeconomic problems. One of the most serious is an increase in the number of deaths due to unintentional overdose. According to the Centers for Disease Control and Prevention, the number of fatal poisonings due to prescription drugs increased 25 % from 1985 to 1995. The number of overdoses due to prescription opioids now surpasses both cocaine and heroin overdoses combined. Paulozzi et al. [5] hypothesized that this increase in fatal poisonings was linked to an increase in opioid prescriptions by physicians. They found that at the end of the 1980s, pain specialists began to argue that the risk of addiction should not prevent opioid analgesics from being prescribed for nonmalignant pain. This increased utilization of opioids for pain was linked to an increase in the sales of opioids and, not surprisingly, the number of deaths due to prescription opioids [5]. However, it is not completely clear that there is a cause and effect relationship. More information and further studies will need to be completed before definitive conclusions can be formed.

Abuse puts a significant strain on society, costing nearly $200 billion dollars a year. This cost comes from medical costs from misuse, crime involved supporting diversion/addiction, loss of productivity and wages, and cost of law enforcement. The illicit drug market was estimated at $322 billion dollars a year [5].

How Will This Affect Your Practice?

In the United States and around the world, pain goes untreated and undertreated every day. This inadequate treatment has been attributed to a lack of knowledge of pain management options, inadequate understanding of addiction, or fears of investigation and sanction by federal, state, and local regulatory agencies [4].

In response to this, multiple advocacy groups and professional organizations have been formed, with the goal of improving pain management. The Joint Committee on Accreditation of Healthcare Organizations labeled pain as the fifth vital sign and suggested hospitals use some form of pain assessment in all patients, allowing for more prompt and thorough treatment [3].

Nearly 90 % of patients being treated in a pain management setting are receiving opioid therapy, with many actually being treated with more than one type of opioid [4]. In order to protect yourself and your patient's well-being, it is vital to understand the laws governing prescribing of these medications. It's also essential to understand addiction, or have a specialist's advice, to help diagnose and adequately treat patients.

Federal Law

In 1973, the DEA was established to serve as the primary federal agency responsible for the enforcement of the Controlled Substances Act, which sets forth the federal law regarding both licit and illicit controlled substances. The Practitioner's Manual is designed to explain the basic federal requirements for prescribing, administering, and dispensing controlled substances to professionals, including physicians, mid-level providers, dentists, and veterinarians. The authors are explicit in explaining that the manual and the laws that guided its writing are not intended to hinder the practitioner's ability to treat pain, but to safeguard society against diversion [7].

In the United States, the Controlled Substances Act (CSA) placed controlled substances into five schedules. Substances are placed into their respective category based on whether they have an accepted medical use and the probability of causing dependence when abused. Schedule I drugs have no accepted medical use, with a very high potential for abuse. Some examples from this class are heroin, lysergic acid diethylamide, marijuana, and peyote. Schedule II substances have a high potential for abuse with severe psychological or physical dependence. Some examples include morphine, codeine, hydromorphone, fentanyl, and meperidine. Schedule III substances have a potential for abuse that is less than schedule II, including narcotics which contain less than 15 mg of hydrocodone and products that contain less than 90 mg of codeine per unit dosage. Schedule IV substances have a lower potential for abuse compared with schedule III and include partial agonist opioids, benzodiazepines, and long-acting barbiturates. Schedule V substances have the lowest potential for abuse and include most of the antitussive, antidiarrheal, and less potent analgesic medications.

In order to prescribe scheduled substances, a practitioner must be registered with the DEA or be considered exempt from the registration process. This registration grants the practitioner authority to handle and prescribe controlled substances and must be renewed every 3 years. In accordance with federal law, the practitioner may only engage in those activities that are authorized under state law for the jurisdiction in which the practice is located. When the state and federal laws conflict, the practitioner must abide by the more stringent aspects of both federal and state laws, in many cases the state laws being stricter. The certificate of registration must be maintained at the registered location in an easily retrievable location should official inspection be needed, and if operating in several states, the practitioner must register with the DEA for each of those states.

Practitioners who are agents or employees of a hospital may use a hospital DEA number to prescribe or administer controlled substances when acting in the usual course of business or employment. Examples include residents, staff physicians, and mid-level practitioners. In order to use the hospital DEA number, the employee must be authorized to do so by the state which they practice, verified by the hospital and acting within the scope of their employment. In 2004, the DEA, in conjunction with the Centers for Medicare and Medicaid Services, instituted an identification number that should be used for all noncontrolled substance prescriptions called the National Provider Identification (NPI). This was formed as a way to allow recognition of prescribers on noncontrolled substances without use of the DEA number, preventing its weakening and overuse.

In order to comply with federal law, a prescription for a controlled substance must be prescribed for a legitimate medical purpose by a practitioner acting in the usual course of professional practice. This prescription must include the drug's name, strength, dosage form, quantity prescribed, directions for use, and number of refills. In addition, all prescriptions must have a signature along with the date the medication was prescribed. Different scheduled medications have different prescribing limitations by the federal (and state) governments. Schedule II substances have no specific federal limitations on quantity and must be written, but cannot be given any refills. In 2007, the DEA passed an amendment that allows schedule II substances to be prescribed for up to 90 days by allowing sequential prescriptions that are written on the same day but, may be filled one at a time, each at 30-day intervals. Schedule III–V substances may be refilled up to five times within 6 months after the initial prescription was issued.

The CSA outlines safeguards that help protect the physician by decreasing diversion. Keeping blank prescriptions in a safe place where they cannot be stolen and limiting the number of prescription pads in use was recommended. Writing out the actual amount prescribed in words in addition to writing the number to help prevent alterations. Never sign out blank prescriptions and use tamper-resistant pads that cannot be photocopied. Each practitioner must maintain meticulous inventories and records of controlled substances. The DEA's Office of Diversion periodically issues informational brochures meant to help decrease the risk of diversion. One such brochure entitled "Don't be Scammed by a Drug Abuser" lists common characteristics of drug abusers. These include:

- Unusual behavior in the waiting room
- Assertive and often demanding personalities
- Strange physical appearance
- Unusual knowledge of controlled substances
- Requesting a specific controlled drug with reluctance to try any other medication
- Cutaneous signs of drug abuse

Patients with abuse problems may demand to be seen right away, request appointments at the end of the business day, call or come in after regular hours, state that they are just "passing through" seeing family members, state that a prescription has been lost or stolen, or pressure the physician by eliciting sympathy or guilt [8]. Any of these signs should tip the physician that the patient may be seeking controlled substances for reasons outside of legitimate pain relief.

When prescribing controlled substances, the practitioner must understand the federal definition of addiction. This definition requires either (a) habitual use that endangers the public morals, health, safety, or welfare or (b) addiction to the use of drugs to the point of loss of self-control over the addiction or (c) the use of narcotic drugs. This definition leaves much up to the practitioner, and some argue that it fails to distinguish psychological from physical dependence, the latter often occurring in chronic pain patients over time [9]. It is important to look for addiction in your practice because frequently when regulatory action is undertaken, it is against the physician, not the patient. The patient will often be given a "deal" that allows escape from prosecution

in exchange for testimony against the prescriber. It would then be up to the prescriber to prove that he/she was acting within the established standard of practice [9]. This is not meant to scare the reader, but to elaborate on the importance of proper prescribing and record keeping.

The federal government amended the Controlled Substance Act in 1974 with the Narcotic Addiction Treatment Act and again in 2000 with the Drug Addiction Treatment Act to provide laws guiding the use of controlled substances in the medical treatment of addiction. These laws established "the approval and licensing of practitioners involved in the treatment of opioid addiction, as well as improving the quality and delivery of treatment to that segment of society." It is very clear that a physician cannot prescribe schedule II maintenance or detoxification treatment, such as methadone, without a separate DEA registration. A practitioner who wants to prescribe schedule III–V medications approved for addiction, such as buprenorphine, may do so if they request a waiver form and fulfill requirements under the Center for Substance Abuse Treatment Program. If there is any question, more information can be found on the DEA's Office of Diversion Control website [7]. It's essential to delineate this from tapering a patient after long-term opioid therapy, which is permitted under federal law. It is therefore up to the practitioner to actively watch for symptoms of addiction and for proper referral of the patient to a proper detoxification clinic if warranted [9].

State Laws

Individual states have different laws for prescriptions of controlled substances. It is extremely important that before prescribing controlled substances, you are familiar with the laws in the state you will be prescribing. Some states have laws which may raise concerns by limiting the amounts of opioids that can be prescribed, requiring special government issues prescriptions, restricting access to patients in pain who have a history of substance abuse, and requiring that opioids be a treatment of last resort [10]. It is impractical in the scope of this chapter to discuss all of the laws of each state. In 1997, the Federation of State Medical Boards undertook an initiative to develop model guidelines to encourage state medical boards and other health-care agencies to adopt unified policies encouraging adequate treatment of pain. The *Model Guidelines for the Use of Controlled Substances for the Treatment of Pain* is now widely distributed and many agencies throughout the health-care world endorse its use.

The first section of the model describes a patient's right to obtain adequate and effective pain relief, which allows for improved quality of life, along with reduction of morbidity and the costs associated with insufficient treatment. Inadequate treatment may result from the physician's lack of knowledge about pain management, fears of investigation, or sanction. The FSMB considers inadequate treatment a departure from the standard of practice; if complaints are filed, it may result in formal investigations. This imparts the importance of a clinician maintaining current knowledge of pain management and treatment modalities. However, they should also remain current with the state and federal laws that pertain to the prescribing of controlled substances. The laws of the state aim to protect public health and safety since improper prescribing of controlled substances may lead to abuse. Accordingly, the FSMB expects physicians to place safeguards to help reduce this potential [2].

The second section gives a basic outline of how a physician should evaluate a patient's pain. The components are:

1. Evaluation of the patient – a thorough medical history and physical exam
2. Treatment plan
3. Informed consent and agreement for treatment
4. Periodic review
5. Consultation
6. Medical records
7. Compliance with controlled substances laws and regulations

Many physicians spend a great deal of time in medical school and residency learning how to accurately obtain a medical history and physical exam. This is the core of what makes us diagnosticians, and it is not surprising that this is an important component of evaluating a patient's pain. This can sometimes be difficult though because we can define in words how the patient's pain feels to them, but we can never truly understand how the pain is affecting them. In Responsible Opioid Prescribing, Dr. Fishman describes this as the physician's paradox, stating: "perhaps one reason that physicians are reluctant to aggressively treat pain has to do with the often frustrating fact that we can't prove that someone is in pain." Pain is an "untreatable hypothesis," and it can be quite difficult to measure a patient's pain, even in the twenty-first century where we have the ability to order complex medical tests and imaging [10]. The FSMB tries to ensure adequate documentation by requiring that the medical record contains the following: nature and intensity of the pain, current and past treatments for pain, underlying or coexisting disease or conditions, the effect of pain on the physical and psychological function, and a history of substance abuse. In addition, the physician should document the presence of one or more recognized indications for or against the use of a controlled substance [2].

A written treatment plan is the second requirement by the FSMB. This will outline objectives that can be used to determine if treatment is a success, i.e., whether the patient benefits from treatment as evidenced by improved physical and psychosocial function. It will also outline whether additional diagnostic evaluation is planned. They recommend that the physician adjust drug therapy to the individual patient and make use of other treatment modalities, such as physical therapy and psychiatric services, when warranted.

Informed consent and agreement for treatment is an essential component of a treatment plan. The FSMB requires that the physician discuss with the patient, or the patient's legal guardian, all of the risks and benefits of using controlled substances. The patient should understand that it is important to only receive controlled substances from one physician and if possible only one pharmacy. If the patient is considered a high risk for abuse, or to protect the patient-physician relationship, a written contract can be formed between the prescriber and patient, defining in writing guidelines what is expected in order to continue the treatment [2]. This type of contract can be called by many different names; most common are "patient agreements," "pain contracts," or "patient care contract." These contracts often stipulate that the patient has urine/serum medication levels when requested, protecting both the patient and prescriber. These contracts offer several advantages, including allowing the patient to participate in the decision-making process, serving as an informed consent, helping to remind the patient of the specific goals of treatment, and preventing any misunderstandings or distortions of understanding [10].

Periodic review of a patient's progress and symptom management during treatment is essential in order to document continued improvements in the patient's condition. The FSMB recommends the clinician to monitor the patient's response to treatment by determining how the pain has changed, both subjective and objective, if the patient has improved quality of life after treatment and if the treatment plan should be altered. The physician should be willing to consult with other clinicians if additional information is needed to adequately treat a specific patient with special attention being given to patients who are at increased risk for abuse or diversion.

Medical records have become an important component of a physician's daily activities, protecting the physician by outlining the thought process behind the treatments undertaken for a patient. The FSMB urges the physician to keep complete and accurate records, something that can be easily neglected in today's busy practice. They recommend having several vital components in your medical record:

1. A complete medical history and comprehensive physical exam
2. Diagnostic, therapeutic, and laboratory results
3. Evaluation and consultations
4. Treatment objectives
5. Discussion of risks and benefits
6. Informed consent
7. Treatments
8. Medications (including date, type, dosage, and quantity prescribed)
9. Instructions and agreements
10. Periodic review

Many states control a practitioner's ability to prescribe opioids for pain with each state being very different. It is essential to know your own states laws. The Texas Medical Practice Act states that physicians cannot prescribe opioids for any patient that has been known to be a habitual user of narcotic drugs. In New York, prescribers are required to report "addicts" to the Commissioner of Public health. In Rhode Island, a practitioner must report the name and ailment of any patient who is being treated with a schedule II substance for more than 3 months. New Jersey limits dispensing of schedule II substances to a 30-day prescription that should not be greater than 120 dosage units [2].

Fear of governmental action has been cited as a possible barrier to proper treatment of pain. A study of medical boards' actions against physicians who prescribe opioids for patients in pain found that the fear is exaggerated compared to the actual risk. In 2006, researchers studied DEA actions for the 2003–2004 year against physicians. They found that of the 963,385 physicians holding DEA licenses, 557 were investigated for possible criminal activity. Three hundred twenty-four physicians lost their DEA number, 116 had the investigation discontinued, and 43 physicians were arrested. A variety of violations resulted in arrest such as prescriptions in exchange for sex, money, and personal use; prescriptions written over the internet without proper medical examination; and prescriptions written without a proper DEA license [11]. These studies suggest that federal agencies do not typically investigate physicians who are prescribing controlled substances appropriately. Although 116 of the 557 investigations resulted in cessation of the investigation, it's unlikely that these physicians were investigated without cause. The small number of investigations resulting in no action proves that the agencies are not out to penalize physicians treating pain. A physician can likely avoid investigation by adhering to proper prescribing laws and keeping meticulous records regarding patients on opioid therapy.

It's worth mentioning again that the practitioner must abide by the more stringent laws, whether that be state or federal. Furthermore, it is the practitioner's responsibility to be familiar with laws at all levels before prescribing opioids.

Assessing the Risk for Abuse

How does a physician adequately screen for patients that may be at risk for addiction or drug abuse? This is certainly not an easy task, and no conclusive answers have come to light. It would go against all of our training and our oath to first do no harm if we assume that all patients will abuse the controlled substances we prescribe, and therefore we should not treat patient's pain adequately. Physicians should remain vigilant and maintain a modicum of suspicion. Often, this may force the prescriber to ask questions the patient may not want to answer. When prescribing controlled substances, it is always essential to determine if abuse is a possibility. Unfortunately, there have not been any conclusive studies allowing us to develop stringent guidelines on which patients are likely to abuse and divert prescribed medications; however, treating everyone with the same diagnostic tests and psychological screens may allow the physician to remain objective with every patient [10].

Guidelines allowing us to determine which patients receiving controlled substances are at risk for abuse are still in their infancy; however, there are certainly risk factors that place a patient at increased risk. Patients with a personal history of substance abuse or a family history of substance abuse are at a much higher risk of misusing the controlled substance they are prescribed compared with patients who do not have these histories. Furthermore, the risk for abuse is higher in younger patients, in those with a history of sexual abuse, mental disease, psychological stress, poor social support, and unclear cause of pain. Additionally, tobacco abuse increases the risk [12].

It seems the most important risk factor for misuse of a prescribed substance is a personal history of substance abuse. Individuals who abuse one substance are seven times more likely to abuse another substance. This makes perfect sense; however, the clinician may need to do some detective work to discover whether a patient has a substance abuse history, because often patients are not forthcoming with this information. This risk increases in patients who have recently abused illicit or licit drugs and may be the highest in those who have abused the prescription medication they are being prescribed. Ives et al. found patients with a history of alcohol, cocaine, or opioid misuse along with those convicted of a DUI or drug offense had a higher rate of abuse when prescribed opioids for chronic pain [13]. The second most important risk factor for abuse is a family history of abuse tendencies. This contributes to increased risk of abuse due to genetic factors that have yet to be elucidated, along with the social ramifications that surround having family members abusing substances. Family attitudes toward misuse of prescription medications can foster a liberal and tolerant environment [12].

Risk factors help determine which patients are in danger of abuse, allowing the clinician to place patients on a hierarchy of potential abuse: high risk, moderate risk, and lower risk of abuse. Depending on which rung the patient is placed will influence how the clinician assesses and monitors the patient.

Assessment through screening tools plays a very important role in determining if a patient is at risk for abusing prescription medications. Unless you are fortunate and have an addiction specialist as part of the pain management care team, a tool will be needed to evaluate patient's risk of abuse. This evaluation should be brief, have easily interpreted results, and must be validated in patients who are suffering from pain.

Most screening tools are designed to find patients at risk for abuse, not diagnose substance abuse. If a patient is found to be at risk through the screening tools, they should have a formal evaluation with a professional trained in diagnosing substance abuse disorders. There are several different screening tools available; some are geared more toward alcohol abuse while others for illicit drugs. Likely the most useful in the clinic will be combined screens which allow the clinician to determine if the patient is at risk for substance abuse for a variety of drugs. A new generation of screening tools has recently been developed specifically tailored to determine if a patient is at risk for opioid misuses [12]. Of course, these tests are not perfect; no test designed thus far has 100 % sensitivity and specificity nor are they able to conclude if a patient is not being forthcoming. They do allow for screening and can help prevent abuse in those with high risk by allowing the clinician to monitor that group of patients more closely. It is important to stress that even if a patient is at high risk for abuse, that patient still has the right to obtain adequate treatment of his pain.

Monitoring patients treated with opioids for chronic pain conditions is a very important step in helping detect abuse during treatment. There are several different guides available, and deciding which to use is a personal preference. The American Academy of Pain Medicine and the American Pain Society set forth five recommended steps of opioid prescribing. The first step is a thorough patient evaluation which should occur at the initial patient visit. Subsequent visits do not need to be as extensive; however, the clinician should be reassessing the patients risk for abuse and how effective the prescribed medications are in treating the patient's pain. Every patient should have an individualized plan tailored to their needs and medical history. Often having the patient actively involved in formulating this plan will solidify what is expected from the relationship. The clinician should obtain consultations when deemed necessary. These can include but are not limited to consultation with psychologists, psychiatrists, physical therapists, and addiction specialists. Finally, appropriate documentation cannot be overemphasized [12]. In addition to the above-mentioned steps, drug screening may be an important tool in detecting abuse. Maintaining doctor-patient trust is important; however, research indicates that relying on a patient's word regarding drug abuse is unwise. Drug screening both for illicit substance use and levels of prescribed medications should be viewed as another diagnostic test similar to blood glucose levels in diabetics. Periodic testing may be used as a deterrent to inappropriate drug use, provide a way to monitor the patient's response to treatment by obtaining levels of prescribed medications, and allowing the clinician to support their medical decisions. At a minimum, clinicians should test patients at the beginning of their therapy and again if any question arises whether the patient could be abusing an illicit substance or misusing the prescribed medicine [12].

The clinician should be aware of pseudoaddiction, a syndrome of abnormal behavior that develops due to inadequate treatment of pain developing tolerance. The three characteristic phases of pseudoaddiction include inadequate treatment with analgesics to meet the primary pain stimuli, escalation of analgesic demands by the patient associated with behavioral changes to convince others of the pain's severity, and crisis of mistrust between the patient and health-care team. This can easily be confused with addictive behaviors and may lead the prescriber to conclude the patient is addicted, instead of in need of higher doses or stronger pain medications [11].

Treating Pain in Patients with Addiction

It is estimated that up to 20–25 % of hospitalized patients have an addictive disorder. Most hospitalized patients will require some form of opioid therapy during their admission, including those with an addictive disorder [3]. In addition, patients in a chronic pain clinic are thought to have addictive disorders with a frequency of around 15 %. These patients can be difficult to manage since the risk of further addiction and diversion is more likely. In 2009, the American Pain Society and American Academy of Pain Medicine formed clinical guidelines for chronic opioid therapy. They recommend a higher level of monitoring and care for high-risk patients: those with a history of drug abuse, psychiatric issues, or serious aberrant drug-related behaviors. These patients will need to have more frequent visits and strict monitoring parameters along with possible consultation with addiction specialists. Furthermore, constant reevaluation should occur to determine if the patient is benefiting from chronic opioid therapy. If drug aberrant behavior occurs, the physician may need to discontinue the opioid therapy completely [14].

Terminating a physician-patient relationship is something that may become necessary when a patient does not adhere to the contract put forth by the provider. No physician should tolerate deviant behavior. Instead, a "zero tolerance" policy should be instituted. It is important that the patient fully understands the reasons that they are being discharged from the practice, and it is advisable to do so in both verbal and written formats. You may want to consider having a witness in the face-to-face conversations. Abandonment must be avoided, and if a physician has no experience with termination of a patient, consultation with professionals such as a bioethics committee or a professional consultant (such as addiction specialists) may help guide them through the process [10].

Prescription Monitoring Programs

Multiple states are adopting prescription monitoring programs, or PMPs, as a way to further prevent diversion of controlled substances. With the advent of computer pharmacy systems and the transition from paper to electronic prescriptions gaining popularity, it has become easier to monitor controlled substance prescribing. The main purpose of PMPs is to reduce diversion. Its objectives typically include not only monitoring but also education, early intervention, and investigative/enforcement arms. It is the goal of a PMP to be as unobtrusive as possible and not hinder the patient-physician relationship. PMPs can benefit the physician immensely when there is a question about prescribing habits (is it of another physician or medication use of the patient? Please clarify), because they allow information to be quickly and efficiently obtained. Additionally, they allow handling of complaints and avoidance of unnecessary investigations [15].

It is important to discuss the legal implications of prescription monitoring programs. To be considered effective, a monitoring system must reduce the abuse of controlled substances, but it also must not interfere with patient privacy or legitimate prescription of controlled substances. Patients are free to obtain prescriptions from any physician and have those prescriptions filled at any pharmacy. Most of the time, physicians and pharmacies do not share the information on what prescriptions are being filled and by whom, which can allow for diversion to easily occur.

Generally, when a state develops a monitoring program, they implement legislation which mandates pharmacies report through electronic databases the dispensing of certain or all controlled substances. The information required to report may vary between states, but the patient's name, physician prescribing the medication, name of the controlled substance, dose, and number dispensed are typically obtained. Once the data is obtained, the agency will do evaluation of the data and determine if certain physicians, pharmacists, or patients are associated with excessive substance prescribing or use. This report also allows physicians and pharmacists to determine if their patients are obtaining medications from other sources [15]. When properly used, the PMPs do their job well; however, there are a few glitches that are still being worked out. One is the accuracy of the data obtained. Some pharmacies provide incomplete or inconsistent data of prescriptions. Furthermore, although infrequent, identity theft occurs in patients on chronic opioid therapy. Both of these inconsistencies could lead to unnecessary investigations. It is important for those involved in gathering and interpreting the data to be looking closely when a question arises about prescribing or obtaining those substances. It should be thoroughly investigated not through the PMP databases alone but uses all other sources available [16].

In 2007, the president signed into law the Food and Drug Administration Amendments Act of 2007 (FDAAA) which authorized the FDA to require pharmaceutical companies to submit proposed risk evaluation and mitigation strategies (REMS) for medications which would ensure the benefits of a drug outweigh the risks. This law applied to both new medications and those already in use. In 2009, the FDA formed a multidisciplinary opioid REMS steering committee which was tasked with reducing the "epidemic" of prescription drug abuse in the United States. The committee revamped education programs for patients taking opioids, while recommending pharmaceutical companies making these medications to be part of this education by distributing information that was written in "consumer friendly language." The FDA also focused on physician education through multiple programs. Additionally, expansion of state prescription monitoring programs and increasing law enforcement to reduce of the number of "pill mills" and doctor shopping was initiated to decrease the excessive amount of opioid medications reaching the public. In 2012, other risk reduction measures such as doctor training and patient counseling are expected to become part of the REMS. These will be required for various "high-risk" medications such as hydromorphone, oxycodone, morphine, methadone, transdermal fentanyl, and oxymorphone [17].

Conclusion

Treatment of pain, both acute and chronic, is a vital part of any physician's practice. There are millions of patients who suffer from pain without getting appropriate treatment. However, the medications we use for this treatment can be fraught with problems such as abuse and addiction. It's important that any physician prescribing these medications distinguish between the signs of addiction and the treatments. Furthermore, a thorough understanding of both the federal and state laws is paramount to proper prescribing.

References

1. Brownstein MJ. A brief history of opiates, opioid peptides, and opioid receptors. Proc Natl Acad Sci. 1993;90:5391–3.
2. Shapiro RS. Legal basis for the control of analgesic drugs. J Pain Symptom Manage. 1994;9(3):153–9.
3. Savage SR, Covington EC, Joranson DE, Heit H, Gilson A. Definitions related to the medical use of opioids: evolution towards universal agreement. J Pain Symptom Manage. 2003;26(1):655–67.
4. Manchikanti L. Prescription drug abuse: what is being done to address this new drug epidemic? Testimony before the subcommittee on criminal justice, drug policy and human resources. Pain Physician. 2006;9(4):287–321.
5. Paulozzi LJ, Budnitz D, Xi Y. Increasing deaths from opioid analgesics in the United States. Pharmacoepidemiol Drug Saf. 2006;15:618–27.

6. Relieving pain in America: a blueprint for transforming prevention, care, education, and research. Washington, DC: National Academies; 2011.

7. Rannazzisi JT, Caverly MW. Practitioner's manual: an informational outline of the controlled substances act. Drug Enforcement Agency. 2006.

8. Publications – don't be scammed by a drug abuser. DEA diversion control program: welcome. 2010. http://www.deadiversion.usdoj.gov/pubs/brochures/drugabuser.htm. 24 Feb. 2010.

9. Clark W, Sees K. Opioids, chronic pain, and the law. J Pain Symptom Manage. 1993;8(5):297–305.

10. Fishman S. Responsible opioid prescribing: a physician's guide. Washington, DC: Waterford Life Sciences; 2009.

11. Jung B, Reidenberg M. The risk of action by the drug enforcement administration against physicians prescribing opioids for pain. Pain Med. 2006;7(4):353–7.

12. Webster LR, Dove B. Avoiding opioid abuse while managing pain: a guide for practitioners. North Branch: Sunrise River; 2007.

13. Ives TJ, Chelminski PR, Hammett-Stabler CA, Malone RM, Perhac SJ, Potisek NM, Shilliday BB, DeWalt DA, Pignone MP. Predictors of opioid misuse in patients with chronic pain: a prospective cohort study. BMC Health Serv Res. 2006;6:46.

14. Chou R, Fanciullo GJ, Fine PG, Adler JA, Ballantyne JC, Davies P, Donovan MI, Fishbain DA, Foley KM, Fundin J, Gilson AM, Kelter A, Mauskop A, O'Connor PG, Passik SD, Pasternak GW, Portenoy RK, Rich BA, Roberts RG, Todd KH, Miaskowski C. Clinical guidelines for the use of chronic opioid therapy in chronic noncancer pain. J Pain. 2009;10(2):113–30.

15. Joranson DE, Carrow GM, Ryan KM, Schaefer L, Gilson AM, Good P, Eadie J, Peine S, Dahl JL. Pain management and prescription monitoring. J Pain Symptom Manage. 2002;23(3):231–8.

16. Brushwood DB. Maximizing the value of electronic prescription monitoring programs. J Law Med Ethics. 2003;31:41–54.

17. FDA Acts to Reduce Harm from Opioid Drugs. U S food and drug administration home page. 2011. http://www.fda.gov/ForConsumers/ConsumerUpdates/ucm251830.htm. N.p., 1 Apr 2011. 27 May 2011.

Methadone for Chronic Pain

Naileshni Singh, Scott M. Fishman, and Kyle Tokarz

Key Points

- Methadone has pharmacological properties that make it unique among opioids including agonist action at mu and delta opioid receptors and antagonist action at NMDA receptors.
- Methadone's lipid solubility, long elimination half-life, high protein binding, and metabolism by the hepatic P450 system make predicting its pharmacokinetics difficult.
- Methadone has known efficacy for a variety of pain syndromes and clinical settings; however, its unstable metabolism, difficulty in predicting equianalgesic dosing, and other adverse effects raise its risk potential and mitigate its usefulness.
- Clinicians prescribing methadone must become familiar with its unique pharmacology and risk profile, including cardiac toxicity and data on rising rates of methadone-related deaths, in order to responsibly weigh risks and benefits of methadone before prescribing.

N. Singh, M.D. (✉)
Department of Anesthesiology, UC-Davis Medical Center, 4860 Y Street, Suite 3020, Sacramento, CA 95817, USA

University of California, Davis School of Medicine, Sacramento, CA, USA
e-mail: naileshni.singh@ucdmc.ucdavis.edu

S.M. Fishman, M.D.
Division of Pain Medicine, Department of Anesthesiology and Pain Medicine, University of California, Davis School of Medicine, 4860 Y Street, Suite 3020, Sacramento, CA 95817, USA
e-mail: smfishman@ucdavis.edu

K. Tokarz, DO
Department of Anesthesiology, Naval Medical Center, San Diego, 2736 West Canyon Ave, San Diego, CA 92123, USA
e-mail: kyle.tokarz@med.navy.mil

Introduction

Methadone use for pain relief has surged over the past two decades. In this time, its special pharmacology has been elucidated which has led to speculation about special properties as well as far greater risks than with other opioid medications. Recently, increasing reports of methadone-related unintended deaths have spurred greater concern about this unique drug. Methadone has many advantages that are now well opposed by many posing serious risks for patients in pain. Advantages include cost, ease of use, and multiple opioid and non-opioid receptor actions. However, risks include metabolic instability related to unique P450 system hepatic clearance that poses drug-drug interactions that differ from other opioids, high protein binding, variable urine clearance, and the potential for cardiac arrhythmia. Thus, this drug that saw a renaissance over the past two decades has now been revealed as more dangerous than previously thought and widely noted to require heightened knowledge and risk management for safe use.

Pharmacology

Methadone, chemically known as 6-dimethylamino-4,4-diphenyl-3-heptanone, is an opioid commonly used in a variety of clinical settings (Fig. 14.1). The pharmacokinetics and unique receptor profile make it distinct from the other commonly used opioids such as morphine or hydromorphone. Methadone was originally created in 1938 in Germany as an alternative to morphine. Following World War II, the drug was manufactured in the United States, but its potential for analgesia was not well appreciated. The first use for methadone was for maintenance of heroin and opioid addiction during the 1950s as a once per day therapy. The use of methadone increased within the last several decades among many medical specialties including primary care and oncology. Also known as Dolophine or Methadose, methadone is now

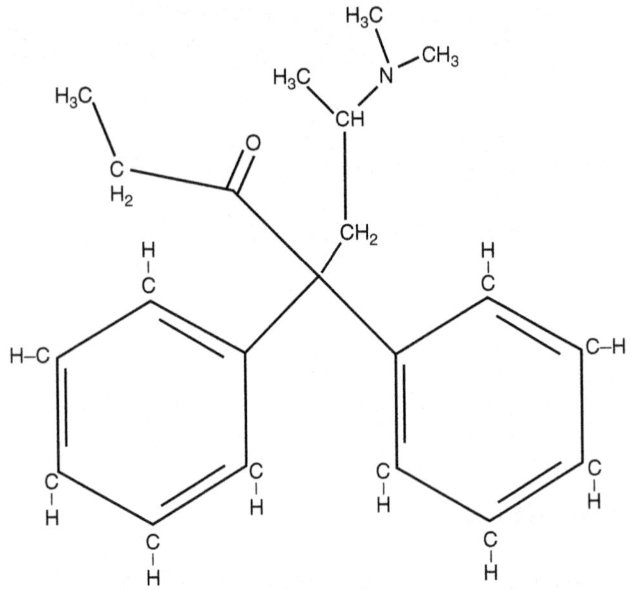

Fig. 14.1 Molecular structure of methadone

one of the most commonly used opioid analgesic therapies in the United States.

Methadone's activity at opioid sub-receptors is unique. Like morphine, methadone has agonist affinity for both the mu and delta opioid receptors. However, in animal studies, methadone has proportionately less mu receptor binding than morphine which may explain its more tolerable side effect profile. It is theorized that when compared to morphine which sensitizes the mu receptor, methadone's pharmacology may desensitize the mu receptor. This, coupled with affinity for the delta mu receptor, may lead some to use methadone to prevent dependence and tolerance. In comparison to other opioids, methadone has action on the serotoninergic and NMDA receptors. Animal and in vitro studies of the NMDA receptor suggest its possible role in neuropathic pain, as well as in tolerance and dependence of opioids. Theoretically, methadone's NMDA antagonist properties may make it better suited than other opioids for neuropathic pain syndromes. How the reuptake inhibition of serotonin and norepinephrine impacts its analgesic effects is currently unclear. Norepinephrine reuptake inhibition has specifically been a target for analgesic drug design in recent years. A medication with a broad ensemble of receptor affinities may have many medical uses. However, rising concerns about potential adverse effects may substantially temper such views.

Methadone has a basic pH and is available as a racemic mixture of enantiomers with different pharmacokinetic properties. The enantiomers, S-methadone (D-isomer) and R-methadone (L-isomer), can be reconstituted from a powder form into oral, rectal, intramuscular, and parenteral formulations. R-methadone acts largely at the mu opioid receptor site, while S-methadone antagonizes the NMDA receptor

and inhibits the reuptake of 5-hydroxytryptamine (serotonin) and norepinephrine. The R isomer is thought to be less cardiotoxic compared to the racemic mixture. The potency of the R enantiomer at the mu opioid receptor is also greater than the S enantiomer.

Methadone has unique pharmacokinetic properties within the opioid class. The drug's high lipophilicity causes it to be stored in fat and released slowly into the plasma to reach a steady state. Elderly people who have higher body fat content may accumulate higher methadone doses and need less frequent dosing. In addition, methadone has a large volume of distribution, ranging from 1.71 to 5.34 l/kg in chronic pain patients and even higher in those with opioid addiction. Methadone is 80 to 90 % protein bound which has repercussions for its duration of action and circulating blood levels. The main binding protein is alpha-1-acid glycoprotein (AAG), an acute phase reactant whose levels can differ in disease states [1]. This fluctuation can predispose to serious variability of circulating methadone levels.

The oral bioavailability of methadone is high, ranging from 40 to 99 %, but is dependent on intestinal transporters. For the oral formulation, time to peak concentration is 2.5 to 4 hours, with a terminal half-life between 24 to 60 hours. The half-life is related to the chronicity of administration with the lower range in chronic methadone therapy versus the upper range in acute dosing. Oral absorption further depends on gastric pH and motility. Rectal bioavailability is similar to parenteral bioavailability with a quick onset of action within 15 to 45 minutes. Methadone, given rectally, is rapidly absorbed through mucosa and has duration of action of up to 10 h. Methadone's plasma concentrations by the intramuscular route will depend on the site of the injection. For example, when compared to administration in the gluteal region, the deltoid muscle offers an increase in peak plasma concentration and improved pain control. Methadone may be used subcutaneously or absorbed through the buccal mucosa due to high lipid solubility.

Methadone's metabolism is largely dependent on the hepatic metabolism. It undergoes N-demethylation in the liver by the P450 CYP enzymes to 2-ethyl-1,5-dimethyl-3,3-diphenylpyrrolinium (EDDP). The main metabolizers are thought to be CYP3A4, CYP2B6, and CYP2C19, while the CYP2B6 enzyme primarily generates EDDP. Other lesser CYP enzymes have varying roles in methadone's metabolism, but of note, certain enzymes may preferentially metabolize the S versus the R enantiomer. Further complicating metabolism is the fact that the type I CYP enzyme system exhibits genetic and ethnic variability in expression, which affects methadone's duration of action between individuals and groups. CYP3A4 is itself unique in being an autoinducible enzyme which brings about methadone's own metabolism over time.

The P450 system can be affected by induction or inhibition by a variety of substrates that are common and medically important. For example, various medications in the treatment of HIV such as ritonavir may prolong methadone action by inhibition of the CYP3A4 and CYP2B6 systems. Many antiepileptic, antibiotic, and antidepressant medications taken concomitantly can influence methadone levels by either inhibition or induction of enzymes. Drug-drug interactions with methadone may make management of complex patients on polypharmacy regimens challenging. In addition, pregnancy does not relate to a state of high gastric pH, elevated AAG; and urine pH < 6.0 can cause methadone to be metabolized faster or decrease its levels. Opioid transporters in the blood-brain barrier also regulate the access of methadone to sites of action. These variables make predicting methadone metabolism and subsequent blood plasma levels difficult.

Methadone use in pregnancy is not uncommon as it has long been recommended for substance abuse treatment and withdrawal prevention. Parturients have a decrease in half-life and an increase in clearance of methadone. Fetuses born to mothers on chronic methadone therapy should be assessed for respiratory depression even though placental transfer and breast milk exposure are thought to be low. Fetal abstinence syndrome has been described in newborns of mothers who were on methadone maintenance therapy. Infant mortality is higher in babies exposed to methadone in utero than for the general parturient population [2]. Methadone has been shown to prolong the QTc interval in human newborns. In addition, the use of opioids in early stages of pregnancy has been linked to birth defects of the cardiovascular system [3].

Methadone is often used in patients with complex medical problems for whom it seems to have certain advantages. The lack of active metabolites is one aspect of methadone's pharmacology that may make it beneficial in some frail patients. Use of methadone in liver disease has been described sparingly. Theoretically, methadone can accumulate in disease states that alter metabolism by the hepatic cytochrome P450 system. Patients in methadone maintenance treatment programs often have a history of intravenous drug use and subsequent chronic hepatitis. Regardless, methadone has been successfully used in patients with chronic hepatitis and cirrhosis.

Elimination of methadone is biphasic, following both an alpha (8 to 12 h) and beta (30 to 60 h) phase (Fig. 14.2). The alpha phase typically corresponds to the analgesic period that is far shorter than the terminal half-life. This alpha phase correlates with the analgesic phase and serves as the rational for 3–4 times a day dosing in chronic pain. The long beta phase prevents withdrawal symptoms but provides for little analgesia. This slow clearance allows for once a day dosing in maintenance therapy programs but dictates careful upward titration [4]. The use of methadone as a breakthrough

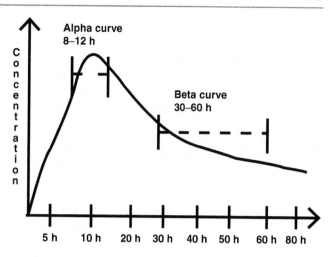

Fig. 14.2 Elimination curve for methadone depicting alpha (8 to 12 h) and beta phase (30 to 60 h)

medication is limited due to the long elimination phase and terminal half-life. Methadone taken in repetitive doses to achieve euphoric effects will often cause accumulation of the drug resulting in subsequent adverse events due to long-lasting pharmacokinetics.

Methadone elimination is largely fecal with some contribution from the renal system. For this reason, it is largely safe for use in renal failure and is insignificantly dialyzed due to high lipid solubility. Patients with renal failure will excrete a vast majority of methadone in the feces. Acidic urine, with a pH < 6, causes more excretion of the unionized total methadone dose. While medications that may alkanize the urine allow methadone to accumulate. Methadone, however, has no neurotoxic metabolites that may accumulate in kidney disease as compared to morphine. This theoretically makes methadone a more tolerable medication in patients with a low glomerular filtration rate.

Clinical Issues

Side effects of methadone are not unlike those of shorter-acting opioids. There is still a serious risk of respiratory depression, sedation, constipation, and pruritis. Many studies attest to methadone having a comparable rate of side effects when compared to morphine. But unique to methadone is the tendency to prolong the QT interval corrected (QTc) for heart rate and predisposition to tachyarrhythmias such as ventricular fibrillation and torsades de pointes. Arrhythmias were originally described in the methadone maintenance population who were presenting with sudden death within weeks of starting the program or after dose escalation. Structural heart disease is often not found among these decedents. The mechanism is thought to be blockade of the cardiac ether-a-go-go-related gene (hERG) coding potassium channel that prevents repolarization during phase III of the cardiac action potential. This channel is the delayed rectifier potassium ion (Ikr) whose blockade causes bradycardia and predisposes to torsades [5]. Methadone, like other opioids, is a negative chronotrope which further slows the heart rate. Several risk factors have been identified for prolongation of the QTc in methadone patients including high dose, concomitant use of other QTc prolonging medications, antidepressants, antibiotics, electrolyte disturbances, congenital long QTc syndrome, structural heart disease, liver or renal disease, and alcohol and benzodiazepine use. Chronic pain patients may be on a variety of medicines that are otherwise potentially cardiotoxic such as tricyclic antidepressants, which theoretically may offer additive toxicity.

How tissue or blood concentrations of methadone exactly cause sudden cardiac death remains unclear. Prolongation of the QTc interval has been seen in patients on low-dose methadone. Unfortunately, in deaths related to methadone, serum blood levels have overlapped those of deaths that were not attributed to methadone, illustrating that a lethal level is difficult to determine [6]. This confusing interaction may be related to methadone's variable pharmacokinetics and the fact that blood concentrations are poor indicators of the potential for toxicity. Several medical organizations such as the American College of Physicians (ACP) recommend discussion of the risks with patients and baseline electrocardiograms prior to treatment initiation. Per ACP recommendations, patients with borderline QTc intervals between 450 and 500 ms should have frequent electrocardiograms during methadone treatment [7]. Cessation of treatment should be considered in patients with QTc intervals greater than 500 ms (Table 14.1). Other authors do not recommend frequent EKGs but do argue for vigilance on the part of the prescribing physician.

In 2006, the Federal Drug Administration issued a warning regarding methadone's potential for prolongation of the QTc interval along with modified dosage instructions. This resulted in a 2006 manufacturer's black box warning regarding the possibility for fatal cardiac arrhythmias. The warning included starting opioid-naïve patients on 2.5 to 10 mg every 8 to 12 h for a maximum daily dose of 30 mg/day. Many patients on methadone therapy are on substantially more medication than recommended with these guidelines.

Respiratory depression in a patient population with a high incidence of sleep apnea is another concerning issue when prescribing medications such as methadone. The rate of sleep apnea is high in methadone maintenance programs, while the overall prevalence is elevated in chronic pain patients. Opioids in general may worsen both obstructive and central sleep apnea by acting on central opioid receptors in the medulla and hypothalamus that regulate breathing and sleep. The dose of opioid agonists and their actions on hypoxic and hypercapnic respiratory drive is another contributing factor. NMDA receptors may also play a key role in multiple areas of the sleep regulatory centers. Combining methadone with other respiratory depressants, such as benzodiazepines, may synergistically contribute to morbidity and even unintended deaths in such a high-risk population. Multiple studies have identified benzodiazepines and other sedating medications in patients who died while on methadone therapy. Whether this is related to sleep apnea, respiratory depression, or cardiac toxicity or as a combination of all three factors or other factors is unknown.

As the popularity of methadone has increased in recent years, so has methadone-related adverse events. Prescribing of methadone increased by almost 400 %, from 1997 to 2002 in the United States [8]. Methadone has become an attractive alternative to other opioids due to the perception that it has low addiction potential combined with its relatively low cost. Increased attention to early and aggressive treatment of cancer pain and increased use of long-acting opioids in patients with noncancer-related pain has likely contributed to escalated prescribing. Due to this methadone has since added to the national epidemic of prescription opioid abuse, misuse, diversion, and addiction. By 2006, the Research Abuse, Diversion and Addiction-Related Surveillance (RADARS) noted methadone to be the second most abused or misused opioid in the United States. Of concern is methadone's particular side effect profile and prolonged duration of action.

Methadone-related deaths have been analyzed in a variety of patient populations to ascertain cause. The National Vital

Table 14.1 ACP recommendations for methadone use and QTc interval screening

Recommendation 1: Disclosure	Clinicians should inform patients of arrhythmia risk
Recommendation 2: history	Clinicians should ask patients about a history of cardiac disease
Recommendation 3: Screening	Obtain a baseline EKG to measure the QTc interval and a follow up 30 days after starting treatment, and then annually
Recommendation 4: Risk stratification	If the QTc interval is greater than 450 ms, then discuss risks of treatment with patients. If the QTc > 500 ms, consider stopping treatment
Recommendation 5: Drug Interactions	Be aware of methadone's interactions with other drugs that may encourage QTc prolongation or methadone accumulation

Adapted from the American College of Physician (2009) [7]

Statistics System (of the United States) noted a 16 % increase in methadone-related deaths between 1999 and 2005, especially among those aged 35 to 54 years old. Of all prescribed opioids and illegal drugs, methadone has had the highest rate of increase in related deaths in recent years. For example, between 2001 and 2006, the state of Florida reported more methadone-related deaths than heroin, and West Virginia saw an increase in unintended overdose deaths during 2007, even in those with valid methadone prescriptions. The U.S. Centers for Disease Control and Prevention (CDC) issued a warning that methadone is implicated in nearly 33% of all prescription opioid deaths [11]. Causes of death in methadone-related scenarios are difficult to assess as many were also taking concomitant drugs, such as illicit substances or benzodiazepines, that could increase the risk of fatal adverse events.

Despite the stated risks, methadone use is widespread. Methadone is often a second- or third-line opioid for chronic pain syndromes in which side effects of other opioids therapies cannot be tolerated or when a less expensive medication is desired. In many settings, methadone has been shown to be as efficacious as long-acting morphine or fentanyl transdermal systems [9]. Additionally, methadone has been used successfully in a variety of pain syndromes including neuropathic and cancer-related pain. Along with oral administration, methadone has been effectively used in patient-controlled analgesia (PCA) delivery systems. Rarely, the medication may be added to intrathecal therapy or used in the IV formulation for intractable pain or intraoperative use. Methadone's high oral availability may be useful in those with "short gut" or "dumping syndrome" who have impaired absorption of medications that depend on the gastrointestinal track. Patients with gastrostomy tubes may benefit from the elixir formulation, while those who are NPO may access the drug through rectal or intramuscular routes. The multiple available formulations and routes of delivery make methadone ideal for end-of-life patients who may have difficulty swallowing or poor intravenous access. Crushing of methadone tablets does not produce a shorter-acting agent, so the potential for abuse from this particular action is theoretically low. Nonetheless, methadone is abused.

Rotation to methadone from another opioid-based therapy can be complicated. Reports of equianalgesic dosing conversion ratios are inconsistent, but typically there is greater potency when patients are being switched from higher dose regimens of other opioids to methadone. Essentially, the more opioid an individual is exposed to prior to starting methadone, the more potent methadone is, mg/mg. For example, studies have recommended ratios between 1 and 4:1 for doses of oral morphine equivalents of less than 100 mg/day, 5:1 for doses greater than 500 mg/day, and up to 20:1 for doses greater than 1,000 mg/day. Conversion from methadone to morphine is equally as challenging; reported

ratios have been up to methadone 1:10 of morphine [10]. The wide variation is thought to be related to individual differences in metabolism, pharmacokinetics, and cross tolerance between opioids. Many now consider methadone conversion to be so inexact as to recommend that practitioners start at the lowest dose and slowly titrate upwards to the effective dose. If the traditional rule of five half-lives is followed, then titration would be no faster than every 5 to 7 days.

Since methadone was initially used for the treatment of addiction, remnants of stigma surrounding its use for chronic or cancer-related pain may remain. Patients may be wary of being on a medication associated with drug addiction. Although practitioners from a variety of medical fields prescribe methadone, rarely is it a first choice medication and many physicians remain hesitant. Recent methadone-related deaths and the emergence of buprenorphine as an alternative long-acting opioid may also deter prescribing among physicians.

The cost of methadone is often substantially less compared to other common opioid therapies. The pharmacoeconomic benefit may be another reason to prescribe methadone over other medications and treatments. The drug is usually far less expensive than other opioids formulations. It should be noted that different formulations may have varying costs. For example, the liquid form is more expensive than the oral form. The oral formulation however remains the commonest form of methadone used often providing for a relative financial advantage.

Conclusions

Although methadone remains an effective analgesia, new information about its adverse event profile must give prescribers pause in evaluating the risk benefit ratio. QTc prolongation is one particular risk that must be kept in mind along with other adverse events such as respiratory depression. Other prescribed and nonprescribed medications, alcohol, and illicit substances concomitantly taken while on methadone therapy may be a confounding factor in assessing risk. Methadone continues to be a compelling choice for some clinicians due to its comparable efficacy to other opioids, attractive multiple pharmacologic actions, low cost, lack of active metabolites, and multiple available formulations. However, the growing body of evidence supporting much greater risks associated with methadone than previously appreciated should temper enthusiasm and heighten risk management required in using methadone for pain. Moreover, clinicians who choose to prescribe methadone must become familiar with its special properties and adverse effects and possess the risk management skills necessary for its safe use.

References

1. Fredheim OM, Moksnes K, Borchgrevink PC, Kaasa S, Dale O. Clinical pharmacology of methadone for pain. Acta Anaesthesiol Scand. 2008;52(7):879–89.
2. Burns L, Conroy E, Mattick RP. Infant mortality among women on a methadone program during pregnancy. Drug Alcohol Rev. 2010;29(5):551–6.
3. Broussard CS, Rasmussen SA, Reefhuis J, et al. Maternal treatment with opioid analgesics and risk for birth defects. Am J Obstet Gynecol. 2011;204(4):314.e1–11.
4. Fishman SM, Wilsey B, Mahajan G, Molina P. Methadone reincarnated: novel clinical applications with related concerns. Pain Med. 2002;3(4):339–48.
5. George S, Moreira K, Fapohunda M. Methadone and the heart: what the clinician needs to know. Curr Drug Abuse Rev. 2008; 1(3):297–302.
6. Gagajewski A, Apple FS. Methadone-related deaths in Hennepin county, Minnesota: 1992–2002. J Forensic Sci. 2003;48(3): 668–71.
7. Krantz MJ, Martin J, Stimmel B, Mehta D, Haigney MC. QTc interval screening in methadone treatment. Ann Intern Med. 2009;150(6):387–95.
8. Paulozzi LJ, Ryan GW. Opioid analgesics and rates of fatal drug poisoning in the United States. Am J Prev Med. 2006;31(6): 506–11.
9. Mercadante S, Porzio G, Ferrera P, et al. Sustained-release oral morphine versus transdermal fentanyl and oral methadone in cancer pain management. Eur J Pain. 2008;12(8):1040–6.
10. Weschules DJ, Bain KT. A systematic review of opioid conversion ratios used with methadone for the treatment of pain. Pain Med. 2008;9(5):595–612.
11. Center for Disease Control & Prevention Prescription Painkiller Overdoses: Methadone. 2012. http://www.cdc.gov/Features/VitalSigns/MethadoneOverdoses/index.html

Toxicology Screening for Opioids

15

Gary L. Horowitz

Key Points
- Screening immunoassays for opiates generate clinically significant false-negative and false-positive results.
- Urine is the specimen of choice for detecting opioids: concentrations are much higher, and opioids can be detected for much longer.
- The patterns and relative concentrations of opioids detected have clinical significance.

Introduction

Monitoring compliance in the field of pain medicine is critically important. The medications that are used are powerful, and the potential for abuse is high. Some patients do not take the prescribed medications in favor of diversion or trafficking [1, 2], and some patients may abuse opioids other than those prescribed. Further complicating matters is that laboratory testing for opioids, though it seems straightforward, can be confusing. Physicians rarely receive adequate training in test ordering and interpretation. Laboratory methods vary tremendously; in addition, laboratorians are rarely consulted and, when they are, may be ill-equipped to answer clinically important questions.

Among the issues covered in this chapter will be the clinical importance of the methods used to detect opioids, the reasons that urine is the preferred sample type, and some of the subtleties related to opioid concentrations and metabolites.

G.L. Horowitz, M.D. (✉)
Department of Pathology, Beth Israel Deaconess Medical Center, 330 Brookline Avenue, Boston, MA 02215, USA

Harvard Medical School, Boston, MA, USA
e-mail: ghorowit@bidmc.harvard.edu

Background

The first question that confronts physicians when contemplating monitoring opioid compliance is what tests to order. Most clinical laboratories offer an "opiate screening assay," but it is often not clear which drugs such screens detect and which drugs they fail to detect. It would be logical, but wrong, to conclude that such screening methods detect all opioids; indeed, very few, if any, can detect all opioids [3]. Furthermore, even if a screening assay is positive, one cannot tell, from the screening assay alone, which opioid was detected, resulting in potentially very misleading, and unfortunate, consequences.

Screening methods were developed principally to help evaluate emergency room patients quickly in order to implement appropriate clinical care rapidly [4]. Traditional analytical methods require combinations of chromatography and mass spectroscopy to generate definitive results. Only specialized laboratories are able to offer such testing, and it often takes several hours to complete an analysis. A major advantage of these methods, though, is that they allow for the identification, and quantitation, of individual drugs (and, frequently, their metabolites).

In contrast, screening immunoassays can be performed by virtually any laboratory, from a physician's office laboratory to a community hospital to an academic medical center. They can be run by ordinary laboratory technologists, on conventional automated equipment used for other routine chemistry tests (such as glucose, creatinine, CK, ALT), and cost remarkably little to perform. When analyses of their clinical performance in the emergency department are compiled, screening immunoassays stand up quite well [5].

Nonetheless, applied to the field of pain medicine, as they so often are, a different picture emerges. In the emergency room, the physician may not care whether a patient is taking morphine versus hydromorphone; he simply needs to know whether there are opioids in the patient's system. For a pain medicine physician, though, the distinction is critical. If she has prescribed hydromorphone, she wants to know whether hydromorphone is present, but she also would like to know if any other opioids are present. With screening immunoassays, one can only say that an opioid is (probably) present. (As we will see later, one cannot be 100 % sure until the result is confirmed by another method based on a different principle.)

In other words, for pain management, screening immunoassays are not sufficient. They can be used, but one needs to ensure that they will detect all the drugs of interest, at relevant concentrations, and that all positive results will be confirmed by a second method.

Scientific Foundation

Methods: Screening Versus Gas Chromatography/Mass Spectroscopy

With chromatographic methods (most commonly, gas chromatography), individual drugs are typically identified by their "retention time," the time it takes them to travel through the system [6]. As reflected in Fig. 15.1, individual opioid drugs each elute from the system at characteristic times. Thus, hydrocodone and morphine elute at roughly 4 and 8 min, respectively. However, it is possible that another drug (or indeed substance of any kind), totally unrelated to hydrocodone (or morphine), could be present in the peak at 4 (or 8) min.

To be absolutely sure that another compound has not "co-eluted" at a given time, the compound(s) eluting at each time is (are) subjected to a second analysis, typically mass spectroscopy. In this technique, each compound presumptively identified by its retention time is ionized, and the resulting fragments, characteristic for the compound, are identified by their mass/charge ratios [7]. A typical mass spectrum for morphine is depicted in Fig. 15.2. If a compound other than morphine eluted at the same time by gas chromatography, it would have an entirely different mass spectrum.

Based on the retention time as well as the mass spectrum, the drug's identity can be assured. As will be seen in the examples later, this is a fundamental principle in clinical toxicology – one must identify each compound by two methods, each of which is based on a distinct analytical principle. It is possible that other compounds could co-elute and/or that other compounds might have the same (or similar) fragmentation patterns, but it is virtually impossible that another molecule would share both characteristics. These methods are the gold standards for identification,

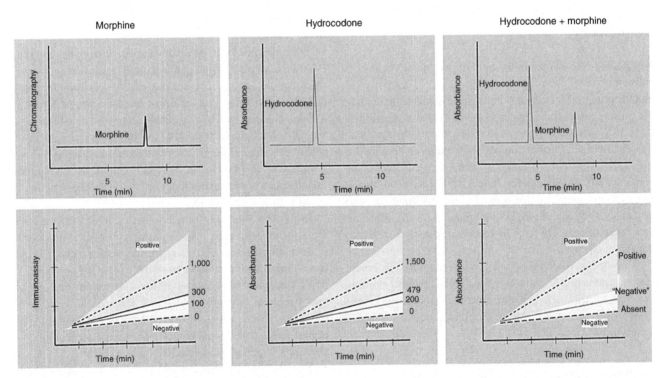

Fig. 15.1 In the top row, the three schematics for gas chromatography show that samples containing morphine, hydrocodone, and a combination of the two can be distinguished from one another because the time it takes the compounds to elute from the system differ. In contrast, in the bottom row, the three schematics show that an immunoassay cannot distinguish among these samples. In each case, the region shaded more darkly represents a positive result; the region shaded less darkly, a negative result. In the leftmost figure, a sample with a morphine concentration of 300 ng/mL is right at the threshold for a positive result; a sample with a morphine concentration of 1000 ng/ml, positive. In the middle figure, because of hydrocodone's reduced cross-reactivity, a hydrocodone concentration of 479 ng/mL is required to reach the positive threshold for the assay. In the right-hand figure, a sample containing both drugs would test positive, but one cannot know whether it represents only morphine, only hydrocodone, or a combination of the two

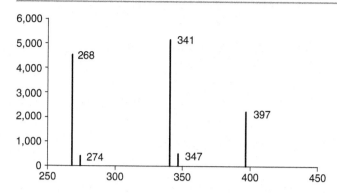

Fig. 15.2 Mass spectrum for morphine. After ionization, morphine is broken down into characteristic fragments, whose relative abundances are plotted against their mass/charge ratios. In this assay, the fragment with a mass/charge ratio of 341 is most abundant, followed by fragments with ratios of 268 and then 397; fragments with ratios of 274 and 347 are much less common. The pattern is unique for morphine

but they both are labor-intensive, demand significant expertise, and require expensive capital equipment.

It is relatively straightforward for the laboratory to determine whether its method can detect a given drug and the smallest concentration it can reliably detect. Thus, the laboratory should be able to provide its users with this data relatively easily. In addition, the laboratory should indicate which drugs are not in its repertoire, and it presumably would be able to offer advice on alternative ways to detect them. The laboratory report should explicitly indicate every individual drug for which the sample was tested, along with the detection limit. Thus, if the "opioid panel" does not explicitly indicate that testing for methadone (or tramadol, or buprenorphine, or fentanyl) was done, then the correct inference is that the test was not done. In most cases, none of these drugs is part of a typical opioid panel [8]. Too often, physicians infer that if a drug is not specifically mentioned, then it was not present.

As noted earlier, opiate screening immunoassays (which include techniques such as EMIT [9], FPIA [10], KIMS [11], CEDIA [12], etc.) can be, and are, performed by virtually any clinical laboratory, often in connection with an emergency toxicology program. Space does not permit a discussion of all the different methods here, but it may help to describe one method, one that is familiar to the author. The salient clinical performance characteristics are very similar for other methods.

In the EMIT assay [13], a small aliquot of a patient's sample is added to a cuvette in which an antibody and an enzyme-labeled drug are present. The drug from the patient and the enzyme-labeled drug compete for the limited sites on the antibody molecules. When the enzyme-labeled drug molecule binds to the antibody, the enzyme activity is inhibited. The more drug present in the patient sample, the less of the enzyme-labeled drug is bound to the antibody (i.e., this is a competitive immunoassay), and therefore, the more enzyme

activity remains in the cuvette [14]. Substrate for the enzyme is added, and the enzyme activity is measured spectrophotometrically as the slope of the line relating absorbance to time, as depicted in Fig. 15.1. If the slope of the line is greater than that of the calibrator (in this case, 300 ng/mL morphine), the result is considered positive; if it is lower, then the result is negative.

As shown in Fig. 15.1, though, the enzyme activity for hydrocodone and the enzyme activity for morphine cannot be distinguished from each other. Each drug with which the antibody reacts will cause an increase in enzyme activity, but it is the same enzyme, and therefore there is nothing unique about the reaction. Thus, one cannot tell from this test which drug is present. In addition, one cannot know if there is one drug, or more than one drug, present. Moreover, one cannot know how much of any given drug is present because the cross-reactivities of the antibody with each drug are not 100 % (see later). In contrast to the case with gas chromatography (even when it is not paired with mass spectroscopy), then, one cannot determine from opiate screening immunoassays which opioids are present nor how much of any drug is present. As a result, it is important, at least in the field of pain management, that positive screening immunoassays be subjected to further analysis to identify which opioids are present.

Another important limitation of opiate screening immunoassays is that a number of important opioids are not detected. Although each assay has its own characteristics, opioids typically not detected include methadone, meperidine, oxycodone, tramadol, buprenorphine, and fentanyl [7]. At this point, it might be worthwhile pointing out that, although people tend to use the terms "opiate" and "opioid" interchangeably, there is a distinction. "Opioids" is the term used to describe all drugs with morphine-like actions; "opiates" are those opioids derived from opium, a group that includes morphine and codeine. Thus, it is perhaps not coincidental that the screening immunoassays are referred to as "opiate immunoassays" rather than "opioid immunoassays"; they are particularly adept at detecting the drugs with structures similar to morphine (see later) [15, 16].

Figure 15.3 provides a flow chart suggesting one way to utilize screening immunoassays effectively in connection with pain management programs; the flow chart needs to be customized to the specific assays available from each laboratory.

Specimen of Choice

Physicians often wonder why laboratories prefer to do opioid measurements on urine, a preference that gives rise to other problems (e.g., sample collection and adulteration). When a blood sample is drawn, one is reasonably certain that one knows the identity of the patient from whom it came and that

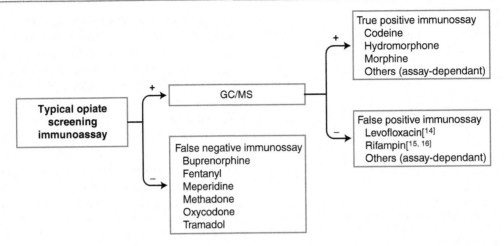

Fig. 15.3 Flow chart for using opiate immunoassays effectively. When using opiate immunoassays as the first step in screening urine samples, it is important to realize that several opioids may not be detected (buprenorphine, fentanyl, meperidine, methadone, oxycodone, and tramadol). Also, all positive results should be confirmed by a second method, such as gas chromatography/mass spectroscopy. If a specific opioid cannot be confirmed, then the original immunoassay result must be considered a false positive. As with all the examples in this chapter, the chart must be customized for each laboratory methods

Table 15.1 Urine versus serum morphine concentrations

Route (amount)	Serum peak (time)	Other serum (time)	Urine peak (time)	Other urine (time)
Intravenous [18] (0.125 mg/kg, ~9 mg)	440 (0.5 min)	20 (2 h)		
Intramuscular [18] (0.125 mg/kg, ~9 mg)	70 (15 min)	20 (4 h)		
By mouth [18] (30-mg tablet)	20 (4 h)			
By mouth [19] (7.5 mg from poppy seeds)	100 (2 h)	6 (24 h)	1,568 (3 h)	720 (24 h)
All concentrations are in ng/mL				

it has not been adulterated in any way, not to mention that one can always get a blood sample from a patient.

There are many reasons for the analytic preference for urine. Drugs are typically concentrated manyfold in the urine, and drugs are present in the urine in relatively high concentrations for many hours [17]. Even in the best case scenario, where one knows exactly which opioid was ingested and when the ingestion occurred, so that one can predict reasonably well when the blood peak concentration will occur, the peak value is manyfold less than the typical urine concentration. For morphine, as shown in Table 15.1, a 0.125 mg/kg intravenous injection will result in a peak concentration in blood of 440 ng/mL after 1 min, which will rapidly decline to just 20 ng/mL at 2 h [18] (and less than that at later times). In contrast, in a study where the peak serum concentration was 100 ng/ml (4.4 fold lower than that just mentioned), the urine concentration averaged 1, 568 ng/mL at 3 h and 720 ng/mL at 24 h [19]. The lesson is clear – if one is trying to detect morphine (or other opioids), it will be easiest to detect it in the urine.

Another reason that most clinical laboratories prefer urine samples is that the assays they use (screening immunoassays) are FDA-approved for use with urine samples only. Laboratories are permitted to run these assays on urine after doing relatively straightforward validation studies. In order to run these same assays on blood, however, laboratories are required to undertake much more extensive validation studies, studies that few laboratories have the resources to do.

Nonetheless, there are a few caveats about using urine samples that are important to keep in mind. As mentioned earlier, specimen collection can be problematic. In the absence of a discrete witnessed voiding, it is possible for patients to substitute pristine urine samples for their own, and it is also possible for patients to add adulterants to a sample of their own urine, adulterants which can interfere with some testing methods [20, 21]. Even with a valid sample from the correct patient, massive hydration, or skipping a drug for several days, can render the concentration so low that it becomes undetectable by some methods [2, 21]. In other words, it is difficult to document conclusively that a patient has not used a drug.

Concentration/Metabolites

As mentioned earlier, with screening immunoassays, it is never clear which opioids are causing the positive reaction; a positive reaction looks the same no matter which opioid

Table 15.2 Immunoassay cross-reactivities

	Assay 1	Assay 2	Assay 3
Morphine	300	300	300
Codeine	50	225	247
Hydrocodone	100	479	364
Hydromorphone	100	620	498
Meperidine	250,000	30,508	>50,000
Oxycodone	1,000	23,166	5,388

Extracted from Magnani [22]

Shown above are the lowest concentrations of selected opioids that will cause a positive immunoassay result with three different commercial assays

All concentrations are in ng/mL

caused it. In truth, it is even a little more complicated. Although each assay is calibrated to turn positive at 300 ng/mL of morphine, other opioids show different amounts of cross-reactivity (Table 15.2) [22]. This is true whether one considers a given manufacturer's assay (columns) or whether one looks at a given opioid across manufacturers (rows). For example, for assay 1, hydrocodone will turn positive at a concentration of 100 ng/mL, but oxycodone will not turn positive until the concentration reaches 1,000 ng/mL; for assay 2, the corresponding figures are 479 and 23,156 ng/mL; and for assay 3, 364 and 5,388 ng/mL. Does this mean a sample with a concentration of 250 ng/mL of hydrocodone will be reported as positive by assay 1 and negative by assays 2 and 3? Absolutely!

As mentioned earlier (and reflected in Table 15.2 for meperidine and oxycodone), none of the opiate screening immunoassays can be relied upon to detect buprenorphine, fentanyl, meperidine, methadone, or oxycodone. This is not entirely unexpected: these opioids have very different chemical structures, so one might predict that antibodies raised to morphine might not "recognize" them (Fig. 15.4).

There is yet another layer of complexity with opiate screening immunoassays. For emergency toxicology purposes, it may be important to prevent false positives by setting the positive threshold at 300 ng/mL, at which concentration morphine is present in potentially clinically significant amounts. But for pain management physicians, the real question is whether it is there at all. Put differently, as just described, a patient whose urine has a hydrocodone concentration of 250 ng/mL will be reported as negative for opiates by assays 2 and 3, but a patient whose urine has a morphine concentration of 200 ng/mL will be reported as negative by all three assays! To make matters even worse, some laboratories are now using as their positive threshold for opiate screening immunoassays a concentration of 2,000 ng/mL [4, 23].

In summary, there are many ways that opiate screening immunoassays may report as negative samples that have concentrations of opioids that would be of interest to the pain management physician: very poor cross-reactivity; thresholds set at levels more appropriate for emergency toxicology; and samples from patients who, by avoiding banned drugs for a few days or by overhydrating themselves, have succeeded in lowering their urine opioid concentrations to very low levels.

When testing is done by gas chromatography/mass spectroscopy, in addition to the specific drug(s) present, you can (and should) consider the expected patterns of metabolism [18]. Assuming your laboratory provides specific data on all the relevant compounds, you should not be surprised to see oxymorphone in the urine of patients on oxycodone therapy since it is a known metabolite. Similarly, since hydromorphone is a metabolite of hydrocodone, it would not be unexpected to find both opioids in a patient taking hydrocodone. In contrast, a patient taking oxymorphone should not have oxycodone in his urine, and a patient taking hydromorphone should not have hydrocodone in his urine because metabolism does not proceed in the reverse direction in either case. These relationships can be confusing, so Table 15.3 is a shortened version of a table the author prepared for use in his institution. As with all the previous examples, much of the data contained therein needs to be customized by each laboratory to take into account the specific assays in use locally.

Clinical Examples

Concrete examples can be very helpful in understanding the principles just described. Each of the examples that follow is based on a real case; indeed, many of them represent relatively common occurrences.

Since most physicians will use laboratories with screening immunoassays, the examples that follow assume that the initial testing is done in that manner. In some of the cases, the initial assay did not prompt an automatic confirmation by another method, which is often the case in practice (though, as described earlier, it should never be the case in pain management).

Clinical Example #1: I Really Am Taking My Oxycodone (False Negative)

A urine sample from a patient on oxycodone therapy is reported as negative for opiates by screening immunoassay. When you talk with your patient about the results and her apparent noncompliance, she is insistent that she has been taking her medication as prescribed.

You call the laboratory and discover that their opiate screening immunoassay, like most such assays, does not cross-react with oxycodone. In order to reliably detect oxycodone, the laboratory recommends using a different test (gas chromatography or an immunoassay specific for oxycodone). Applied to your patient's original sample, these methods indicate that oxycodone is indeed present.

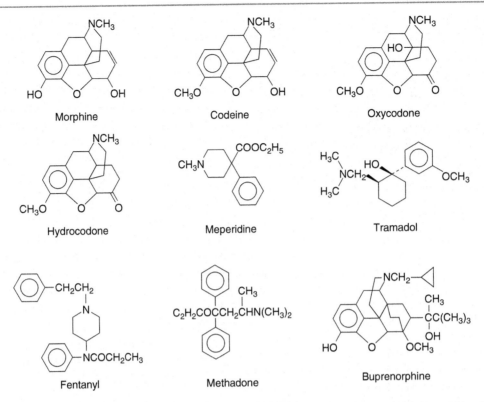

Fig. 15.4 Chemical structures of common opioids. The antibodies used in immunoassays are designed to detect morphine. One might predict that these antibodies would cross-react with codeine and hydrocodone, as their structures are so similar. By the same token, it is not surprising that these antibodies typically do not cross-react with meperidine, tramadol, fentanyl, methadone, and buprenor-phine, whose structures are so different. Although, at first blush, oxycodone looks very similar to morphine, the presence of the (relatively large) hydroxyl (–OH) group in the center of the diagram must be sufficient to limit the cross-reactivity because few opiate immunoassays detect oxycodone (All structures were adapted from Magnani [22])

Clinical Example #2: Methadone Does Not Cause a Positive Opiate Immunoassay

A urine sample from a patient on methadone therapy is reported as positive for opiates by screening immunoas-say from your laboratory. In this case, no confirmatory testing was done. In addition, you ordered a methadone immunoassay on the sample, which was also reported as positive.

When you discuss these findings with the patient, he explains that his methadone is responsible for the positive reaction and that the test proves he is taking his medication as prescribed.

Because of its structure, which is very different from mor-phine (Fig. 15.4), methadone is not detected by opiate screening immunoassays. Indeed, this is the reason that a separate immunoassay is needed for its detection [8, 24, 25].

To prove that the positive opiate screening immunoassay result was not related to methadone, the specimen was referred for confirmatory testing by gas chromatography/mass spectroscopy, which came back positive for morphine.

Clinical Example #3: A True Positive Unrelated to Drug Use

A urine sample from a patient on oxycodone therapy is reported as positive for opiates by screening immunoassay from your laboratory. As requested, the laboratory refers the sample for confirmatory testing, which comes back positive for morphine by gas chromatography/mass spectrometry. There is no indica-tion on the report that oxycodone is present.

If oxycodone is not mentioned, do not assume that it is not present. Good laboratories will report present or absent for each drug tested, often along with their detection limits. In this case, oxycodone was not part of the testing laboratory's opioid panel. One would have to request it specifically in order to have it done.

Fortunately, specific immunoassays are becoming avail-able that make testing for oxycodone as easy as it is to test for methadone [26].

As to the morphine, the patient denied using morphine. A careful history taken after the fact revealed that she had consumed a large number of poppy seed crackers a few hours

Table 15.3 Laboratory facts about opioid tests (applicable only at hospital XYZ)

| Opioid | In-house (rapid TAT) opiate screening immunoassay | | | Gas chromatography/mass spectroscopy | | | |
	Detected	Detection limit ng/mL	Included in GC panel?	Detection limit ng/mL	Metabolites	Typical window of detection (days)
Buprenorphine	No		No (order as individual test)	5	Norbuprenorphine	0.5–1
Codeine	Yes (not specifically identified)	224	Yes	50	Morphine (minor metabolite)	1–2
Fentanyl	No		No (order as individual test)	0.5	Norfentanyl	1 (3 for metabolite)
Hydrocodone	Probably (not specifically identified)	1,100	Yes	50	Hydromorphone dihydrocodeine	1–2
Hydromorphone	Probably (not specifically identified)	1,425	Yes	50	–	1–2
Meperidine	No		Yes	50	Normeperidine	0.5–1
Methadone	No (order methadone immunoassay)		No (order as individual test)	100	–	3–11
Morphine	Yes (not specifically identified)	300	Yes	50		1–2
Oxycodone	No		Yes	50	Oxymorphone noroxycodone	1–1.5 (3 for controlled release)
Tramadol	No		No (order as individual test)	500	–	0.5–1.5

Some information taken from White and Black [24]

Note that opiate immunoassay will not specifically identify any drug

Note that GC/MS detection limits are consistently much lower and that individual drugs are identified

before submitting her urine sample. Although many people believe that poppy seeds cause a false-positive reaction for morphine, poppy seeds in fact contain genuine morphine. It has been well documented that ingestion of realistic numbers of crackers containing poppy seeds can cause true positive results for morphine (Fig. 15.5) [27].

Clinical Example #4: I Really Am Taking My Morphine (False Negative)

A urine sample from a patient on morphine therapy is reported as negative for opiates by screening immunoassay. Although the laboratory does refer samples that test positive for confirmation, this sample underwent no further testing.

When you discuss the apparent lack of compliance with your patient, she maintains that she has been taking the drug regularly. You call the laboratory to discuss the test results, and you discover that the patient's sample showed more reactivity than most negative samples (Fig. 15.1) but less than that required to be called positive. You ask that the sample be referred for more definitive testing. Gas chromatography/mass spectroscopy confirms that morphine is present at a concentration of 200 ng/mL. Most patients on morphine therapy will have urine concentrations far above the 300 ng/mL threshold. But it is possible for urine

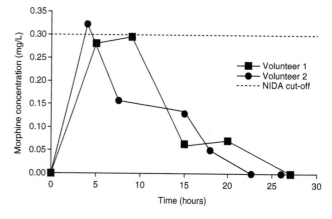

Fig. 15.5 Morphine concentration in urine after eating poppy seed crackers. At several time intervals after eating poppy seed crackers, two volunteers submitted urine samples to determine the morphine concentrations by gas chromatography/mass spectroscopy. As noted, samples from both individuals in the 5–10-h range had values that approached or exceeded the positive threshold (0.30 mg/L (300 ng/mL) (With permission from McCutcheon and Wood [27])

from patients who skip doses (sometimes a sign of bingeing) [2] or from patients who overhydrate themselves [21] to have lower levels. As a result, it is important to note that screening immunoassays are usually calibrated to turn positive at 300 ng/mL of morphine and that lower levels will be called negative.

Clinical Example #5: I Really Am Taking My Hydromorphone (False Negative)

A urine sample from a patient on hydromorphone is reported as negative for opiates by screening immunoassay. When you call the laboratory for clarification, they assure you that their assay can detect the drug (in contrast to methadone and oxycodone). You insist that the sample be sent for a specific assay for hydromorphone, which comes back positive for hydromorphone at a concentration of 350 ng/mL.

Remember that opiate screening immunoassays are calibrated to turn positive at 300 ng/mL of morphine. Because of differences in cross-reactivity, it typically requires higher concentrations of hydrocodone to show this amount of reactivity (Table 15.2). Your patient's sample had 350 ng/mL and was therefore screen negative, but the drug was clearly present.

Clinical Example #6: It's Just Pneumonia (False Positive)

A patient on chronic methadone therapy has been compliant for many years. As his pain medicine consultant, you test him regularly for opiates as well as methadone (separate assay). His methadone test is always positive, and until this most recent test, his opiate screening immunoassay has been negative, just as you expect.

You share the positive opiate screening immunoassay test results with him, telling him how disappointed you are, but he assures you that he has not taken any opioids other than methadone. You arrange to have the sample retested by gas chromatography/mass spectroscopy to identify the specific opiate involved, but no opioid could be identified by the more definitive technique. The opiate screening immunoassay must have been a false positive.

After sharing the good news with the patient, you review his history in more detail, and you uncover the fact that the week before he submitted his urine sample for testing, his primary care physician had started him on a course of levofloxacin for community-acquired pneumonia. Checking the literature, you discover quinolones have been reported to cause false-positive results with opiate screening immunoassays (Fig. 15.6) [14].

Clinical Example #7: When Two Opioids Are Present

A urine sample from a patient on hydromorphone tests positive for opiates by screening immunoassay. Your laboratory has a policy that all samples with positive screening tests be confirmed by gas chromatography/mass spectroscopy. This sample turns out to contain not only hydromorphone but also morphine.

In the absence of the gas chromatography/mass spectroscopy analysis, you would not have been aware of the noncompliance problem (i.e., that this patient is ingesting morphine as well as hydromorphone). With immunoassay

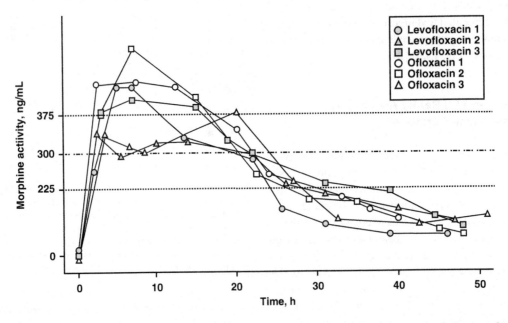

Fig. 15.6 False-positive opiate immunoassays following antibiotic ingestion. At several time intervals after single doses of levofloxacin or ofloxacin, three volunteers submitted urine samples for opiate screening by immunoassay. In every case, these urine samples tested positive for a prolonged period (roughly 24 h) (With permission from Baden et al. [14])

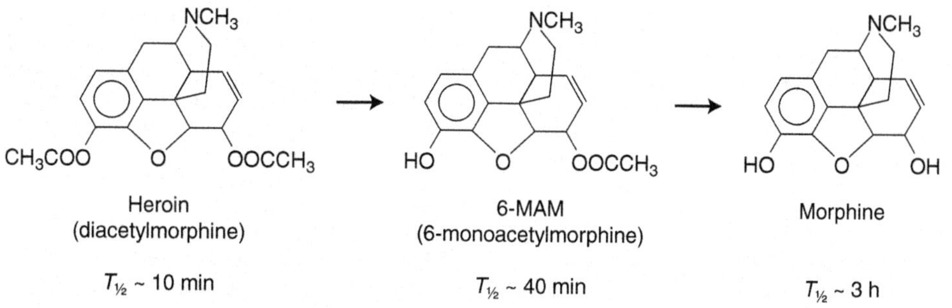

Fig. 15.7 Metabolic pathways relating heroin and morphine. Heroin (diacetyl morphine) is rapidly broken down to 6-monoacetylmorphine (6-MAM), which is then converted to morphine. The half-lives of the three compounds are roughly 10, 40, and 180 min. Thus, if a patient uses heroin, one may only find morphine in the urine; if one does find 6-MAM in addition to morphine, though, it is proof that heroin was the source of the morphine (Adapted from Baselt [18])

screening, you do not know which, or how many, opioids are present in a sample.

Clinical Example #8: Understanding Metabolites #1

A patient on morphine therapy tests positive for opiates by screening immunoassay, and the confirmatory tests always show the presence of morphine only. On his most recent sample, the screening immunoassay is positive again, but the gas chromatography/mass spectroscopy report indicates the presence of a low concentration of hydromorphone (Dilaudid®).

You suspect that the patient has begun using hydromorphone illicitly. When you discuss your suspicion with him, he maintains that he has not used any opioids other than the morphine you prescribe for him.

Further investigation reveals that hydromorphone may be a minor metabolite of morphine and that the results from this sample do not conclusively prove that the patient ingested hydromorphone in addition to his prescribed morphine [28].

Clinical Example #9: Understanding Metabolites #2

A urine sample from a patient on oxycodone was referred to a laboratory for analysis by gas chromatography/mass spectroscopy. The report shows results for both oxycodone (positive) and oxymorphone (absent). Since you know that oxymorphone is a metabolite of oxycodone, you worry that the patient is not taking her oxycodone regularly, diverting the majority of her prescription, and crushing a tablet into her urine sample in order to test positive and remain under your care.

Even though oxymorphone is indeed a metabolite of oxycodone, whether or not it should be detected in urine samples is controversial [29, 30]. Possible explanations include the fact that some patients may not metabolize oxycodone efficiently and that the detection limits of some assays may not be sufficiently low enough. In any case, if pill crushing is a concern, one might decide to revert to a witnessed collection procedure [1].

Clinical Example #10: Understanding Metabolites #3

A patient on morphine therapy always tests positive for opiates by screening immunoassay, and the confirmatory tests always show the presence of morphine only. On his most recent sample, the screening immunoassay is positive again, but the gas chromatography/mass spectroscopy report indicates the presence of 6-monoacetylmorphine (6-MAM) as well as morphine.

You call the laboratory to find out what that means. As indicated in Fig. 15.7, heroin (diacetylmorphine) is metabolized to 6-MAM, which is then metabolized to morphine. The half-lives of heroin and 6-MAM are short (9 and 38 min, respectively), so they do not persist for long in patient samples. If 6-MAM is detected, it is proof that heroin has been taken [31]; morphine is not metabolized to 6-MAM. Its absence does not prove that heroin was not ingested; because of its short half-life, it is present in urine samples for a relatively short time. This patient may have been using heroin all along, but it was only on this sample that traces of the heroin metabolite (and morphine precursor) were found.

Recommendations

Know your laboratory! Compile a list of all the drugs you want to be able to detect in your patients and review it with your lab. Together, put together a set of test orders that will detect all the drugs you want. Common error includes thinking that methadone and oxycodone will be detected by opiate screening immunoassays; they will not!

Insist that all drugs detected by opiate screening immunoassay be confirmed by a second method so as to absolutely eliminate false positives.

Use urine as the preferred specimen to be sure you get the highest concentrations, but be aware of specimen integrity issues.

Concentrations, at least relative concentrations, as well as patterns of drugs detected can be helpful.

References

1. Braithwaite RA, Jarvie DR, Minty PS, et al. Screening for drugs of abuse (I): opiates, amphetamines and cocaine. Ann Clin Biochem. 1995;32:123–53.

2. Gourlay D, Heit HA, Caplan YH. Urine drug testing in primary care. Dispelling the myths & designing strategies. Monograph for California Academy of family Physicians. 2002. http://www.alaskaafp.org/udt.pdf. Accessed on 24 Aug 2012.

3. Hammett-Stabler CA, Pesce AJ, Cannon DJ. Urine drug screening in the medical setting. Clin Chim Acta. 2002;315:125–35.

4. Wu AHB, McKay C, Broussard LA, et al. Laboratory medicine practice guidelines: recommendations for the use of laboratory tests to support poisoned patients who present to the emergency department. Clin Chem. 2003;49:357–9.

5. Bailey DN. Results of limited versus comprehensive toxicology screening in a university medical center. Am J Clin Pathol. 1996; 105:572–5.

6. Annesley TM, Rockwood AL, Sherman NE. Chromatography. In: Burtis CA, Ashwood ER, Bruns DE, editors. Tietz fundamentals of clinical chemistry. 6th ed. St. Louis: Saunders Elsevier; 2008. p. 112–27.

7. Annesley TM, Rockwood AL, Sherman NE. Mass spectrometry. In: Burtis CA, Ashwood ER, Bruns DE, editors. Tietz fundamentals of clinical chemistry. 6th ed. St. Louis: Saunders Elsevier; 2008. p. 128–39.

8. Heit HA, Gourlay D. Urine drug testing in pain medicine. J Pain Symptom Manage. 2004;27:260–7.

9. Rubenstein KE, Schneider RS, Ullman EF. "Homogeneous" enzyme immunoassay: new immunochemical technique. Biochem Biophys Res Commun. 1972;47:846–51.

10. Caplan YH, Levine B, Goldberger B. Fluorescence polarization immunoassay evaluated for screening amphetamine and methamphetamine in urine. Clin Chem. 1987;33:1200–2.

11. Adler FL, Liu CT. Detection of morphine by hemagglutination-inhibition. J Immunol. 1971;106:1684–5.

12. Henderson DR, Friedman SB, Harris JD, et al. CEDIA, a new homogeneous immunoassay system. Clin Chem. 1986;32:1637–41.

13. Kricka LJ. Principles of immunochemical techniques. In: Burtis CA, Ashwood ER, Bruns DE, editors. Tietz fundamentals of clinical chemistry. 6th ed. St. Louis: Saunders Elsevier; 2008. p. 155–70.

14. Baden LR, Horowitz G, Jacoby H, Eliopoulos GM. Quinolones and false-positive urine screening for opiates by immunoassay technology. JAMA. 2001;286:3115–9.

15. van As H, Stolk LM. Rifampicin cross-reacts with opiate immunoassay. J Anal Toxicol. 1999;23:71.

16. Daher R, Haidar JH, Al-Amin H. Rifampin interference with opiate immunoassays. Clin Chem. 2002;48:203–4.

17. Wolff K, Farrell M, Marsden J, et al. A review of biological indicators of illicit drug use, practical considerations and clinical usefulness. Addiction. 1999;94:1279–98.

18. Baselt RC. Disposition of toxic drugs and chemicals in man. 7th ed. Foster City: Biomedical Publications; 2004. p. 759–63.

19. Hayes LW, Krasselt WG, Mueggler PA. Concentrations of morphine and codeine in serum and urine after ingestion of poppy seeds. Clin Chem. 1987;33:806–8.

20. Cook JD, Caplan YH, LoDico CP, Bush DM. The characterization of human urine for specimen validity determination in workplace drug testing: a review. J Anal Toxicol. 2000;24:579–88.

21. Wu AHB. Urine adulteration before testing for drugs of abuse. In: Shaw LM, Kwong TC, editors. The clinical toxicology laboratory. Washington D.C.: AACC Press; 2001. p. 157–72.

22. Magnani B. Concentrations of compounds that produce positive results. In: Shaw LM, Kwong TC, editors. The clinical toxicology laboratory. Washington D.C.: AACC Press; 2001. p. 491–2.

23. Lee PR, Shahala DE. Changes to the cutoff levels for opiates for federal workplace drug testing programs. Substance abuse and mental health services administration. Fed Regist. 1995;60:575–85.

24. White RM, Black ML. Pain management. Washington D.C.: AACC Press; 2007.

25. Simpson D, Braithwaite RA, Jarvie DR, et al. Screening for drugs of abuse (II): cannabinoids, lysergic acid diethylamide, buprenorphine, methadone, barbiturates, benzodiazepines, and other drugs. Ann Clin Biochem. 1997;34:460–510.

26. Backer RC, Monforte JR, Poklis A. Evaluation of the DRI® oxycodone immunoassay for the detection of oxycodone in urine. J Anal Toxicol. 2005;29:675–7.

27. McCutcheon JR, Wood PG. Snack crackers yield opiate-positive urine. Clin Chem. 1995;41:769–70.

28. Reisfeld GM, Chronister CW, Goldberger BA, Bertholf RL. Unexpected urine drug testing results in a hospice patient on high-dose morphine therapy. Clin Chem. 2009;55:1765–9.

29. Smith HS. Opioid metabolism. Mayo Clin Proc. 2009;84:613–24.

30. Schneider J, Miller A. Oxycodone to oxymorphone metabolism. Pract Pain Manag. 2009;7:71–3.

31. von Euler M, Villen T, Svensson J-O, Stahle L. Interpretation of the presence of 6-monoacetylmorphine in the absence of morphine-3-glucuronide in urine samples: evidence of heroin abuse. Ther Drug Monit. 2003;25:645–8.

Monitoring Drug Use and Abuse: The Evolution of a Paradigm

Steven D. Passik and Kenneth L. Kirsh

16

Key Points

- If a prescriber decides that a patient is a candidate for an opioid trial, the equally important decision of how opioid therapy is to be delivered in an individualized fashion must also be made.
- An opioid trial should be preceded by a risk assessment, and opioid therapy should be delivered in a fashion matched to the risk level of the individual.
- Once a trial is initiated and an initial risk assessment is completed, the job of monitoring and evaluating is not over; prescribers need to perform ongoing checkups and evaluations, including documentation in the domains of the 4 A's: analgesia, activities of daily living, adverse side effects, and potentially aberrant drug-taking behaviors.
- Many tools can be used in this initial and ongoing effort, including urine screening, use of prescription monitoring program reports, and creating a visit schedule tailored to the individual.

Introduction

Contrary to reports in the popular media that tend to focus solely on the recent problems of prescription drug abuse, our country faces two, not one, worrisome public health crises. The first is the problem of poorly treated chronic pain,

S.D. Passik, Ph.D. (✉)
Psychiatry and Anesthesiology, Vanderbilt University Medical Center, Psychosomatic Medicine, 1103 Oxford House, Nashville, TN 37232, USA
e-mail: passiks@mskcc.org

K.L. Kirsh, Ph.D.
Department of Behavioral Medicine, The Pain Treatment Center of the Bluegrass, 2416 Regency Road, Lexington, KY 40503, USA
e-mail: doctorken@windstream.net

and the second is the problem of prescription drug abuse. Pain clinicians do not have the luxury of focusing on only one of these two and instead have to attempt to find a balance in their practice that allows them to treat pain with controlled substances as needed and take reasonable steps to prevent drug abuse and diversion.

Affecting approximately 75 million Americans, poorly treated chronic pain causes losses of productivity that amount to more than 60 billion dollars per year while undermining quality of life for patients and families [1–4]. Indeed, chronic pain affects physical, psychological, and social well-being, and patients frequently experience sleep disturbance, depression, and anxiety [5]. Thus, despite advances in the knowledge of pain pathophysiology, understanding of treatments, and development of multidisciplinary approaches to pain management, pain care is still inadequate, and the problem is only expected to grow as the population continues to age.

Understanding Undertreatment

Why is pain still so poorly treated? The treatment of pain is complicated and often requires a multidisciplinary approach, which is becoming increasingly difficult to provide with poor reimbursement from managed care organizations. In addition, chronic pain is not usually associated with sympathetic arousal, and, therefore, the objective signs of physiological stress are often absent. Patients with chronic pain may not appear to be in physical pain, sometimes leading to skepticism by observers, which is particularly true when past histories of substance problems or the potential use of opioid medications are involved. Finally, with increasing regulatory scrutiny and the growth of prescription drug abuse, there has been a trend for clinicians to shy away from using opioids, and this fear reflects that the treatment of pain has become all the more controversial and undesirable [6, 7].

In truth, at the beginning of what became a massive expansion of opioid prescribing, there was a marked tendency to trivialize the risk of drug abuse and addiction, and we are now "playing catch-up." A new paradigm has emerged, one that attempts to incorporate the principles of addiction medicine into pain management, in a manner and fashion that is appropriate to each individual patient. Several instruments have been created to help with screening and ongoing documentation and management of pain patients being considered for or treated with opioid therapy. This does not answer all of the needs, however, and a novel set of guidelines and criteria are proposed that clinicians can use to determine whether they should apply routine or more intensive monitoring and documentation, given the risk level of the patient in question and within the guideposts of peer prescribing.

The Interface of Pain and Drug Abuse

Poorly treated chronic pain persists despite a massive increase of opioid prescribing in the country. Almost every class of analgesics has had substantial increases in prescribing during the last 3 years, with hydrocodone compounds being the most widely prescribed medication in the United States [8]. With the wider availability of opioids has also come a much larger concern about public abuse. From 2002 to 2005, there were 190 million prescriptions for opioids in the United States resulting in 9.4 billion doses [9]. In 2005, for the first time, opioids displaced marijuana to become the new illicit drug of choice [10]. A year later, the National Survey on Drug Use and Health data showed a minimum of 430 million abused doses [11]. Thus, clinicians are placed in a difficult position wherein they acknowledge on one hand that opioids are effective, but are faced with the potential that they might be contributing to drug abuse and diversion on the other. Unlike any other medication class, opioid prescribing requires documentation of informed consent or a treatment agreement.

With the dilemma of treating pain while avoiding abuse and diversion, it is crucial that proper assessments be performed to take reasonable steps to guard against abuse and diversion and to assure that patients are being treated safely and effectively – with gains not only in terms of pain relief but also in terms of stabilization or improvement in their functional status. While clearly a chronic pain assessment should include a detailed assessment of the pain itself, including intensity, quality, location, and radiation of pain, identification of factors that increase and decrease the pain should be elicited as well as a review of the effectiveness of various interventions that have been tried to relieve the pain, and of course, the impact of pain on sleep, mood, level of stress, and function in work, relationships, and recreational activities should be assessed, since improvement in these areas may be a goal of pain treatment and a measure of the efficacy of interventions. To aid in this endeavor, a number of general screening instruments, such as the Brief Pain Inventory, already exist for the clinical setting [12–14].

While these tools are useful for a good generalized assessment, we have been sorely in need of screening instruments designed specifically for identifying patients who are more likely to misuse their opioid medications. To answer this, many researchers have recently flooded the literature with a wide variety of assessment tools to examine potential risk when prescribing opioid analgesics. A few of the more promising measures are discussed below.

Tools for Predicting Risk of Misuse and Abuse in Pain Patients

Most of the recent research has focused on screening tools that can be used to prescreen patients to determine level of risk when considering opioids as part of the treatment regimen. Safe opioid prescribing demands proper risk stratification and the accommodation of that risk into a treatment plan. In addition, we must always keep in mind that a spectrum of nonadherence exists and that this spectrum is distinct for pain patients versus those who use these medications for nonmedical purposes. Nonmedical users can be seen as self-treating personal issues, purely as recreational users, or as having a more severe and consistent substance use disorder or addiction. On the other hand, pain patients are more complex, and their behaviors might range from strict adherence to chemically coping to a frank addiction. Thus, scores indicating increased risk on the following tools do not necessarily indicate addiction, but might be uncovering some of the grey areas of noncompliance.

Screener and Opioid Assessment for Patients With Pain

The Screener and Opioid Assessment for Patients with Pain (SOAPP) is a self-report measure with 14 items utilizing a 5-point scale (0 = never, to 4 = very often) and can be completed by patients while they are in the waiting room. Scores from each item are summed to create a total score, with a cutoff score of 8 or greater suggesting as the cut point to determine risk [15, 16]. The SOAPP has undergone a number of iterations, and the relatively low cutoff score of 8 or greater was chosen partially to account for the underreporting of behaviors. The SOAPP is an accurate tool for assessing abuse potential in patients considered for opioid therapy and has good psychometric properties, although the data available to date are correlational and not causal in nature. In addition, few demographic and medical data were recorded in the validation of the SOAPP, raising the chance for differences to exist in the cutoff scores among different subpopulations.

Despite this, the SOAPP has an active research program behind it and will likely emerge as a clinically relevant tool for years to come.

Opioid Risk Tool

The Opioid Risk Tool (ORT) is made up of 5 yes-or-no self-report items, covering issues such as family and personal history of substance abuse, age, history of preadolescent sexual abuse, and psychological disease [17]. A self-report version is available so that patients can complete it in the waiting room. Alternately, the clinician form can be completed during the patient visit and can be done briefly as part of the patient intake. Positive endorsements are given a score based on patient gender (i.e., a family history of alcoholism equates to a score of 3 for male patients and 1 for female patients), and then, the scores are summed for a total score. Scores of 0–3 are associated with low risk, 4–7 with moderate risk, and 8 or more with high risk for addiction. The ORT was tested on 185 consecutive patients and displayed excellent discriminatory ability in both men and women for identifying patients who will go on to abuse their medications or develop an addiction, with observed c statistic values of 0.82 and 0.85, respectively. The ORT is useful due to its brevity and ease of scoring, but the face-valid nature of the ORT brings up the issue of susceptibility to deception. For many, this will be an acceptable risk tool, but may not be sufficient for all.

Pain Assessment and Documentation Tool

To initiate follow-up once a patient has been started on opioid therapy, it is important to consider four major domains. These domains have been labeled the "4 A's" (analgesia, activities of daily living, adverse effects, and aberrant drug-related behaviors) for teaching purposes [18]. The last "A," aberrant drug-taking behaviors, is perhaps the most salient when considering whether a patient should remain a candidate for opioid therapy. In short, aberrant drug-taking behaviors is a term encompassing a range of behaviors that may or may not be indicative of addiction in a patient, but definitely account for behaviors that need to be addressed and corrected. Examples of aberrant drug-taking behaviors less indicative of addiction can include increase in medication dose without authorization, requesting frequent early renewals, and appearing unkempt. More egregious aberrant drug-taking behaviors include doctor shopping, changing route of administration of medications, and forging prescriptions.

In application, Passik and colleagues [19, 20] set out to field test a short form that could be used as a charting note. The Pain Assessment and Documentation Tool (PADT) is a simple charting device based on the 4 A's that focuses on key outcomes and provides a consistent way to document progress in pain management therapy over time. The PADT is a two-sided chart note that can be easily included in the patient's medical record. It is designed to be intuitive, pragmatic, and adaptable to clinical situations. With regard to time burden, it took clinicians between 10 and 20 min to complete the original tool, and the revised PADT is substantially shorter and only requires a few minutes to complete. The PADT does not provide strict scoring criteria, as it is meant as a charting tool, but evidence from the trials suggests that four or more aberrant behaviors in a 6-month period predicts abuse and possibly true addiction.

Prescribing Outside the Bounds of Typical Practice

Should the prescriber decide that a patient appears to be an acceptable risk for opioid therapy based off one or more of the above screening tools along with clinical judgment, another set of criteria should come into play. Medicine is a peer-practiced art and science and thus requires that some thought be given to what other physicians are doing in their own practices. Where possible, some form of consensus should be established as standards of care while still acknowledging that a great deal of variability exists between physician philosophies and patients' responses and analgesic requirements.

The concept of monitoring opioid prescribing proposes that prescribing patterns can be viewed as either in the normal range of peer-related prescribing or outside of these norms. Prescribing in a normal range refers to the prescribing of opioids in a usual and customary fashion similar to that of their colleagues. Conversely, prescribing outside this zone refers to prescribing opioids in a manner which deviates from the usual prescribing habits of the majority of physicians writing opioid prescriptions. It is important to realize that there is nothing inherently wrong with prescribing outside these loose norms and there may be excellent reasons to do so. However, this concept may be helpful as a mechanism to alert certain prescribers to the fact that they are no longer in line with the usual prescribing practice of the majority of their colleagues, and so may decide to increase the degree, amount, or rigor of documentation.

It may be extremely appropriate to prescribe outside the bounds of typical practice long term for many decades on any given individual patient. The purpose of this label is not to highlight a prescriber as doing something wrong or aberrant, but to help notify prescribers that they are prescribing outside typical bounds for a given patient to ensure that they are aware of this so that they can choose to act (only if appropriate) or do nothing. Although experienced experts in pain medicine may know when they are doing this, novices and health-care providers from other disciplines of medicine may not.

Factors That Define Prescribing Outside the Scope of Normal Practice

Five factors may be important in defining whether a clinician is prescribing outside the scope of normal practice. Some of the factors have clear cut points, while others do not. The first thing to consider is the type of pain complaint; is it controversial or less common when considering opioid therapy (e.g., headaches)? Another thing is whether or not the patient has active psychiatric or substance abuse issues. While not all psychiatric disorders will be complicating factors, things such as depression, bipolar disorder, impulse control disorders, and substance use disorders will complicate care and may indicate prescribing outside the scope of normal practice. A third factor to consider is whether the patient has a significant amount of contact with nonmedical users of opioids. While difficult to determine at times, physicians learning of this social influence need to consider whether this pushes prescribing into a different category. The fourth factor is patient age. While exceptions definitely exist, problems of abuse and addiction are usually associated with younger adults, and this age group does increase risk of outside the box prescribing. Finally, the amount of opioid prescribed is the final factor to consider.

Of all the factors mentioned above, opioid dose is perhaps the most clear-cut (i.e., can be backed by prescribing statistics) but also the most controversial. The doses used in controlled studies are generally in the moderate range (up to 180 mg of morphine or a morphine equivalent per day), although a few patients received higher doses [21–23]. Daily doses above 180 mg of morphine or a morphine equivalent duration involving patients with chronic noncancer pain have not been validated in clinical trials of significant size and thus may be considered the high watermark for appropriate prescribing among peer physicians as reported in the literature (see Table 16.1) [21, 24–26].

Prescribing outside the scope of normal practice for any particular individual patient should not necessarily spark efforts to alter one's prescribing. Although no specific action is necessary when prescribing in this realm, actions which prescribers may choose to take include (a) consultation or referral to a pain specialist, (b) close reevaluation of the patient's clinical situation (e.g., repeat comprehensive history and physical examination and consideration for further medical work-up), (c) careful review of how the prescribing became outside the scope of normal practice and over what period of time, (d) investigation into the patient's home and social environment as well as their contacts with nonmedical users and where their pain medications are stored (e.g., whether they are secured in a locked space and who may have access), or (e) increase the degree of documentation and/or patient monitoring. Certain prescribers such as pain specialists who care for complex challenging patients with persistent pain may appropriately prescribe beyond normal bounds quite often.

If after careful consideration of the individual patient's situation or discussion with a pain specialist a prescriber chooses to attempt to reduce dosing to more modest levels, potential therapeutic options which may be helpful include the opioid rotation, the addition of other medications (e.g., anti-inflammatory agents, adjuvants such as antidepressants and antiepileptic drugs), the addition of behavioral medicine treatment approaches, the addition of physical medicine treatment approaches, the addition of interventional treatment approaches, the addition of neuromodulation treatment approaches, a change to opioid administration intraspinally (with or without additional agents) [27], and/or the addition of complementary and alternative medicine treatment approaches.

Table 16.1 Listing of factors that may lead to opioid prescribing outside the scope of normal practice

#	Factor which may lead to increased medication dosing
1	Progression of the patient's painful condition
2	Development of a new painful condition
3	Aberrant drug-taking behavior
4	Chemical coping (or using medications to treat life stress while not rising to the level of an addiction)
5	Development of opioid tolerance/hyperalgesia
6	Pharmacokinetic phenomena (e.g., ultrarapid metabolizers) [26]
7	Increased spiritual/emotional or socioeconomic suffering
8	"Prescriber style" (e.g., aggressive opioid titration, perhaps with intent to entirely eliminate pain)
9	Pharmodynamic phenomena (e.g., decreased efficiency of the signaling processes of the opioid receptor) [26]
10	Pseudotolerance (e.g., increased physical activity, drug interactions) – a situation in which opioid dose escalation occurs and appears consistent with pharmacological tolerance but, after a thoughtful evaluation, is better explained by a variety of other variables [25]
11	Pseudoaddiction – drug-seeking behavior for the appropriate purpose of pain relief, rather than abuse or substance misuse [24]. It is characterized by a demand for more medication for analgesic purposes, as well as by behaviors that appear similar to those seen in addicted patients (e.g., anger, hostility). Pseudoaddiction can be differentiated from drug misuse by increasing the dose by an appropriate amount and determining whether the complaints abate

Applying a Risk Management Package

Opioid abuse can have harmful consequences, such as stigmatization, opiophobia, and the undertreatment of pain [28]. Hence, it is important that the practice of opioid prescribing strikes a balance between the extremes of widespread opioid use and opioid avoidance, wherein risk stratification is used for patient selection and the principles of addiction medicine are applied during ongoing treatment. Exposure to drugs does not create drug addicts. Rather, only vulnerable individuals who are exposed to drugs have a risk of addiction. Only individuals exposed to alcohol or opioids, who have the genetic, social, and/or psychological predisposition to addiction, actually develop a problem. There is no problem inherent to the chemical nature of opioids; rather, the growing problem of prescription drug abuse is due to the increasing use of prescription drugs among individuals not screened for risk of drug abuse. The recent problems associated with oxycodone have stemmed from the prescription of the opioid to individuals who were not assessed for their risk of drug abuse and then were treated in the context of a low-risk drug treatment paradigm. The sustained-release preparation of oxycodone approved by the Food and Drug Administration (FDA) in 1995 was thought to have much lower abuse potential, leading to the unsubstantiated belief that the risk of opioid addiction was obviated with this slower-release oxycodone [6]. Truly, abuse deterrence is only tested and proven on the streets once the product is made available.

Opioid risk management techniques must be implemented to understand the risk of drug abuse of an individual in order to better guide the decision of whether or not opioids should be used for pain control and, if so, how best to deliver the analgesic and to tailor therapy accordingly. The assessment is directed at determining whether an individual will likely take their medication as prescribed and derive better function from the ~30–60 % pain relief that the opioids provide or whether the opioid will be used as a coping mechanism for other issues and will not lead to psychosocial gains. If the individual has a penchant for recreational drug use, prescription of opioids could lead to the abuse and or diversion of the analgesics and, at worst, addiction. Several patient factors have been found to be predictive of a patient's risk for opioid misuse or abuse. A mental health disorder is a moderately strong predictor of opioid abuse, while a history of illicit drug and alcohol abuse or legal problems is also predictive of future aberrant drug behaviors according to a survey of 145 patients being treated for chronic pain and a systematic review of the literature [29, 30]. Tobacco use is highly prevalent among substance misusers, and the Screening Instrument for Substance Abuse Potential (SISAP) and the Screener and Opioid Assessment for Patients with Pain (SOAPP) include

tobacco use as a factor in determining risk [16, 31]. While smoking has been found to increase the desire to abuse drugs in an addict population ($N = 160$), alternatively, smoking can be used as a form of substance replacement in those trying to abstain from drug use [32, 33]. Furthermore, individuals who have chronic pain smoke at higher rates than the general population [34]. Cigarette use has been correlated with nonspecific low back pain, fibromyalgia, and headache disorders [35–37].

All patients being considered for opioid therapy need an individualized risk assessment. Patients considered for opioid therapy to treat chronic pain need to be assessed for risk of addiction with a validated tool; there have been many devices developed to assess addiction risk in order to help clinicians make better informed decisions regarding treatment for their patients [38]. As described above, the ORT and SOAPP are good choices for many clinics [15–17]. However, whatever tool may be chosen, it is important to approach this with patient from a standpoint that there are no right or wrong answers and that this is an important step in determining a treatment plan.

Delivering opioid therapy at a lower risk begins with learning how to document cases well. Chart reviews of primary care patients in pain management indicate that oftentimes the notes are not complete enough to support continuing opioid treatment. Typical notations such as "pain stable; renew hydrocodone #240" need to be modified to include the 4 A's of pain treatment outcomes discussed above in reference to the PADT [18–20]. This approach helps to broaden the focus of opioid effects beyond analgesia to other important aspects such as physical functioning. An example of a good chart note is, "Mr. Jones is taking hydrocodone for his chronic low back pain. His pain has reduced from severe to moderate and he is now able to attend church with his wife and help with household chores. Constipation had been noted, but he is responding to a bowel regimen; there is no evidence of aberrant drug-related behaviors." This documentation, along with a pain-focused physical examination and corroboration from a source other than self-report such as a significant other, caregiver, urine toxicology screen, or prescription monitoring report, is enough to thoroughly support pain management with opioids.

Addiction is a disorder characterized by craving, continued use despite harm, and compulsive and out-of-control behaviors. Behaviors that are common and sometimes ambiguous can be clearly associated with addiction when they continually reoccur. Fleming demonstrated in a primary care patient population that patients who self-report four or more aberrant drug behaviors over a lifetime are more likely to have a current substance use disorder [39]. Therefore, it is important to document the occurrence of even less predictive aberrant drug behaviors, because additively, they may indicate an addiction problem. Toward this end, there is a tool available called the Addiction Behaviors Checklist that has been designed and validated to longitudinally track behaviors potentially suggestive of addiction in patients taking long-term opioid therapy for chronic pain [40]. In the meantime, the available data suggests that patients should be given a second chance when one of these behaviors less predictive of addiction is noted; only when the problem reoccurs over a 6–12 month period should opioid therapy discontinuation or a referral be considered. Some individuals with chronic pain are treatable by primary care physicians, while others may require comanagement with a specialist or complete management by a clinician with addiction medicine training.

Aberrant behaviors can be due to several different etiologies, such as pseudoaddiction, in which poorly treated pain causes patients desperate for relief to appear as if they are addicted to their medication. Although pseudoaddiction was a concept first reported in the literature as a case study two decades ago, it has *not* been empirically validated, and it has been overextended. Moreover, sometimes in the face of circumstances that could be due to pseudoaddiction, dosages are escalated to unsafe levels. Instead, in cases where patients exhibit aberrant behaviors and complain of unrelieved pain, alternative approaches to pain control can be pursued instead of continued dose escalation [24, 41]. For example, for a patient who is seemingly unable to take their oxycodone as prescribed due to unrelieved pain, they can instead be prescribed a drug with a lower street value, such as sustained-release morphine. In addition, the patient could be given a urine toxicology screen and scheduled for an appointment with a psychologist in order to address the behavioral problems in opioid drug taking. Pseudoaddiction is a behavioral syndrome that needs to be addressed along with improving pain control. On the other hand, other individuals exhibit aberrant drug-taking behaviors when self-medicating to address a psychiatric issue, while still others may be selling their opioid medications. Individuals involved in drug diversion will be negative for opioids in a urine toxicology screen and will have no medicine to show when called in early for a pill count.

Tolerance and physiological dependence are *not* signs of addiction in an individual exposed to opioids for medical purposes. Although there are many behaviors that can be indicative of a developing drug addiction, such as stealing another patient's drugs or injecting an oral opioid formulation, most of these obvious signs are not reported by patients [42]. Meanwhile, other types of behaviors, such as early dosing, drug hoarding, and increasing the dose without physician's consent, are less predictive of addiction and very common. Opioid drug studies indicate that approximately 15–20 % of patients exhibit multiple behaviors possibly indicative of addiction. Therefore, with higher risk patients who are prone to engaging in aberrant behaviors, other systems of monitoring should be incorporated within their pain management program.

Once opioid treatment has begun, prescription monitoring program data can be an invaluable way to identify patients who are "doctor shopping"; however, this type of data varies in accessibility and quality from state to state, with many states now having operational prescription drug monitoring programs [43]. Still, a high-quality national database is yet needed to monitor opioid prescriptions in order to identify patients who doctor-shop across state lines. Prescribers who do not have the availability of a statewide program to track controlled substance prescriptions should at minimum develop a system to minimize duplicate prescriptions within their group practice.

Compliance monitoring with urine toxicology screens is also needed to corroborate patient claims due to the well-recognized unreliability of self-reported information [44]. The results of this drug testing can indicate whether the patient is taking their opioid medications as prescribed, whether they are obtaining controlled substances from another source, and whether they are concurrently taking illicit drugs. Urine toxicology screens are used for long-term monitoring in order to reduce the risk of a potentially serious adverse event, such as addiction or medication misuse, but are not intended to police patients. With chronic pain management, as with other chronic conditions such as heart disease and cancer, the ongoing consequences of treatment must be monitored to ensure safety. Observations of only patient behaviors are often not enough information to clearly indicate the presence or absence of drug misuse or abuse. Even pain and addiction specialists fail to identify a problem in one in five patients as indicated by surprise urine testing that showed drug use outside of the prescribed opioid and dose [44]. New technology developed for urine screening provides results in <5 min for 12 illicit or controlled substances at the point of care. The Federation of State Medical Board furnishes a strong foundation for support of the reimbursement of urine toxicology screening costs. Their model policy strongly recommends urine toxicology screens in patients who are considered high risk for nonadherence to taking their medications as prescribed and as an occasional screening tool to corroborate patient reports.

Due to the high prevalence of procurement of opioids from a family or friend, even adherent patients should be educated about drug storage and inventorying; "self-treaters" often have the misconception that sharing prescription medications is safe. Indeed, education regarding drug storage and sharing is another aspect of due diligence needed in comprehensive opioid risk management. Opioids should be locked away. New devices are being developed that allow the patient only to have access to medications on a schedule programmed by the clinician and, if tampered with, sends a notification email to the prescriber. When prescribing a pain reliever for a high-risk patient, it may be best not to initiate therapy with an opioid with a high abuse rate.

Furthermore, highly structured approaches to therapy should be implemented for these patients. This type of strategy was assessed in a primary care population at a Veterans Affairs hospital in 335 patients who were referred due to aberrant drug behaviors [45]. Once enrolled in the "opioid renewal clinic," they signed an opioid treatment agreement, underwent frequent doctor visits, prescribed limited amounts of opioids on a short-term basis (either weekly or bi-weekly), and were given random urine toxicology screens and pill counts. When needed, the patients were given counseling and comanagement with addiction services. With this type of structured care intervention, 45 % of patients stopped abusing their opioids and pharmacy cost savings were noted [45]. Another study of 500 patients enrolled in an adherence monitoring program with similar structured care elements noted a 50 % reduction in the incidence of opioid abuse [46]. For actively drug-abusing patients with severe pain resulting in functional interference, a methadone-based program combined with adherence, motivational, and cognitive-behavioral therapies has been applied with positive outcomes [47]. A National Institute on Drug Abuse study of these interventions for 40 opioid-abusing patients with pain found significant reductions in positive tests for nonprescribed opioids and reductions in illicit drugs, along with positive tests for methadone after 6 months of treatment.

Conclusion and Future Directions

While the psychometrics of various screening tools still require further evaluation and the in/out of the box concept needs further refinement, we must remember that good pain management should lead to some decreases in pain perception for the patient combined with a corresponding increase in ability to function. By reviewing these tools and proposed novel guidelines for in/out of the box prescribing and adopting them into practice as appropriate, the physician will take a significant step in providing effective pain management for their pain patient while minimizing risk of opioid misuse.

References

1. ABC News/USA Today/Stanford University Medical Center Poll: Pain. Broad experience with pain sparks a search for relief. 2011. Available at: http://www.abcnews.go.com/images/Politics/979a1T heFightAgainstPain.pdf. Accessed 11 Jan 2011.
2. American Pain Foundation. Annual report. 2006. http://www.painfoundation.org/About/2006AnnualReport.pdf. Accessed 10 May 2010.
3. McCarberg BH, Billington R. Consequences of neuropathic pain: quality-of-life issues and associated costs. Am J Manag Care. 2006;12(9 Suppl):S263–8.
4. Stewart WF, Ricci JA, Chee E, Morganstein D, Lipton R. Lost productive time and cost due to common pain conditions in the US workforce. JAMA. 2003;290:2443–54.
5. Argoff CE. The coexistence of neuropathic pain, sleep, and psychiatric disorders: a novel treatment approach. Clin J Pain. 2007; 23(1):15–22.
6. Cicero TJ, Inciardi JA, Munoz A. Trends in abuse of Oxycontin and other opioid analgesics in the United States: 2002–2004. J Pain. 2005;6(10):662–72.
7. Lipman AG. Does the DEA truly seek balance in pain medicine? J Pain Palliat Care Pharmacother. 2005;19(1):7–9.
8. Volkow ND. Scientific research on prescription drug abuse, before the Subcommittee on Crime and Drugs, Committee on the Judiciary and the Caucus on International Narcotics Control United States Senate. 2008. Available at: http://www.drugabuse.gov/Testimony/3-12-08Testimony.html. Accessed 10 May 2010.
9. SAMHSA. The NSDUH report: patterns and trends in nonmedical prescription pain reliever use: 2002 to 2005. Substance Abuse and Mental Health Services Administration, Department of Health and Human Services; 2007.
10. SAMHSA. Office of Applied Studies of the Substance Abuse and Mental Health Services Administration. Results from the 2005 National Survey on Drug Use and Health: National Findings. Department of Health and Human Services. Publication No. SMA 06-4194. Available at: http://www.oas.samhsa.gov/ NSDUH/2k5NSDUH/2k5results.htm. Accessed 10 May 2010.
11. SAMHSA. Office of Applied Studies of the Substance Abuse and Mental Health Services Administration. Results from the 2006 National Survey on Drug Use and Health: National Findings. Department of Health and Human Services. Available at: http:// www.oas.samhsa.gov/nsduh/2k6nsduh/2k6Results.pdf. Accessed 10 May 2010.
12. Cleveland CS, Ryan KM. Pain assessment: global use of the brief pain inventory. Ann Acad Med Singapore. 1994;23(2):129–38.
13. Kroenke K, Spitzer RL, Williams JB. The PHQ-9: validity of a brief depression severity measure. J Gen Intern Med. 2001;16(9):606–13.
14. Stratford PW, Binkley J, Solomon P, Finch E, Gill C, Moreland J. Defining the minimum level of detectable change for the Roland-Morris questionnaire. Phys Ther. 1996;76(4):359–65.
15. Akbik H, Butler SF, Budman SH, et al. Validation and clinical application of the screener and opioid assessment for patients with pain (SOAPP). J Pain Symptom Manage. 2006;32:287–93.
16. Butler SF, Budman SH, Fernandez K, Jamison RN. Validation of a screener and opioid assessment measure for patients with chronic pain. Pain. 2004;112:65–75.
17. Webster LR, Webster RM. Predicting aberrant behaviors in opioid-treated patients: preliminary validation of the opioid risk tool. Pain Med. 2005;6:432–42.
18. Passik SD, Weinreb HJ. Managing chronic nonmalignant pain: overcoming obstacles to the use of opioids. Adv Ther. 2000;17:70–83.
19. Passik SD, Kirsh KL, Whitcomb LA, Portenoy RK, Katz N, Kleinman L, Dodd S, Schein J. A new tool to assess and document pain outcomes in chronic pain patients receiving opioid therapy. Clin Ther. 2004;26(4):552–61.
20. Passik SD, Kirsh KL, Whitcomb LA, Schein JR, Kaplan M, Dodd S, Kleinman L, Katz NP, Portenoy RK. Monitoring outcomes during long-term opioid therapy for non-cancer pain: results with the pain assessment and documentation tool. J Opioid Manag. 2005; 1(5):257–66.
21. Ballantyne JC, Mao J. Opioid therapy for chronic pain. N Engl J Med. 2003;349:1943–53.
22. Haythornthwaite JA, Menefee LA, Quatrano-Piacentini AL, Pappagallo M. Outcome of chronic opioid therapy for non-cancer pain. J Pain Symptom Manage. 1998;15:185–94.
23. Raja SN, Haythornthwaite JA, Pappagallo M, Clark MR, Travison TG, Sabeen S, Royall RM, Max MB. Opioids versus antidepressants in postherpetic neuralgia. A randomized, placebo-controlled trial. Neurology. 2002;59:1015–21.
24. Weissman DE, Haddox JD. Opioid pseudoaddiction – an iatrogenic syndrome. Pain. 1989;36:363–6.

25. Pappagallo M. The concept of pseudotolerance to opioids. J Pharm Care Pain Symptom Control. 1998;6:95–8.

26. Smith HS. Variations in opioid responsiveness. Pain Physician. 2008;11:237–48.

27. Smith HS, Deer T, Staats P, Singh V, Sehgal N, Cordner H. Intrathecal drug delivery: a focused review. Pain Physician. 2008;11:S89–104.

28. Zacny J, Bigelow G, Compton P, et al. College on problems of drug dependence taskforce on prescription opioid non-medical use and abuse: position statement. Drug Alcohol Depend. 2003;69(3):215–32.

29. Edlund MJ, Steffick D, Hudson T, et al. Risk factors for clinically recognized opioid abuse and dependence among veterans using opioids for chronic non-cancer pain. Pain. 2007;129(3):355–62.

30. Michna E, Ross EL, Hynes WL, et al. Predicting aberrant drug behavior in patients treated for chronic pain: importance of abuse history. J Pain Symptom Manage. 2004;28(3):250–8.

31. Coambs RB, Jarry JL, Santhiapillai AC, et al. The SISAP: a new screening instrument for identifying potential opioid abusers in the management of chronic malignant pain within general medical practice. Pain Res Manag. 1996;1(3):155–62.

32. Rohsenow DJ, Colby SM, Martin RA, et al. Nicotine and other substance interaction expectancies questionnaire: relationship of expectancies to substance use. Addict Behav. 2005;30(4):629–41.

33. Conner BT, Stein JA, Longshore D, et al. Associations between drug abuse treatment and cigarette use: evidence of substance replacement. Exp Clin Psychopharmacol. 1999;7(1):64–71.

34. Hahn EJ, Rayens MK, Kirsh KL, et al. Brief report: pain and readiness to quit smoking cigarettes. Nicotine Tob Res. 2006;8(3):473–80.

35. Jamison RN, Stetson BA, Parris WC. The relationship between cigarette smoking and chronic low back pain. Addict Behav. 1991; 16(3–4):103–10.

36. Yunus MB, Arslan S, Aldag JC. Relationship between fibromyalgia features and smoking. Scand J Rheumatol. 2002;31(5):301–5.

37. Payne TJ, Stetson B, Stevens VM, et al. The impact of cigarette smoking on headache activity in headache patients. Headache. 1991;31(5):329–32.

38. Passik SD, Kirsh KL, Casper D. Addiction-related assessment tools and pain management: instruments for screening, treatment planning, and monitoring compliance. Pain Med. 2008; 9(S2):S145–66.

39. Fleming MF, Davis J, Passik SD. Reported lifetime aberrant drug-taking behaviors are predictive of current substance use and mental health problems in primary care patients. Pain Med. 2008;9(8): 1098–106.

40. Wu SM, Compton P, Bolus R, et al. The addiction behaviors checklist: validation of a new clinician-based measure of inappropriate opioid use in chronic pain. J Pain Symptom Manage. 2006;32(4): 342–51.

41. Passik SD, Webster L, Kirsh KL. Pseudoaddiction revisited: a commentary on clinical and historical considerations. Pain Manag. 2011;1(3):239–48.

42. Passik SD, Portenoy RK, Ricketts PL. Substance abuse issues in cancer patients. Part 1: prevalence and diagnosis. Oncology (Williston Park). 1998;12(4):517–21, 524.

43. Office of Diversion Control. State prescription drug monitoring programs. http://www.deadiversion.usdoj.gov/faq/rx_monitor.htm.

44. Katz N, Fanciullo GJ. Role of urine toxicology testing in the management of chronic opioid therapy. Clin J Pain. 2002;18(4 suppl): S76–82.

45. Wiedemer NL, Harden PS, Arndt IO, et al. The opioid renewal clinic: a primary care, managed approach to opioid therapy in chronic pain patients at risk for substance abuse. Pain Med. 2007; 8(7):573–84.

46. Manchikanti L, Manchukonda R, Damron KS, et al. Does adherence monitoring reduce controlled substance abuse in chronic pain patients? Pain Physician. 2006;9(1):57–60.

47. Bethea A, Acosta M, Haller D. Role of the therapeutic alliance in the treatment of pain patients who abuse prescription opioids. "PROJECT PAIN." NIDA (Grant #R01DA1369). In: Paper presented at: College on problems of drug dependence, Scottsdale, 17–22 June 2006.

Polypharmacy and Drug Interaction

17

Christopher A. Steel and Jill Eckert

Key Points

- When prescribing multiple drugs, consider the following:
  - The desired effect of each drug being administered, the clinical goal, or end point for each
  - Side effect profile of each of the drugs being administered and how they may be potentiated by an additional drug
  - Each of the drug effects on the metabolism of other drugs being administered
  - Impact of systemic illness such as renal or hepatic failure on specific drug levels
  - Likely risks of toxicity and which signs or symptoms to monitor for closely

Introduction

In days past, a basic understanding of a drug's mechanism of action was sufficient for the purpose of prescribing a medication to treat the vast majority of patients and their conditions. Those days are long gone with 48 % of Medicare beneficiaries over the age of 65 having three or more chronic medical conditions and 21 % having five or more of these conditions [1]. It has been estimated that the likelihood of a drug interaction in a patient taking only two different medications is

only 6 %, whereas when the number of medication increases to ten, the likelihood of drug interaction increases to 100 % [2]. With this virtual certainty of frequently dealing with drug interaction, a physician must have a solid understanding of polypharmacy along with drug interactions.

Background

Not only has the increase in prescription medication influenced the need for understanding drug interactions; recent research has identified which specific enzymes are inhibited or induced by drugs and which drugs are substrates for these enzymes. This knowledge allows physicians to anticipate an added drug's likely pharmacokinetic response when administered to a patient already taking a variety of medications.

Pain physicians use a variety of medications and must therefore have a vast armamentarium of different drug groups and individual drugs. They must possess knowledge of not only what the drug does to target sites in the body (pharmacodynamics) but also how the body metabolizes and eliminates the drug (pharmacokinetics). Combining this information with reported adverse events and known side effects, a physician can dramatically reduce the chances of prescribing or administering a medication which will result in an adverse drug interaction. This chapter will discuss some of the more pertinent potential interactions; please refer to specific prescribing information for a specific medication to obtain a complete list of interactions and side effects.

Anticonvulsants

Anticonvulsant drugs exert their effect on pain via multiple pathways. Those felt to contribute greatly in the treatment of chronic pain include calcium channel blockade, depressed glutamate transmission, sodium channel blockade, and gamma-aminobutyric acid (GABA) potentiation [3].

C.A. Steel, M.D. (✉)
Department of Anesthesiology, Pennsylvania State University Milton S. Hershey Medical Center, 500 University Drive, 850, Hershey, PA 17033, USA
e-mail: chris_a_steel@yahoo.com

J. Eckert, DO
Department of Anesthesiology, Pennsylvania State University Milton S. Hershey Medical Center, 500 University Drive, 850, Hershey, PA 17033, USA

Pennsylvania State University College of Medicine, Hershey, PA, USA
e-mail: jeckert@psu.edu

T.R. Deer et al. (eds.), *Treatment of Chronic Pain by Medical Approaches: the AMERICAN ACADEMY of PAIN MEDICINE Textbook on Patient Management*, DOI 10.1007/978-1-4939-1818-8_17,
© American Academy of Pain Medicine 2015

Anticonvulsant drugs are classified in two main groups: first generation and second generation. The first-generation drugs include benzodiazepines, carbamazepine, ethosuximide, phenobarbital, phenytoin, primidone, and valproic acid. The second generation consists of felbamate, gabapentin, lamotrigine, oxcarbazepine, pregabalin, tiagabine, topiramate, vigabatrin, and zonisamide. Of the above drugs, only those commonly used for the treatment of chronic pain will be discussed in detail.

First-generation drugs unfortunately exhibit high toxicity along with multiple drug interactions. This group has continued to be utilized due to its proven efficacy and low cost [4, 5]. To safely use this group of drugs, a practitioner must understand the pharmacodynamics including the mechanism of action of each drug, pharmacokinetics, and adverse effects to fully appreciate the implications of its use on the other medications being used by a patient.

Phenytoin

The effect of this medication is mediated via slowing of the recovery rate of the voltage-activated sodium channels even at low levels of this drug. At higher levels, potentiation of GABA and decreased glutamate transmission can be detected [3, 6]. Phenytoin is approximately 90 % bound by plasma proteins which allows small changes in albumin levels or competition with other drugs to greatly affect the free phenytoin level. The plasma half-life of phenytoin increases as the plasma concentration increases.

The drug interactions are due to the metabolism of phenytoin by certain liver enzymes and the induction of certain liver enzymes. Phenytoin is known to increase (or induce) the metabolism of drugs which are metabolized by CYP2C and CYP3A enzymes, and this maximum induction takes place 1–2 weeks after initiation of the drug [7]. This causes a decrease in the level of many drug groups including antiepileptic drugs (AEDs) and antidepressants. Oral contraceptive pills are known to be unreliable when phenytoin started. Notably, there is a decrease in the ethinylestradiol component of birth control when phenytoin is implemented, requiring at least 50 mcg ethinylestradiol in the patient's oral contraceptive and a warning to report any abnormal bleeding patterns [8]. Phenytoin is a substrate for CYP2C9, considering warfarin is also a substrate for this enzyme; addition of phenytoin to a stable warfarin regimen has led to significant bleeding problems.

The drug level of phenytoin can be increased or decreased when certain drugs are used with it simultaneously. Fluoxetine inhibits CYP2C19 enzyme for which phenytoin is a substrate, so the phenytoin level increases when fluoxetine is added to the regimen. Valproic acid is an inhibitor of the CYP2C9 enzyme which metabolizes phenytoin, so addition of valproic acid may increase the level of phenytoin. However, valproic acid also displaces phenytoin from albumin, so addition of valproic acid to a stable phenytoin regimen may increase, decrease, or not alter the phenytoin level [7]. The drug level of phenytoin is increased when these following drugs are coadministered: oxcarbazepine and topiramate [7–9]. Levetiracetam has been shown to cause no change in phenytoin levels [10]. The drug levels of phenytoin and carbamazepine are usually both decreased when they are used together [7].

Considering phenytoin is metabolized by the liver, hepatic disease can increase plasma phenytoin levels, and dose must be adjusted accordingly. It is known to only be 5 % excreted in the kidneys, so renal disease will not require dosing changes [11]. Toxic side effects include sedation, anorexia, nausea, megaloblastic anemia, gingival hyperplasia, osteomalacia, and hirsutism. Allergic reactions are thought to be responsible for serious skin, liver, and bone marrow effects. It is recommended to monitor complete blood count (CBC), electroencephalogram (EEG), liver function tests (LFTs), mean corpuscular volume (MCV), serum albumin level, and serum phenytoin level [11].

Valproic Acid

Valproic acid has been shown to block voltage-dependent sodium channels and to increase GABA levels, which are effective for the treatment of neuropathic pain. Calcium channels may also be blocked by this drug, but it requires a much higher drug level [12, 13].

Valproic acid is metabolized via hepatic glucuronidation and oxidation by CYP2A6, CYP2C9, and CYP2C19 and UGT [11, 14]. It is known to inhibit UGT and CYP2C9, thereby increasing the levels of phenytoin if it was being used, due to phenytoin's metabolism by CYP2C9. Valproic acid is also 90 % bound to albumin, which displaces other AEDs such as carbamazepine and phenytoin when used concurrently [7]. Cotherapy with valproic acid and topiramate causes a 17 % decrease in topiramate plasma concentrations and a 13 % increase in topiramate clearance [9]. Valproic acid does not, however, affect the use of birth control like other first-generation anticonvulsants due to its lack of action on the CYP3A enzyme [7].

Valproic acid is also affected by the use of other drugs. Felbamate inhibits the beta-oxidation pathway, thereby inhibiting the metabolism of valproic acid [7]. Topiramate is known to induce beta-oxidation and therefore decreases stable valproic acid levels by 11 % and increases its clearance, though the change is thought not to be clinically significant [9]. Carbamazepine and phenytoin both induce CYP2 enzymes which are responsible for valproic acid's metabolism, so both of these drugs will decrease stable valproic acid levels if added to a regimen [9].

Drug clearance can be affected by up to 50 % in hepatic dysfunction and with the possible change in serum albumin that can occur with severe liver disease; valproic acid levels should be dosed accordingly and followed closely [11]. It is 30–50 % excreted by the kidneys in the form of glucuronide conjugate and 3 % unchanged. Considering the significant changes that occur in protein binding in renal failure, valproic acid levels must be monitored closely. Common side effects noted with the use of valproic acid include nausea, sedation, peripheral edema, ataxia, diplopia, and nystagmus. In severe sedation, a physician must consider valproate-associated hyperammonemic encephalopathy (VHE) which has been reported [15, 16]. Some physicians follow blood tests due to reported thrombocytopenia and blood dyscrasias which occur in 0.4 % of patients [17, 18]. Other recommended monitoring tests include CBC including platelets, LFTs, serum ammonia levels, and serum valproic acid levels [11].

Carbamazepine

Carbamazepine has been implicated to work on a number of receptors and via number of mechanisms including sodium channels, calcium channels, potassium channels, adenosine receptors, release of serotonin, increase dopaminergic transmission, inhibition of glutamate release, interaction with peripheral-type benzodiazepine receptors, and decrease of basal and stimulated cAMP levels [19]. Pain relief has been attributed to disruption of synaptic transmission in the trigeminal nucleus [11]. Carbamazepine is known to induce metabolism not only of other drugs but also of itself, doubling its plasma clearance over the first few weeks of administration. This is due to the fact that it induces CYP3A4, which is one of the enzymes for which it is a substrate for (the other enzymes are CYP1A2, CYP2C8, and CYP2C9) [14]. As exhibited by phenytoin, carbamazepine decreases the levels of many other drugs. Carbamazepine also induces the enzyme which breaks down tricyclic antidepressants (TCAs), causing a decrease in TCA plasma concentration and an increase in metabolite concentration [7]. With the induction of CYP3A4, acetaminophen and codeine, which are broken down by this enzyme, have decreased levels due to their increased breakdown when used in coordination with carbamazepine [20]. Carbamazepine has a similar effect on oral contraceptives as was described with phenytoin [8]. It also can intensify the anticoagulant effect of warfarin as exhibited by phenytoin [21].

The interaction between carbamazepine and phenytoin is unpredictable as discussed earlier. Fluoxetine coadministration increases the level of carbamazepine. Also, the addition of valproic acid to a carbamazepine regimen can cause either no change or an increase in carbamazepine levels [7].

Stevens-Johnson syndrome (SJS) and another form of SJS known as toxic epidermal necrolysis only occur in 1–6 in 10,000 new carbamazepine users in this country, but can be up to ten times more prevalent in patients with Asian ancestry. These patients should undergo a test for HLA-B*1502 prior to starting this drug, and if the patient has this allelic variant, they should not start this medication [18]. Carbamazepine has a number of other side effects including severe hematologic disorders, antidiuretic effect, hepatic failure, hyperlipidemia, vertigo, drowsiness, and ataxia [6, 18, 22]. The latter being an important matter to consider in the elderly [12]. Blood dyscrasias are serious side effects and occur in 2.1 % of patients, causing most physicians to monitor blood tests on a weekly basis for the first 4–6 weeks [17]. Other significant labs to monitor include CBC, LFTs, serum carbamazepine level, and cholesterol profile [11, 18, 22, 23].

Second-Generation Anticonvulsants

Oxcarbazepine

Oxcarbazepine has been shown to inhibit sodium channels, potassium channels, calcium channels, and adenosine receptors and exhibit a dopaminergic effect. The other mechanisms of carbamazepine such as effects on peripheral-type benzodiazepine receptors, serotonergic effect, and the decrease in cAMP system have not yet been shown in oxcarbazepine. The main effect of both of the above agents, however, is their inhibition of the voltage-dependent sodium channels [19]. Oxcarbazepine is eliminated via glucuronide conjugation via glucuronyl transferases primarily and secondarily by renal excretion [21]. It is metabolized via CYP3A4 and shows mild inhibition of CYP2C19 [14]. Compared to carbamazepine, it has less metabolism via P450, no production of epoxide metabolite, and less protein binding, therefore leading most to believe it is more tolerable and has fewer drug interactions [24].

Oxcarbazepine induces the metabolism of oral contraceptives and requires the same precautions noted as with phenytoin. Doses of up to 900 mg/day have been shown not to affect the anticoagulant effect of warfarin, unlike carbamazepine [21]. Oxcarbazepine does increase stable phenytoin levels when added.

Approximately, 95 % of the drug is excreted by the kidneys, so requires dose decrease in renal failure, but no significant changes are need in hepatic failure [11]. Common side effects include dizziness, headache, diplopia, ataxia, nausea, and vomiting, which are less frequent and severe compared to carbamazepine. However, there is an increased risk of hyponatremia compared to carbamazepine [24]. Though side effects are noted, this drug does not require monitoring of laboratory tests compared to first-generation antiepileptics [11, 18].

Gabapentin

Gabapentin is structurally related to GABA, but does not directly interact with GABA receptors, though $GABA_B$ may be activated. It has shown to block hydroxy-5-methyl-4-isoxazolepropionic acid (AMPA) receptor-mediated transmission, enhance N-methyl-D-aspartate (NMDA) current at GABA interneurons, activate adenosine triphosphate-sensitive potassium channels, and modulate voltage-dependent calcium channels. It thereby inhibits the release of glutamate, aspartate, substance P, and calcitonin gene-related peptide (CGRP) [13, 25]. It is minimally metabolized and therefore excreted unchanged in the urine. Due to its renal excretion and lack of induction of hepatic enzymes, it has significantly fewer drug interactions. In the setting of renal failure with a creatinine clearance less than 60 ml/min, the dose of the medication will need to be reduced, and reduction should continue as renal function worsens [18]. It has been shown to act synergistically with NSAIDs and morphine, and that morphine can increase its area under the curve (AUC) [26, 27]. Side effects include somnolence, dizziness, peripheral edema, headache, and nausea, no interference with oral contraceptives [21].

Pregabalin

Pregabalin is a similar structure and is thought to have a similar mechanism of action as compared to gabapentin [28]. The main difference between pregabalin and gabapentin is that pregabalin has a uniform absorption from the GI tract whereas gabapentin demonstrates a decrease in absorption with escalating dosages [28]. In the setting of renal failure, the area under the curve (AUC) and half-life are increased, so it is recommended to decrease the dose by 50 % for creatinine clearance less than 60 ml/min [29]. Side effects are similar to gabapentin which include dizziness, somnolence, and peripheral edema. Due to the lack of metabolism and low protein binding, there are no significant drug interactions noted with the use of pregabalin [28]. No interference with oral contraceptives is also noted from pregabalin [21].

Topiramate

Topiramate inhibits sodium and calcium currents, blocks glutamate receptor at AMPA, and enhances GABA-mediated chloride channels [13]. Topiramate is approximately 15 % bound to plasma protein. It shows minimal CYP2C19 inhibition [14]. Adding either phenytoin or carbamazepine to a topiramate regimen can decrease the level of topiramate by approximately 40–50 %, whereas adding valproic acid to a topiramate regimen will decrease the topiramate level by only

approximately 15 %. When topiramate is used with phenytoin, the phenytoin level is increased up to 25 % [7, 30]. Topiramate induces the metabolism of oral contraceptives, and similar precautions used with phenytoin should be employed [21].

Side effects of topiramate include psychomotor slowing, fatigue, and sedation. An observed increase in the rate of kidney stone formation was noted and found to be due to an increase in urinary bicarbonate excretion and urine pH along with a lower amount of citrate in the urine and the serum bicarbonate level. Also, metabolic acidosis, acute myopia, and oligohydrosis with hyperthermia have been rarely reported [18]. Considering this drug is excreted in the kidneys, the dose is usually decreased by 50 % in the setting of moderate to severe renal failure [11]. No specific recommendations have been made for prescribing in the setting of hepatic impairment [18]. For these reasons, serum electrolytes must be monitored, and the risk of kidney stone must be explained to patients [31].

Zonisamide

Zonisamide blocks sodium and calcium channels and also may inhibit monoamine release and metabolism. It also inhibits carbonic anhydrase [11, 13]. No interference with oral contraceptives is noted [21]. Zonisamide is a substrate for CYP3A4, UGT, and CYP2C19. It is not to inhibit or induce any CYP450 enzymes [11]. Therefore, its levels are significantly decreased with the concurrent use of phenytoin and carbamazepine, whereas the addition of valproic acid does not change the level of zonisamide. Phenytoin levels are increased by 16 % with the addition of zonisamide, and the carbamazepine levels have been variable in different studies with the addition of zonisamide [30].

In the setting of hepatic disease, zonisamide dose must be decreased due to its metabolism by the P450 system. In the setting of renal failure, there is an increase in the risk of metabolic acidosis which is thought to be due to the loss of bicarbonate via the inhibition of carbonic anhydrase. The dose is decreased in mild to moderate renal failure and should not be used with GFR < 50 ml/min [18]. Side effects include increased hepatic enzymes, azotemia, sedation, dizziness, metabolic acidosis, anorexia, and renal stones. It is recommended to monitor CBC, LFTs, serum bicarbonate, serum blood urea nitrogen (BUN) and serum creatinine, and urinalysis [11].

Levetiracetam

Levetiracetam is felt to bind to a specific site on the synaptic plasma membrane, though the exact mechanism of action is unknown [13]. It is not dependent on the CYP450 system for metabolism and is 66 % excreted unchanged in the urine and 27 % as inactive metabolites [11, 30]. Levetiracetam does not have any significant impact on other drug level, and no other drugs cause changes in levetiracetam levels [30]. There is no known interference with oral contraceptives [21].

Liver disease has little effect on this drug unless severe failure is present, in which the renal component will likely exert the greatest impact on the drug. In the setting of renal failure, the drug dose will need to be reduced accordingly [11]. Side effects include somnolence, dizziness, and fatigue. Serum BUN and serum creatinine are monitored due to extensive drug excretion [11].

Antidepressants

Selective Serotonin Reuptake Inhibitors (SSRIs)

The mechanism of action of SSRIs, as their name implies, is by blocking the reuptake of serotonin. The increased level of serotonin has been helpful in treating depression and OCD, in addition to other off-label uses. Side effects include sedation and sexual dysfunction [32]. Some specific agents do have significant drug interactions which must be considered.

Several SSRIs have been shown to increase warfarin levels due to inhibition of CYP2C9 and CYP3A4 and carbamazepine levels via inhibition of CYP3A4 [14, 20, 33]. The adverse effect of serotonin syndrome should lead practitioners to avoid combining MAOIs and SSRIs. One should also allow a 7-day washout period before starting MAOIs, and a 14-day washout period should be permitted prior to initiation of SSRI therapy after MAOIs have been used. Serotonin syndrome can occur when combined with triptans (naratriptan, rizatriptan, sumatriptan, and zolmitriptan) [34]. When combined with tramadol, there is an increased potential for seizures, and serotonin syndrome should be monitored [25]. SSRIs which inhibit CYP2D6 increase the concentration of TCAs when combined, and anticholinergic excess can occur [14, 34]. For SSRIs, no laboratory monitoring is absolutely required, though the inquiring into the presence of side effects will aid clinicians in determining when laboratory tests may be applicable [35].

Fluoxetine

Fluoxetine is metabolized by CYP2C9, CYP2C19, CYP2D6, and CYP3A4. It primarily inhibits enzyme CYP2D6, but also to lesser extent inhibits CYP2A1, CYP3A4, and CYP2C19 [20, 33]. It is known to significantly increase TCA levels when used in combination, which is ascribed to CYP2D6 inhibition. It can also increase the phenytoin level by almost twofold, which requires following phenytoin levels when implementing fluoxetine [33].

In the setting of the hepatic failure, the dose of this drug will need to be reduced, in contrast to renal failure which will not require a dose adjustment. Common side effects include somnolence, gastrointestinal dysfunction, headache, and sexual dysfunction. Rarely, hyponatremia occurs typically due to syndrome of inappropriate antidiuretic hormone secretion (SIADH) [36]. Weight loss, sexual dysfunction, hypothyroidism, hepatic disease, decreased bone growth, suicidal ideation, hyperglycemia, and impaired platelet aggregation have also been described [11, 18, 37, 38]. Therefore, monitoring has been recommended to include CBC with differential, LFTs, and thyroid function tests (TFTs), only if symptoms warrant these tests [11, 35, 39].

Sertraline

Sertraline is metabolized by CYP2B6, CYP2C9, CYP2C19, CYP2D6, and CYP3A4 and primarily inhibits CYP2D6, CYP1A2, CYP2C9, and CYP3A4. It has less of an impact on drug interactions compared to fluoxetine and paroxetine [14, 20, 33].

In patients with hepatic disease, sertraline doses will need to be decreased, as opposed to in the setting of renal failure, when the dose does not need to be changed. Side effects include hyponatremia, sexual dysfunction, and impaired platelet aggregation. Rarely, hypothyroidism and elevated liver transaminases are caused, and therefore, LFTs are monitored and baseline thyroid function tests (TFTs) are obtained [11, 23]. For this reason, monitoring has been recommended to include electrolytes, TFTs and LFTs, which should be obtained if signs or symptoms suggest derangements in these tests [11, 18, 23, 35].

Paroxetine

Paroxetine is metabolized by CYP2D6 and is the most potent SSRI for inhibition of enzyme CYP2D6, but is also known to inhibit CYP1A2 and CYP3A4 [14, 20, 33]. This leads to a dramatic increase in TCA levels when used in combination [20]. Specifically, desipramine plasma levels were increased 400 % by the addition of paroxetine [33]. Clinically, significant bleeding has been noted in patients who were taking warfarin when paroxetine was added, so monitoring INR would be prudent [33].

In mild to moderate renal failure and in hepatic failure, paroxetine plasma concentration is increased two times its normal value, whereas in severe renal failure, it can be up to four times the normal value. For this reason, dose adjustment for these dysfunctions is recommended [11, 18, 23]. Side effects including headache, somnolence, sexual dysfunction, and weight loss. Rarely, hypothyroidism, hepatic disease, and renal impairment occur, so it is recommended to monitor LFTs, TFTs, and serum BUN and creatinine, if signs and symptoms suggest possible derangements in these values [11, 23, 35].

Fluvoxamine

Fluvoxamine is metabolized by CYP1A2 and CYP2D6 and known to inhibit CYP1A2, CYP2C19, CYP3A4, and CYP2D6 [14, 20]. Of all the SSRIs, it is the most potent inhibitor of CYP 1A2 and likely CYP2C19. Due to its CYP enzyme inhibition, it has been shown to dramatically increase TCA levels. It can also increase warfarin levels, so INR levels should be monitored when this drug is added to chronic warfarin therapy [33].

In the setting of severe hepatic failure, the half-life is increased from 15 to 24 h, and dose frequency should be adjusted accordingly. There is no significant change in the half-life, and drug level in the setting of renal failure and dose and frequency of medication should not necessarily be changed. Side effects include headache, nausea, and sexual dysfunction. Rarely, hypothyroidism and elevated liver transaminases are caused, and therefore, LFTs are monitored and baseline TFTs are obtained, if signs and symptoms warrant these tests [11, 23, 35].

Citalopram

Citalopram is metabolized via CYP2C19 and CYP2D6 and possible CYP3A4 and is a weak inhibitor of CYP2D6, though this exerts less of an effect than other SSRIs [20, 40]. It has not shown to cause the same decrease in metabolism of TCAs, as seen with other SSRIs, but its breakdown products may decrease TCA metabolism [20]. In the setting of hepatic failure, clearance is decreased and the half-life is increased, so adjusting the dose accordingly may be warranted. In the setting of mild to moderate renal failure, no dose change will be needed, but in severe renal failure, a close monitoring and dose adjustment may be warranted [11, 23]. Side effects include somnolence, nausea, diaphoresis, and sexual dysfunction, which is less prominent than seen with some other SSRIs, along with the change of elevated liver enzymes and hypothyroidism. Therefore, signs and symptoms may prompt a clinician to perform lab tests such as LFTs and TFTs.

Escitalopram

Escitalopram is metabolized by CYP2C19, CYP2D6, and CYP3A4 and is a mild inhibitor of CYP2D6.

In the setting of hepatic failure, clearance is decreased and half-life is increased, so adjusting the dose accordingly may be warranted. In the setting of mild to moderate renal failure, no dose change will be needed, but in severe renal failure, a close monitoring and dose adjustment may be warranted [11, 23]. Side effects include headache, nausea, and sexual dysfunction. More rare side effects such as hypothyroidism, bleeding disorder, and elevated LFTs should prompt a clinician to obtain labs such as LFTs or TFTs if deemed clinically necessary [11, 23, 35].

Serotonin-Norepinephrine Reuptake Inhibitors (SNRIs)

Milnacipran

Milnacipran blocks the reuptake of norepinephrine and serotonin with preference given to the former. It is only 13 % protein bound. It minimally interacts with the P450 system and has little inhibition or induction on these enzymes. Severe reactions such as autonomic changes, muscle rigidity, and neuroleptic malignant syndrome can occur when MAO inhibitors are combined with milnacipran. Serotonin syndrome can occur when milnacipran is combined with SSRIs and other SNRIs. In the setting of severe hepatic failure, the half-life is increased by 55 % and area under the curve (AUC) increased by 31 %, therefore requiring a slight decrease in dosing in these patients. In the setting of severe renal failure, the half-life is increased by 122 %, and the AUC is increased 199 %, requiring significant dose reductions. Side effects include headache, hot flashes, and nausea.

Venlafaxine

Venlafaxine blocks the reuptake of serotonin, norepinephrine, and dopamine. This drug was created in attempt to provide the benefits of TCAs without the adverse side effects. It has been shown to have great efficacy in many chronic pain disorders while providing a more tolerable side effect profile as compared to TCAs and SSRIs [41]. It is metabolized by CYP2D6, and inhibition of this enzyme is mild compared to other agents. Combined with its low protein binding of 25–30 %, it has shown much fewer drug interactions than many of the TCAs and SSRIs. The adverse effect of serotonin syndrome should be avoided via observation of washout periods after discontinuation of MAOIs or starting of MAOIs described in the SSRI section [42]. Serotonin syndrome due to the combination of venlafaxine and MAOIs has been reported leading to death [43].

In the setting of renal failure, the dose should be reduced 25 %, and if the patient is undergoing hemodialysis, the dose should be reduced 50 %. This is because in renal failure, the clearance is decreased by 24 %, and the half-life is increased 50 %. In dialysis, in one study of six patients on maintenance hemodialysis, a 4-h dialysis treatment removed only about 5 % of a single 50 mg dose of venlafaxine [44]. In the setting of hepatic failure, the dose should be reduced by 50 % since the half-life is increased by 30 %, and the clearance is decreased by 50 %. Side effects include headache, nausea, insomnia, somnolence, gastrointestinal distress, and inhibition of sexual function [11, 23, 41]. Elevation of blood pressure and cholesterol is a potential side effect of this medication [11, 35].

Duloxetine

Duloxetine is a balanced inhibitor of serotonin and norepinephrine reuptake. The resultant increase in these levels is felt to play a significant role in treating neuropathic pain along with treating depression [41]. Duloxetine is metabolized by CYP1A2 and CYP2D6 and inhibits CYP2D6 [14]. Side effects include nausea, headache, sexual dysfunction, dry mouth, and insomnia. Since 1 % of these patients develop an elevated ALT, consider checking LFTs after initiation [11, 35]. Duloxetine should not be prescribed to patients with preexisting liver disease due to the risk of exacerbating this condition. In the setting of mild to moderate renal failure with a creatinine clearance of greater than 30 ml/min, there should be no adjustments made to this medication; however, it should not be administered to patients with creatinine clearance less than 30 ml/min [18].

Tricyclic Antidepressants (TCAs)

Tricyclic antidepressants are composed of secondary amines and tertiary amines. Secondary amines include desipramine and nortriptyline, and tertiary amines include amitriptyline, clomipramine, and imipramine, among others. The major difference between the groups is the increase in norepinephrine reuptake inhibition seen in the secondary amines versus their tertiary amine counterparts [45].

TCAs inhibit the reuptake of 5-HT and norepinephrine and exert postsynaptic antagonism of the H1, alpha-1, muscarinic, and 5-HT2a receptors, all to varying degrees [46]. The most potent property is that of H1 antagonism, which is intuitive, considering TCAs were developed from antihistamines in the 1950s [46].

Secondary amines are metabolized primarily by CYP2D6 followed to a lesser extent by CYP2C19 and CYP1A2 and is not affected by CYP 3A4 in nortriptyline [47]. Tertiary amines are metabolized by CYP2C19, CYP1A2, CYP3A4, and CYP2D6. The inhibition of CYP2C19 is significant. They have a moderate effect on CYP1A2 and CYP3A4 and a clinically insignificant effect on CYP2D6 [46]. TCA levels are known to be increased when combined with SSRIs [34]. When combined with MAOIs, they have been reported to cause serotonin syndrome and death [43]. Side effects stem from anticholinergic muscarinic (dry mouth, xerostomia, sinus tachycardia, and urinary retention), alpha-2 blockade (postural hypotension), dopaminergic blockade (extrapyramidal side effects and neuroleptic malignant syndrome), and histamine blockade (sedation) [48]. TCAs are known to cause various ECG changes including tachycardia; ventricular tachycardia; ventricular fibrillation; supraventricular tachycardia; sinus arrest; QRS, PR, and QT prolongation; AV block; and bundle branch block. With this in mind, it is recommended to obtain a baseline ECG prior to starting these medications. For long-term monitoring, if the patient fails to respond or shows signs or symptoms of TCA toxicity, some recommend obtaining TCA level to rule out toxic levels or to help guide therapy [35, 49, 50]. In the setting of renal or hepatic failure, TCAs should be used with caution, with little literature to guide their use currently in these patient settings [51].

Monoamine Oxidase Inhibitors (MAOIs)

Monoamine oxidase is an enzyme which metabolizes 5-HT, histamine, dopamine, norepinephrine, and epinephrine. MAOIs inhibit this enzyme which causes an increase in the level of these substances [52]. First created were hydrazine derivative MAOIs, but due to liver toxicity, bleeding, and hypertensive crises, non-hydrazine derivatives were created. Unfortunately, non-hydrazine MAOIs still were implicated in hypertensive crises, though the liver problems were avoided. The hypertension eventually was coined as the "cheese reaction" caused by combination of MAOIs with tyramine-containing foods including fermented cheese. Individual reversible and irreversible MAO A and MAO B inhibitors were designed, along with multiple nonselective inhibitors [52].

Side effects of MAOIs include orthostatic hypotension, weight gain, drowsiness, and dizziness.

When combined with SSRIs, they have been documented to causes serotonin syndrome and death [43].

Opioids

Opioids exert action via the opioid receptors by acting as opioid agonists. Most opioids exert their effects via the OP1 (delta), OP2 (kappa), and OP3 (mu). This group of medications all exhibit similar side effects including but not limited to constipation, nausea/vomiting, dizziness, respiratory depression, hypotension, urticaria, urinary retention, and drowsiness. Long-term use can lead to physical dependence, hyperalgesia, hormonal abnormalities, and impairment of the immune system [53, 54]. If compliance becomes an issue or the patient experiences signs or symptoms indicative of toxicity, the clinician should test for the specifically prescribed opioid level [55].

Codeine

The major metabolite of codeine is codeine-6-glucuronide which is produced via glucuronidation by UGT2B7. Two minor metabolites are morphine and norcodeine which are formed by O-demethylation by CYP2D6 and N-demethylation by CYP3A4, respectively. Usually, less than 10 % of codeine is converted into morphine, but in the presence of a CYP2D6 or CYP3A4 inhibitor or CYP2D6 genetic polymorphism, the residual morphine level may be higher or lower [56]. Baseline creatinine levels have been recommended to obtain prior to long-term therapy [51].

Morphine

Morphine predominantly exerts its effect on the opioid receptors via the mu-opioid receptors [57]. Morphine is metabolized via glucuronidation by UGT2B7 into morphine-6-glucuronide and morphine-3-glucuronide. The former possesses 2–3 times more analgesic properties than morphine, while the latter does not bind to opioid receptors [58, 59]. In the setting of hepatic or renal failure, morphine dose should be decreased and monitored closely for signs or symptoms of toxicity. Baseline creatinine levels have been recommended to obtain prior to long-term therapy [51].

Fentanyl

Fentanyl is a mu-agonist with a high lipid solubility and low molecular weight, which makes it very attractive for the use of transdermal formulations. Unfortunately, the absorption has been shown to decrease after 48–72 in cachectic patients when compared to normal patients, making it less attractive for patients in this condition [60]. Fentanyl is metabolized by CYP3A4 into norfentanyl, which has no analgesic activity itself [59, 61]. In the setting of hepatic or renal failure, fentanyl dose should be decreased and monitored closely for signs or symptoms of toxicity [18]. In patients who are taking a CYP3A4 inducer or inhibitor, they could have a higher or lower metabolism of fentanyl and require an increase or decrease in frequency of dosing, respectively.

Oxycodone

Oxycodone exerts an agonist effect on the mu-, kappa-, and delta-opioid receptors, causing inhibition on adenylyl cyclase, hyperpolarization of neurons, and decreased excitability. It is known to work via the kappa receptor, more than the mu and delta receptors. Morphine, on the other hand, has more of an effect on the mu receptors than oxycodone, and it is less metabolized and therefore has less bioavailability. O-demethylation by CYP2D6 occurs which converts oxycodone to oxymorphone (a potent analgesic) which is excreted by the kidneys [57, 62]. N-demethylation of oxycodone to noroxycodone (a weak analgesic) takes place via CYP3A5 and CYP3A4, and noroxycodone is then excreted via the

kidneys [63]. In the setting of renal and hepatic impairment, the dose should be reduced and patient monitored closely [18]. Baseline creatinine levels have been recommended to obtain prior to long-term therapy [51].

Methadone

Methadone is an opioid agonist with a predominant effect on the mu-opioid receptor [64]. Methadone is also known to block the NMDA receptor which may aid in blocking the windup mechanism thought to be responsible for chronic pain [65]. Methadone is a racemic mixture of R- and S-methadone. R-methadone has a 10–50-fold greater affinity for the mu and delta-opioid receptors when compared to S-methadone. Methadone has a half-life of approximately 22 h, which only produces 6 h of analgesia on initiation of drug, but increases to 8–12 h of analgesia after repeated dosing [66]. R-methadone is predominantly metabolized by CYP3A4, and also metabolized by CYP2C8 and CYP2D6 to a lesser extent. S-methadone is metabolized by CYP3A4 and CYP2C8 equally and to a lesser extent by CYP2D6. The breakdown product of methadone is EDDP (2-ethylidene-1,5-dimethyl-3,3-diphenylpyrrolidine), although at least six others have been identified, and all are inactive [67]. Methadone has been shown to prolong the QT interval even in small doses and to a greater extent in higher doses even resulting in torsades de pointes. For this reason, a baseline ECG should be taken prior to methadone induction and again after a stabilized dose is reached. If the corrected QT interval (QT_c) is increased by 40 ms above baseline or the total QT_c is 500 ms or greater, the patient would be considered to be at risk for torsades de pointes, and the dose should be reduced or discontinued. Also if the patient is prone to electrolyte abnormalities, electrolytes should be checked more frequently due to risk of electrolyte abnormalities further prolonging the QT_c [68]. In addition to prolongation of QT interval, other side effects include respiratory depression, sedation, and anxiety. In the setting of renal or hepatic failure, the dose should be decreased and patient monitored closely for signs and symptoms of toxicity [18].

Opioid Combinations

Tramadol

Tramadol is a mu-opioid receptor agonist and a norepinephrine and serotonin reuptake inhibitor. Considering it has a similar mechanism of action to MAOIs, when it is combined with MAOIs or other antidepressants, serotonin syndrome has been reported, and possible fatalities due to this interaction have been reported [43, 69]. Considering tramadol is 60 %

metabolized via hepatic metabolism via CYP2D6, CYP2B6, and CYP3A4 and excreted via renal excretion, in the setting of liver of renal failure, tramadol doses should be decreased by approximately 50 % [11, 62, 69]. Enzyme inducers of CYP2D6 (carbamazepine) cause approximately a 50 % decrease in tramadol levels [70].

Tramadol should be avoided in patients with codeine or other opioid allergy due to the risk of anaphylacticreaction from cross-reactivity. Side effects include dizziness, nausea, headache, seizures, and constipation [11, 18].

Agonist/Antagonist

Buprenorphine

Buprenorphine is a mixed agonist antagonist, with partial agonism of the mu-opioid receptor and antagonism of the kappa-opioid receptor. At low doses, the mu-agonist effect predominates, allowing pain control with a potency of 25–40 times that of morphine. In contrast to morphine, however, at higher doses, there is a ceiling effect due to the antagonistic properties. This is advantageous to avoid respiratory depression, yet the medication may be lacking in treatment of severe pain [71]. This drug is 96 % protein bound and is metabolized to its active metabolite norbuprenorphine via multiple enzymes including CYP3A4, CYP2C8, CYP2C9, CYP2C18, and CYP2C19. Of all of these enzymes, CYP3A4 is responsible for 65 % of the metabolite, and CYP2C8 creates 30 % of the metabolite [62, 72]. In the setting of renal failure, buprenorphine levels are not significantly affected. However, in the setting of hepatic failure, the risk of increased LFTs has been noted and warrants obtaining baseline LFTs and periodic monitoring of LFTs [73].

Side effects including headache, insomnia, anxiety, nausea, weakness, sedation with rare instances of hypotension, and respiratory depression. The risk of increased LFTs has been noted and warrants obtaining baseline LFTs and periodic monitoring of LFTs.

Muscle Relaxants

Baclofen

Baclofen works directly on the spinal cord by blocking afferent pathways traveling from the brain to the skeletal muscles. Considering baclofen is an analog of gamma-aminobutyric acid (GABA), it also may have GABA-like effects in decreasing the release of excitatory neurotransmitters such as aspartate and glutamate. Baclofen is only 15 % metabolized in the liver, and 70–85 % is excreted unchanged in the urine, and it is poorly dialyzable. For these reasons, hepatic failure should

not significantly affect dosing, whereas in renal failure or dialysis dependence, the dose should be reduced [11, 23, 74]. Side effects include drowsiness, ataxia, insomnia, slurred speech, seizures, and weakness, which can also be signs of toxicity [23].

Cyclobenzaprine

Cyclobenzaprine is close in chemical structure to amitriptyline and has some similar effects of TCAs like anticholinergic activity. It is felt to relieve muscle spasms via some central action and not directly at the neuromuscular junction. Cyclobenzaprine is a substrate for CYP3A4 and CYP1A2 and to a lesser extent CYP2D6. It is then excreted as inactive metabolites by the kidneys. Even in mild hepatic impairment, the AUC can be increased by up to 100 %, requiring dose reduction. Dosing in the elderly should also be reduced and titrated slowly. Side effects include drowsiness, headache, dizziness, and xerostomia [11, 18, 23].

Tizanidine

Tizanidine is an alpha-2 agonist which has antinociceptive and antispasmotic properties. It is metabolized via the enzyme CYP1A2. Therefore, inhibitors of CYP1A2 can lead to toxic levels of tizanidine. Of clinical significance is fluvoxamine which is contraindicated with tizanidine due to its being shown to increase the plasma level of tizanidine 12-fold. Other CYP1A2 inhibitors including but not limited to oral contraceptives and ciprofloxacin are discouraged in their use with tizanidine [75]. In the setting of hepatic impairment, this drug should be avoided if possible, or significant drug reduction should be used. In the setting of renal dysfunction, the dose should be decreased. Side effects include hypotension, somnolence, and weakness. Occasionally, hepatic dysfunction has been reported. It is recommended to obtain baseline LFTs and BUN/creatinine, along with periodic LFTs, BUN/creatinine, and blood pressure measurements [18, 51].

Clonidine

Clonidine is an alpha-2 agonist which exerts its effects on peripheral nerves, spinal cord, and brain stem. It is used as an alternative in the setting of refractory neuropathic pain. It can also be administered in a variety of ways including transdermal, intrathecal, epidural, perineural, intravenous, and per os [51]. Fifty percent of clonidine undergoes hepatic metabolism via CYP2D6, and other minor hepatic enzymes, and much of the remainder is excreted unchanged in the urine [76, 77]. With this in mind, in the setting of renal or hepatic failure, the dose should be decreased [18]. Side effects include drowsiness, hypotension, rebound hypertension, xerostomia, skin rash, decreased intraocular pressure, and decreased retinal blood flow. Blood pressure should be monitored, and the patient should receive periodic eye exams [18, 78].

Metaxalone

Metaxalone is a skeletal muscle relaxant which acts centrally without working directly on the skeletal muscles but instead possesses sedative properties which indirectly relax the muscles [23]. It is metabolized by CYP1A2, CYP2D6, CYP2E1, and CYP3A4 and to a lesser extent by CYP2C8, CYP2C9, and CYP2C19. In the setting of hepatic failure, LFTs should be followed and dose should be decreased. In patients with renal disease, the dose should also be decreased. Side effects include drowsiness, dizziness, headache, nausea, GI irritability, seizure exacerbation, and increased liver transaminases [11, 18, 23].

Carisoprodol

Carisoprodol is a skeletal muscle relaxant which acts centrally without working directly on the skeletal muscles but instead possesses sedative properties which indirectly relax the muscles [79]. It is broken down by CYP2C19 into its major active metabolite meprobamate. Meprobamate is equipotent with carisoprodol and has a significantly longer half-life compared to its parent compound carisoprodol. Since CYP2C19 exhibits genetic polymorphisms, different races may metabolize carisoprodrol at different rate, which should be considered. In the setting of hepatic and renal failure, the dosage should be reduced. Obtaining baseline BUN/creatinine may aid in identifying underlying renal dysfunction [23]. The main side effect is drowsiness though its dose poses the risk of abuse, which must be considered prior to prescribing this medication [79]. Other side effects include GI irritability, nausea, seizures, pancytopenia, and adverse skin reactions [51].

The Future of Polypharmacy

The future of limiting polypharmacy and drug interaction lies in pharmacogenomics. Of the P450 enzymes, 40 % of the metabolic function takes place by polymorphic enzymes CYP2A6, CYP2C9, CYP2C19, and CYP2D6 [80]. Unfortunately, these polymorphisms lead to interpatient variability, which makes prescribing and administering certain drugs an inexact science at its best. This contributes highly to the reported two million hospitalized patients annually who have severe adverse drug reactions [81].

In December of 2004, the FDA approved AmpliChip CYP450 test. This test uses microarrays to determine if a patient possesses a genetic polymorphism for CYP2D6 or CYP2C19. It will provide information whether a patient is a slow metabolizer versus an ultrarapid metabolizer [82]. This will undoubtedly aid clinicians in dosing and avoid many adverse drug reactions. Future research will give clinicians similar tests to accurately predict drug levels in the setting of polypharmacy and individual genetic polymorphisms.

References

1. Boyd C, et al. Clinical practice guidelines and quality of care for older patients with multiple comorbid diseases, implications for pay for performance. JAMA. 2005;294(6):716–24.
2. Lin P. Drug interactions and polypharmacy in the elderly. Can Alzheimer Dis Rev. 2003;10–4.
3. Gilron I. The role of anticonvulsant drugs in postoperative pain management: a bench-to-bedside perspective. Can J Anaesth. 2006;53:562–71.
4. Misra UK, Kalita J, Rathore C. Phenytoin and carbamazepine cross reactivity: report of a case and review of literature. Postgrad Med J. 2003;79:703–4.
5. Wadzinski J, Franks R, Roane D, Bayard M. Valproate-associated hyperammonemic encephalopathy. J Am Board Fam Med. 2007;20:499–502.
6. McNamara J. Pharmacotherapies of the epilepsies. Goodman & Gilman's the pharmacological basis of therapeutics. 11th ed. USA: McGraw Hill; 2006.
7. Anderson G. A mechanistic approach to antiepileptic drug interactions. Ann Pharmacother. 1998;32:554–63.
8. Crawford P. Interactions between antiepileptic drugs and hormonal contraception. CNS Drugs. 2002;16(4):263–72.
9. Garnett WR. Clinical pharmacology of topiramate: a review. Epilepsia. 2000;41:S61–5.
10. Browne TR, Szabo GK, Leppik IE, Josephs E, Paz J, Baltes E, Jensen CM. Absence of pharmacokinetic drug interaction of levetiracetam with phenytoin in patients with epilepsy determined by new technique. J Clin Pharmacol. 2000;40:590.
11. Elsevier Health. MD consult web site. Drugs. 2010. Available at: http://www.mdconsult.com/das/pharm/lookup/134025550-4?type=alldrugs. Accessed June 2010.
12. Jensen T. Anticonvulsants in neuropathic pain: rationale and clinical evidence. Eur J Pain. 2002;6:A61–8.
13. Kwan P, Sills GJ, Brodie MJ. The mechanisms of action of commonly used antiepileptic drugs. Pharmacol Ther. 2001;90:21–34.
14. Kutscher EC, Alexander B. A review of the drug interactions with psychiatric medicines for the pharmacy practitioner. J Pharm Pract. 2007;20(4):327–33.
15. Wadzinski J, Franks R, Roane D, Bayard M. Valproate-associated hyperammonemic encephalopathy. JABFM. 2007;20(5):499–502.
16. Mattson RH, Cramer JA, Williamson PD, Novelly RA. Valproic acid in epilepsy: clinical and pharmacological effects. Ann Neurol. 1978;3:20–5.
17. Tohen M, Castillo J, Baldessarini RJ, Zarate Jr C, Kando JC. Blood dyscrasias with carbamazepine and valproate: a pharmacoepidemiological study of 2,228 patients at risk. Am J Psychiatry. 1995;152(3):413–8.

18. Lexi-Comp Online™, Pediatric Lexi-Drugs Online™, Hudson, Ohio: Lexi-Comp, Inc. 2007; 2010.

19. Ambrosio A, Soares-da-Silva P, Carvalho CM, Carvalho AP. Mechanisms of action of carbamazepine and its derivatives, oxcarbazepine, BIA 2-093, and BIA 2-024. Neurochem Res. 2002; 27:121–30.

20. Baker GB, Fang J, Sinha S, Coutis RT. Metabolic drug interactions with selective serotonin reuptake inhibitor (SSRI) antidepressants. Neurosci Biobehav Rev. 1998;22(2):325–33.

21. Perucca E. Clinically relevant drug interactions with antiepileptic drugs. Br J Clin Pharmacol. 2005;61:246–55.

22. Kumar P, et al. Effect of anticonvulsant drugs on lipid profile in epileptic patients. Int J Neurol. 2004;3(1).

23. Basow DS, editor. UpToDate web site. 2010. Available at: http://utdol.com/online/content/search.do. Accessed June 2010.

24. Kalis MM, Huff NA. Oxcarbazepine, an antiepileptic agent. Clin Ther. 2001;23(5):680–700.

25. Kong VKF, Irwin MG. Gabapentin: a multimodal perioperative drug? Br J Anesth. 2007;99(6):775–86.

26. Hurley R, et al. Gabapentin and pregabalin can interact synergistically with naproxen to produce anti-hyperalgesia. Anesthesiology. 2002;97(5):1263–73.

27. Gilron I, et al. Morphine, gabapentin, or their combination for neuropathic pain. N Engl J Med. 2005;352:1324–34.

28. Stacey BR, Swift JN. Pregabalin for neuropathic pain based recent clinical trials. Curr Pain Headache Rep. 2006;10:179–84.

29. Randinitis EJ, et al. Pharmacokinetics of pregabalin in subjects with various degrees of renal function. J Clin Pharmacol. 2003; 43:277–83.

30. Hachad H, Ragueneau-Majlessi I, Levy RH. New antiepileptic drugs: review on drug interactions. Ther Drug Monit. 2002;24: 91–103.

31. Welsh BJ, Graybeal D, Moe OW, et al. Biochemical and stone-risk profiles with topiramate treatment. Am J Kidney Dis. 2006;48(4): 555–63.

32. Remick RA. Diagnosis and management of depression in primary care: a clinical update and review. CMAJ. 2002;167(11):1253–60.

33. Elliot R. Pharmacokinetic drug interactions of new antidepressants: a review of the effects on the metabolism of other drugs. Mayo Clin Proc. 1997;72:835–47.

34. Ament PW, Bertolino JG, Liszewski JL. Clinically significant drug interactions. Am Fam Physician. 2000;61:1745–54.

35. Carlat D. Laboratory monitoring when prescribing psychotropics. Carlat Psychiatry Rep. 2007;5(8):1, 3, 6, 8.

36. Liu BA, Mittmann N, Knowles SR, Shear NH. Hyponatremia and the syndrome of inappropriate secretion of antidiuretic hormone associated with the use of selective serotonin reuptake inhibitors: review of spontaneous reports. CMAJ. 1996;155:519–27.

37. Christodoulou C, et al. Extrapyramidal side effects and suicidal ideation under fluoxetine treatment: a case report. Ann Gen Psychiatry. 2010;9(5):1–3.

38. Warden S, et al. Inhibition of the serotonin (5-hydroxytryptamine) transporter reduces bone growth accrual during growth. Endocrinology. 2005;146:685–93.

39. The Merck Manual. Unbound Medicine, Inc.; 2010.

40. Herrlin K, et al. Metabolism of citalopram enantiomers in CYP2C19/CYP2D6 phenotyped panels of healthy Swedes. Br J Clin Pharmacol. 2003;56:415–21.

41. Lyengar S, Webster AA, Hemrick-Luecke SK, Xu JY, Simmons RMA. Efficacy of duloxetine, a potent and balanced serotonin-norepinephrine reuptake inhibitor in persistent pain models in rats. JPET. 2004;311(2):576–84.

42. Barkin RL, Fawcett J. The management challenges of chronic pain: the role of antidepressants. Am J Ther. 2000;7:31–47.

43. Gillman PK. Monoamine oxidase inhibitors, opioid analgesics and serotonin toxicity. Br J Anaesth. 2005;95:434–41.

44. Troy SM, Schultz RW, Parker VD, Chiang ST, Blum RA. The effect of renal disease on the disposition of venlafaxine. Clin Pharmacol Ther. 1994;56:14–21.

45. Petroianu G, Schmitt A. First line symptomatic therapy for painful diabetic neuropathy: a tricyclic antidepressant or gabapentin? Int J Diab Metab. 2002;10:1–13.

46. Gillman PK. Tricyclic antidepressant pharmacology and therapeutic drug interactions updated. Br J Pharmacol. 2007;151:737–48.

47. Oleson OV, Linnet K. Hydroxylation and demethylation of the tricyclic antidepressant nortriptyline by cDNA-expressed human cytochrome P-450 isozymes. Drug Metab Dispos. 1997;25(6): 740–4.

48. Barkin RL, Barkin D. Pharmacologic management of acute and chronic pain: focus on drug interactions and patient specific pharmacotherapeutic selection. South Med J. 2001;94(8):756–70.

49. Harrigan R, Brady W. ECG abnormalities in tricyclic antidepressant ingestion. Am J Emerg Med. 1999;17:387–93.

50. Wiechers I, Smith F, Stern T. A guide to the judicious use of laboratory tests and diagnostic procedures in psychiatric practice. Psychiatric Times. 2010.

51. Eisenach JC, De Kock M, Klimscha W. Alpha sub 2 -adrenergic agonists for regional anesthesia: a clinical review of clonidine (1984–1995). Anesthesiology. 1996;85(3):655–74.

52. Youdim MBH, Edmondson D, Tipton KF. The therapeutic potential of monoamine oxidase inhibitors. Nat Rev. 2006;7:295–309.

53. Furlan AD, Sandoval JA, Mailis-Gagnon A, Tunks E. Opioid for chronic noncancer pain: a meta-analysis of effectiveness and side effects. CMAJ. 2006;174(11):1589–94.

54. Ballantyne JC, Mao J. Opioid therapy for chronic pain. N Engl J Med. 2003;349:1943–53.

55. White S, Wong S. Standards of laboratory practice: analgesic drug monitoring. Clin Chem. 1998;45(5):1110–23.

56. Caraco Y, Tateishi T, Guengerich FP, Wood AJJ. Microsomal codeine n-demethylation: cosegregation with cytochrome P4503A4 activity. Drug Metab Dispos. 1996;24(7):761–4.

57. Gallego AO, Baron MG, Arranz EE. Oxycodone: a pharmacological and clinical review. Clin Transl Oncol. 2007;9:298–307.

58. Coffman BL, King CD, Rios GR, Tephly TR. The glucuronidation of opioid, other xenobiotics, and androgens by human UGT2B7Y(268) and UGT2B7H(268). Drug Metab Dispos. 1998; 26(1):73–7.

59. Miser AW, Narang PK, Dothage JA, Young RC, Sindelar W, Miser JS. Transdermal fentanyl for pain control in patients with cancer. Pain. 1989;39:15–21.

60. Heiskanen T, Matzke S, Haakana S, Gergov M, Vuori E, Kalso E. Transdermal fentanyl in cachectic cancer patients. Pain. 2009;144:218–22.

61. Feierman DE, Lasker JM. Metabolism of fentanyl, a synthetic opioid analgesic, by human liver microsomes. Drug Metab Dispos. 1996;24(9):932–9.

62. Pergolizzi J, et al. Opioids and the management of chronic severe pain in the elderly: consensus statement of an international expert panel with focus on the six clinically most often used world health organization step III opioids (buprenorphine, fentanyl, hydromorphone, methadone, morphine, oxycodone). Pain Pract. 2008;8(4):287–313.

63. Lalovic B, Phillips B, Risler LL, Howald W, Shen DD. Quantitative contribution of CYP2D6 and CYP3A to oxycodone metabolism in human liver and intestinal microsomes. Drug Metab Dispos. 2004;32(4):447–54.

64. Ripamonti C, Zecca E, Bruera E. An update on the clinical use of methadone for cancer pain. Pain. 1997;70:109–15.

65. Andersen S, Dickenson AH, Kohn M, Reeve A, Rahman W, Ebert B. The opioid ketobemidone has a NMDA blocking effect. Pain. 1996;67:369–74.

66. Toombs J, Kral L. Methadone treatments for pain states. Am Fam Physician. 2005;71:1353–8.

67. Wang J, DeVane CL. Involvement of CYP3A4, CYP2C8, and CYP2D6 in the metabolism of (R)- and (S)-methadone in vitro. Pain. 2003;31(6):742–7.

68. Martell BA, Arnsten JH, Ray B, et al. The impact of methadone induction on cardiac conduction in opiate users. Ann Intern Med. 2003;139(2):154–5.

69. Klotz U. Tramadol – the impact of its pharmacokinetic and pharmacodynamic properties on the clinical management of pain. Arzneim Forsch Drug Res. 2003;53(10):681–7.

70. Grond S, Sablotzki A. Clinical pharmacology of tramadol. Clin Pharmacokinet. 2004;43(13):879–923.

71. Sporer KA. Buprenorphine: a primer for emergency physicians. Ann Emerg Med. 2004;43:580–4.

72. Picard N, Cresteil T, Djebli N, Marquet P. In vitro metabolism study of buprenorphine: evidence for new metabolic pathways. Drug Metab Dispos. 2005;33:689–95.

73. Taikato M, et al. What every psychiatrist should know about buprenorphine in substance misuse. Psychiatr Bull. 2005;29:225–7.

74. Addolorato G, et al. Effectiveness and safety of baclofen for maintenance of alcohol abstinence in alcohol-dependent patients with liver cirrhosis: randomized, double-blind controlled study. Lancet. 2007;370:1915–22.

75. Granfors MT, et al. Fluvoxamine drastically increases concentrations and effects of tizanidine: a potentially hazardous interaction. Clin Pharmacol Ther. 2004;75:331–41.

76. Abraham BK, Adithan C. Genetic polymorphism of CYP2D6. Indian J Pharmacol. 2001;33:147–69.

77. Elliot JA. α_2-Agonists. In: Smith HS, editor. Current therapy in pain. Philadelphia: Saunders; 2009. p. 476–9. Print.

78. Weigert G, Resch H, Luksch A, et al. Intravenous administration of clonidine reduces intraocular pressure and alters ocular blood flow. Br J Ophthalmol. 2007;91:1354–8.

79. Toth P, Urtis J. Commonly used muscle relaxant therapies for acute low back pain: a review of carisoprodol, cyclobenzaprine hydrochloride, and metaxalone. Clin Ther. 2004;26(9):1355–67.

80. Ingelman-Sundberg M, Oscarson M, McLellan R. Polymorphic human cytochrome P450 enzymes: an opportunity for individualized drug treatment. Trends Pharmacol Sci. 1999;20(8):342–9.

81. Phillips K, et al. Potential role of pharmacogenomics in reducing adverse drug reactions: a systematic review. JAMA. 2001;286(18):2270–9.

82. AmpliChip CYP450 test package insert. Roche Molecular Systems, Inc.; 2009.

Role of Cannabinoids in Pain Management

Ethan B. Russo and Andrea G. Hohmann

Key Points

- Cannabinoids are pharmacological agents of endogenous (endocannabinoids), botanical (phytocannabinoids), or synthetic origin.
- Cannabinoids alleviate pain through a variety of receptor and non-receptor mechanisms including direct analgesic and anti-inflammatory effects, modulatory actions on neurotransmitters, and interactions with endogenous and administered opioids.
- Cannabinoid agents are currently available in various countries for pain treatment, and even cannabinoids of botanical origin may be approvable by FDA, although this is distinctly unlikely for smoked cannabis.
- An impressive body of literature supports cannabinoid analgesia, and recently, this has been supplemented by an increasing number of phase I–III clinical trials.

Introduction

Plants and Pain

It is a curious fact that we owe a great deal of our insight into pharmacological treatment of pain to the plant world [1]. Willow bark from *Salix* spp. led to development of aspirin and eventual elucidation of the analgesic effects of prostaglandins and their role in inflammation. The opium poppy (*Papaver somniferum*) provided the prototypic narcotic analgesic morphine, the first alkaloid discovered, and stimulated the much later discovery of the endorphin and enkephalin systems. Similarly, the pharmacological properties of cannabis (*Cannabis sativa*) prompted the isolation of Δ^9-tetrahydrocannabinol (THC), the major psychoactive ingredient in cannabis, in 1964 [2]. It is this breakthrough that subsequently prompted the more recent discovery of the body's own cannabis-like system, the endocannabinoid system (ECS), which modulates pain under physiological conditions. Pro-nociceptive mechanisms of the endovanilloid system were similarly revealed by phytochemistry of capsaicin, the pungent ingredient in hot chile peppers (*Capsicum annuum* etc.), which activates transient receptor potential vanilloid receptor-1 (TRPV1). Additional plant products such as the mints and mustards activate other TRP channels to produce their physiological effects.

The Endocannabinoid System

There are three recognized types of cannabinoids: (1) the phytocannabinoids [3] derived from the cannabis plant, (2) synthetic cannabinoids (e.g., ajulemic acid, nabilone, CP55940, WIN55, 212-2) based upon the chemical structure of THC or other ligands which bind cannabinoid receptors, and (3) the endogenous cannabinoids or endocannabinoids. Endocannabinoids are natural chemicals such as anandamide (AEA) and 2-arachidonoylglycerol (2-AG) found in animals whose basic functions are "relax, eat, sleep, forget, and protect" [4]. The endocannabinoid system encompasses the endocannabinoids themselves, their biosynthetic and catabolic enzymes, and their corresponding receptors [5]. AEA is hydrolyzed by the enzyme fatty-acid amide hydrolase (FAAH) into breakdown products arachidonic acid and ethanolamine [6]. By contrast, 2-AG is hydrolyzed primarily by the enzyme monoacylglycerol lipase (MGL) into breakdown

E.B. Russo, M.D. (✉)
GW Pharmaceuticals, 20402 81st Avenue SW,
Vashon, WA 98070, USA

Pharmaceutical Sciences, University of Montana,
Missoula, MT, USA
e-mail: ethanrusso@comcast.net

A.G. Hohmann, Ph.D.
Department of Psychological and Brain Sciences, Indiana
University, 101 East 10th Street, Bloomington, IN 47405, USA
e-mail: hohmanna@indiana.edu

T.R. Deer et al. (eds.), *Treatment of Chronic Pain by Medical Approaches: the AMERICAN ACADEMY of PAIN MEDICINE Textbook on Patient Management*, DOI 10.1007/978-1-4939-1818-8_18,
© American Academy of Pain Medicine 2015

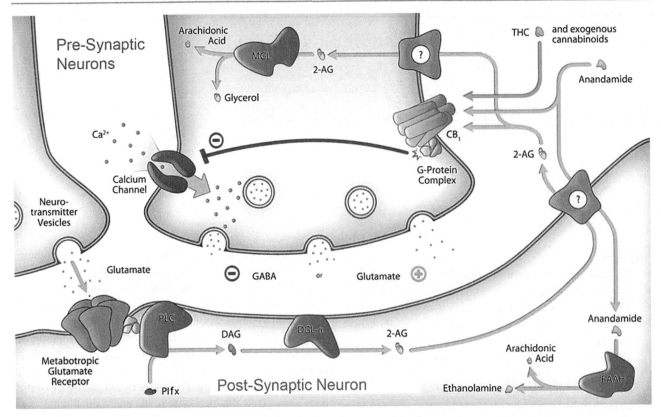

Fig. 18.1 Putative mechanism of endocannabinoid-mediated retrograde signaling in the nervous system. Activation of metabotropic glutamate receptors (*mGluR*) by glutamate triggers the activation of the phospholipase C (*PLC*)-diacylglycerol lipase (*DGL*) pathway to generate the endocannabinoid 2-arachidonoylglycerol (*2-AG*). First, the 2-AG precursor diacylglycerol (*DAG*) is formed from PLC-mediated hydrolysis of membrane phospholipid precursors (*PIPx*). DAG is then hydrolyzed by the enzyme DGL-α to generate 2-AG. 2-AG is released from the postsynaptic neuron and acts as a retrograde signaling molecule. Endocannabinoids activate presynaptic CB₁ receptors which reside on terminals of glutamatergic and GABAergic neurons. Activation of CB₁ by 2-AG, anandamide, or exogenous cannabinoids (e.g., tetrahydrocannabinol, *THC*) inhibits calcium influx in the presynaptic terminal, thereby inhibiting release of the primary neurotransmitter (i.e., glutamate or GABA) from the synaptic vesicle. Endocannabinoids are then rapidly deactivated by transport into cells (via a putative endocannabinoid transporter) followed by intracellular hydrolysis. 2-AG is metabolized by the enzyme monoacylglycerol lipase (*MGL*), whereas anandamide is metabolized by a distinct enzyme, fatty-acid amide hydrolase (*FAAH*). Note that MGL co-localizes with CB₁ in the presynaptic terminal, whereas FAAH is localized to postsynaptic sites. The existence of an endocannabinoid transporter remains controversial. Pharmacological inhibitors of either endocannabinoid deactivation (e.g., FAAH and MGL inhibitors) or transport (i.e., uptake inhibitors) have been developed to exploit the therapeutic potential of the endocannabinoid signaling system in the treatment of pain (Figure by authors with kind assistance of James Brodie, GW Pharmaceuticals)

products arachidonic acid and glycerol [7] and to a lesser extent by the enzymes ABHD6 and ABHD12. FAAH, a postsynaptic enzyme, may control anandamide levels near sites of synthesis, whereas MGL, a presynaptic enzyme [8], may terminate 2-AG signaling following CB₁ receptor activation. These enzymes also represent therapeutic targets because inhibition of endocannabinoid deactivation will increase levels of endocannabinoids at sites with ongoing synthesis and release [9]. The pathways controlling formation of AEA remain poorly understood. However, 2-AG is believed to be formed from membrane phospholipid precursors through the sequential activation of two distinct enzymes, phospholipase C and diacylglycerol lipase-α. First, PLC catalyzes formation of the 2-AG precursor diacylglycerol (DAG) from membrane phosphoinositides. Then, DAG is hydrolyzed by the enzyme diacylglycerol lipase-α (DGL-α) to generate 2-AG [199].

There are currently two well-defined cannabinoid receptors, although additional candidate cannabinoid receptors have also been postulated. CB₁, a seven transmembrane spanning G-protein-coupled receptor inhibiting cyclic AMP release, was identified in 1988 [10]. CB₁ is the primary neuromodulatory receptor accounting for psychopharmacological effects of THC and most of its analgesic effects [11]. Endocannabinoids are produced on demand in postsynaptic cells and engage presynaptic CB₁ receptors through a retrograde mechanism [12]. Activation of presynaptic CB₁ receptors then acts as a synaptic circuit breaker to inhibit neurotransmitter release (either excitatory or inhibitory) from the presynaptic neuron (*vide infra*) (Fig. 18.1). CB₂ was identified in 1992, and while thought of primarily as a peripheral immunomodulatory receptor, it also has important effects on pain. The role of CB₂ in modulating persistent inflammatory and neuropathic pain [13] has been recently reviewed [14, 15]. Activation of CB_2 suppresses neuropathic pain mechanisms through nonneuronal (i.e., microglia and astrocytes) and neuronal mechanisms that may involve interferon-gamma [16]. THC, the prototypical classical cannabinoid, is a weak partial agonist at both CB_1 and CB_2 receptors. Transgenic mice lacking cannabinoid receptors (CB_1, CB_2, GPR55), enzymes controlling endocannabinoid breakdown (FAAH, MGL, ABHD6), and endocannabinoid synthesis (DGL-α, DGL-β) have been generated [17]. These knockouts have helped elucidate the role of the endocannabinoid system in controlling nociceptive processing and facilitated development of inhibitors of endocannabinoid breakdown (FAAH, MGL) as novel classes of analgesics.

A Brief Scientific History of Cannabis and Pain

Centuries of Citations

Cannabis has been utilized in one form or another for treatment of pain for longer than written history [18–21]. Although this documentation has been a major preoccupation of the lead author [22–25], and such information can provide provocative direction to inform modern research on treatment of pain and other conditions, it does not represent evidence of form, content, or degree that is commonly acceptable to governmental regulatory bodies with respect to pharmaceutical development.

Anecdotes Versus Modern Proof of Concept

While thousands of compelling stories of efficacy of cannabis in pain treatment certainly underline the importance of properly harnessing cannabinoid mechanisms therapeutically [26, 27], prescription analgesics in the United States necessitate Food and Drug Administration (FDA) approval. This requires a rigorous development program proving consistency, quality, efficacy, and safety as defined by basic scientific studies and randomized controlled trials (RCT) [28] and generally adhering to recent IMMPACT recommendations [29], provoking our next question.

Can a Botanical Agent Become a Prescription Medicine?

Most modern physicians fail to recognize that pharmacognosy (study of medicinal plants) has led directly or indirectly to an estimated 25 % of modern pharmaceuticals [30]. While the plethora of available herbal agents yield an indecipherable cacophony to most clinicians and consumers alike, it is certainly possible to standardize botanical agents and facilitate their recommendation based on sound science [31]. Botanical medicines can even fulfill the rigorous dictates of the FDA and attain prescription drug status via a clear roadmap in the form of a blueprint document [32], henceforth termed the *Botanical Guidance*: http://www.fda.gov/downloads/Drugs/GuidanceComplianceRegulatoryInformation/Guidances/ucm070491.pdf. To be successful and clinically valuable, botanicals, including cannabis-based medicines, must demonstrate the same quality, clinical analgesic benefit, and appropriately safe adverse event profile as available new chemical entities (NCE) [28].

The Biochemical and Neurophysiological Basis of Pain Control by Cannabinoids

Neuropathic Pain

Thorough reviews of therapeutic effects of cannabinoids in preclinical and clinical domains have recently been published [33, 34]. In essence, the endocannabinoid system (ECS) is active throughout the CNS and PNS in modulating pain at spinal, supraspinal, and peripheral levels. Endocannabinoids are produced on demand in the CNS to dampen sensitivity to pain [35]. The endocannabinoid system is operative in such key integrative pain centers as the periaqueductal grey matter [36, 37], the ventroposterolateral nucleus of the thalamus [38], and the spinal cord [39, 40]. Endocannabinoids are endogenous mediators of stress-induced analgesia and fear-conditioned analgesia and suppress pain-related phenomena such as windup [41] and allodynia [42]. In the periphery and PNS [13], the ECS has key effects in suppressing both hyperalgesia and allodynia via CB_1 [43] and CB_2 mechanisms (Fig. 18.2). Indeed, pathological pain states have been postulated to arise, at least in part, from a dysregulation of the endocannabinoid system.

Antinociceptive and Anti-inflammatory Pain Mechanisms

Beyond the mechanisms previously mentioned, the ECS plays a critical role in peripheral pain, inflammation, and hyperalgesia [43] through both CB_1 and CB_2 mechanisms. CB_1 and CB_2 mechanisms are also implicated in regulation of contact dermatitis and pruritus [44]. A role for spinal CB_2 mechanisms, mediated by microglia and/or astrocytes, is also revealed under conditions of inflammation [45]. Both THC and cannabidiol (CBD), a non-euphoriant phytocannabinoid common in certain cannabis strains, are potent

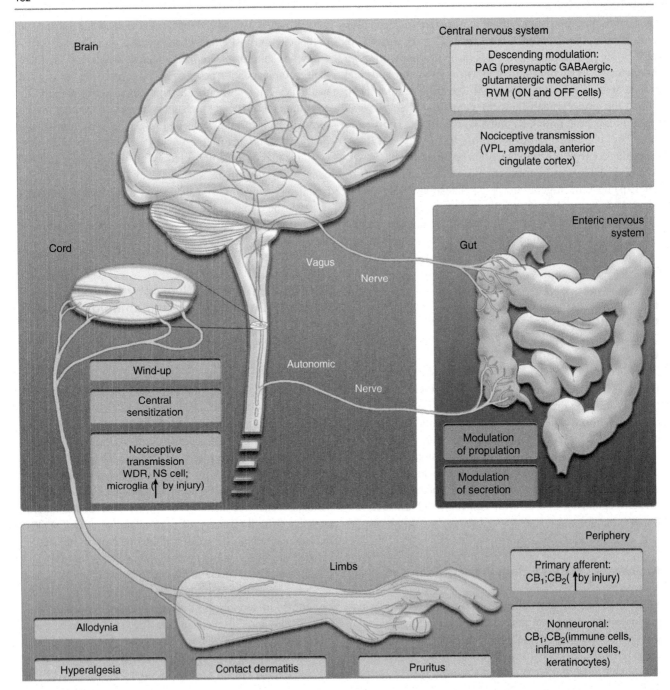

Fig. 18.2 Cannabinoids suppress pain and other pathophysiological (e.g., contact dermatitis, pruritis) and physiological (e.g., gastrointestinal transit and secretion) processes through multiple mechanisms involving CB_1 and CB_2 receptors. Peripheral, spinal, and supraspinal sites of cannabinoid actions are shown. In the periphery, cannabinoids act through both neuronal and nonneuronal mechanisms to control inflammation, allodynia, and hyperalgesia. CB_1 and CB_2 have been localized to both primary afferents and nonneuronal cells (e.g., keratinocytes, microglia), and expression can be regulated by injury. In the spinal cord, cannabinoids suppress nociceptive transmission, windup, and central sensitization by modulating activity in the ascending pain pathway of the spinothalamic tract, including responses of wide dynamic range (*WDR*) and nociceptive specific (*NS*) cells. Similar processes are observed at rostral levels of the neuraxis (e.g., ventroposterolateral nucleus of the thalamus, amygdala, anterior cingulate cortex). Cannabinoids also actively modulate pain through descending mechanisms. In the periaqueductal gray, cannabinoids act through presynaptic glutamatergic and GABAergic mechanisms to control nociception. In the rostral ventromedial medulla, cannabinoids suppress activity in ON cells and inhibit the firing pause of OFF cells, in response to noxious stimulation to produce antinociception (Figure by authors with kind assistance of James Brodie, GW Pharmaceuticals)

anti-inflammatory antioxidants with activity exceeding that of vitamins C and E via non-cannabinoid mechanisms [46]. THC inhibits prostaglandin E-2 synthesis [47] and stimulates lipooxygenase [48]. Neither THC nor CBD affects COX-1 or COX-2 at relevant pharmacological dosages [49].

While THC is inactive at vanilloid receptors, CBD, like AEA, is a $TRPV_1$ agonist. Like capsaicin, CBD is capable of inhibiting fatty-acid amide hydrolase (FAAH), the enzyme which hydrolyzes AEA and other fatty-acid amides that do not bind to cannabinoid receptors. CBD additionally inhibits AEA reuptake [50] though not potently. Thus, CBD acts as an endocannabinoid modulator [51], a mechanism that various pharmaceutical firms hope to emulate with new chemical entities (NCEs). CBD inhibits hepatic metabolism of THC to 11-hydroxy-THC, which is possibly more psychoactive, and prolongs its half-life, reducing its psychoactivity and attenuating attendant anxiety and tachycardia [51]; antagonizes psychotic symptoms [52]; and attenuates appetitive effects of THC [53] as well as its effects on short-term memory [54]. CBD also inhibits tumor necrosis factor-alpha (TNF-α) in a rodent model of rheumatoid arthritis [55]. Recently, CBD has been demonstrated to enhance adenosine receptor A2A signaling via inhibition of the adenosine transporter [56].

Recently, GPR18 has been proposed as a putative CBD receptor whose function relates to cellular migration [57]. Antagonism of GPR18 (by agents such as CBD) may be efficacious in treating pain of endometriosis, among other conditions, especially considering that such pain may be endocannabinoid-mediated [58]. Cannabinoids are also very active in various gastrointestinal and visceral sites mediating pain responses [59, 60].

Cannabinoid Interactions with Other Neurotransmitters Pertinent to Pain

As alluded to above, the ECS modulates neurotransmitter release via retrograde inhibition. This is particularly important in NMDA-glutamatergic mechanisms that become hyperresponsive in chronic pain states. Cannabinoids specifically inhibit glutamate release in the hippocampus [61]. THC reduces NMDA responses by 30–40 % [46]. Secondary and tertiary hyperalgesia mediated by NMDA [62] and by calcitonin gene-related peptide [40] may well be targets of cannabinoid therapy in disorders such as migraine, fibromyalgia, and idiopathic bowel syndrome wherein these mechanisms seem to operate pathophysiologically [63], prompting the hypothesis of a "clinical endocannabinoid deficiency." Endocannabinoid modulators may therefore restore homeostasis, leading to normalization of function in these pathophysiological conditions. THC also has numerous effects on serotonergic systems germane to migraine [64], increasing its production in the cerebrum while decreasing reuptake [65].

In fact, the ECS seems to modulate the trigeminovascular system of migraine pathogenesis at vascular and neurochemical levels [66–68].

Cannabinoid-Opioid Interactions

Although endocannabinoids do not bind to opioid receptors, the ECS may nonetheless work in parallel with the endogenous opioid system with numerous areas of overlap and interaction. Pertinent mechanisms include stimulation of beta-endorphin by THC [69] as well as its ability to demonstrate experimental opiate sparing [70], prevent opioid tolerance and withdrawal [71], and rekindle opioid analgesia after loss of effect [72]. Adjunctive treatments that combine opioids with cannabinoids may enhance the analgesic effects of either agent. Such strategies may permit lower doses of analgesics to be employed for therapeutic benefit in a manner that minimizes incidence or severity of adverse side effects.

Clinical Trials, Utility, and Pitfalls of Cannabinoids in Pain

Evidence for Synthetic Cannabinoids

Oral dronabinol (THC) has been available as the synthetic Marinol® since 1985 and is indicated for nausea associated with chemotherapy and appetite stimulation in HIV/AIDS. Issues with its cost, titration difficulties, delayed onset, and propensity to induce intoxicating and dysphoric effects have limited clinical application [73]. It was employed in two open-label studies of chronic neuropathic pain in case studies in 7 [74] and 8 patients [75], but no significant benefit was evident and side effects led to prominent dropout rates (average doses 15–16.6 mg THC). Dronabinol produced benefit in pain in multiple sclerosis [76], but none was evident in postoperative pain (Table 18.1) [77]. Dronabinol was reported to relieve pruritus in three case-report subjects with cholestatic jaundice [78]. Dronabinol was assessed in 30 chronic non-cancer pain patients on opioids in double-blind crossover single-day sessions vs. placebo with improvement [79], followed by a 4-week open-label trial with continued improvement (Table 18.1). Associated adverse events were prominent. Methodological issues included lack of prescreening for cannabinoids, 4 placebo subjects with positive THC assays, and 58 % of subjects correctly guessing Marinol dose on test day. An open-label comparison in polyneuropathy examined nabilone patients with 6 obtaining 22.6 % mean pain relief after 3 months, and 5 achieving 28.6 % relief after 6 months, comparable to conventional agents [80]. A pilot study of

Table 18.1 Randomized controlled trials of cannabinoids in pain

Agent	N =	Indication	Duration/type	Outcomes/reference
Ajulemic acid	21	Neuropathic pain	7 day crossover	Visual analogue pain scales improved over placebo ($p = 0.02$)/Karst et al. [92]
Cannabis, smoked	50	HIV neuropathy	5 days/DB	Decreased daily pain ($p = 0.03$) and hyperalgesia ($p = 0.05$), 52 % with >30 % pain reduction vs. placebo ($p = 0.04$)/Abrams et al. [94]
Cannabis, smoked	23	Chronic neuropathic pain	5 days/DB	Decreased pain vs. placebo only at 9.4 % THC level ($p = 0.023$)/Ware et al. [98]
Cannabis, smoked	38	Neuropathic pain	Single dose/DBC	NSD in pain except at highest cannabis dose ($p = 0.02$), with prominent psychoactive effects/Wilsey et al. [95]
Cannabis, smoked	34	HIV neuropathy	5 days /DB	DDS improved over placebo ($p = 0.016$), 46 % vs. 18 % improved >30 %, 2 cases toxic psychosis/Ellis et al. [97]
Cannabis, vaporized	21	Chronic pain on opioids	5 days/DB	27 % decrement in pain/Abrams et al. [118]
Cannador	419	Pain due to spasm in MS	15 weeks	Improvement over placebo in subjective pain associated with spasm ($p = 0.003$)/Zajicek et al. [120]
Cannador	65	Postherpetic neuralgia	4 weeks	No benefit observed/Ernst et al. [122]
Cannador	30	Postoperative pain	Single doses, daily	Decreasing pain intensity with increased dose ($p = 0.01$)/Holdcroft et al. [123]
Marinol	24	Neuropathic pain in MS	15–21 days/DBC	Median numerical pain ($p = 0.02$), median pain relief improved ($p = 0.035$) over placebo/Svendsen et al. [76]
Marinol	40	Postoperative pain	Single dose/DB	No benefit observed over placebo/Buggy et al. [77]
Marinol	30	Chronic pain	3 doses, 1 day/DBC	Total pain relief improved with 10 mg ($p < 0.05$) and 20 mg ($p < 0.01$) with opioids, AE prominent/Narang et al. [79]
Nabilone	41	Postoperative pain	3 doses in 24 h/DB	NSD morphine consumption. Increased pain at rest and on movement with nabilone 1 or 2 mg/Beaulieu [85]
Nabilone	31	Fibromyalgia	2 weeks/DBC	Compared to amitriptyline, nabilone improved sleep, decrease wakefulness, had no effect on pain, and increased AE/Ware et al. [90]
Nabilone	96	Neuropathic pain	14 weeks/DBC vs. dihydrocodeine	Dihydrocodeine more effective with fewer AE/Frank et al. [88]
Nabilone	13	Spasticity pain	9 weeks/DBC	NRS decreased 2 points for nabilone ($p < 0.05$)/Wissel et al. [87]
Nabilone	40	Fibromyalgia	4 weeks/DBC	VAS decreased in pain, Fibromyalgia Impact Questionnaire, and anxiety over placebo (all, $p < 0.02$)/Skrabek et al. [89]
Sativex	20	Neurogenic pain	Series of 2-week N-of-1 crossover blocks	Improvement with Tetranabinex and Sativex on VAS pain vs. placebo ($p < 0.05$), symptom control best with Sativex ($p < 0.0001$)/Wade et al. [132]
Sativex	24	Chronic intractable pain	12 weeks, series of N-of-1 crossover blocks	VAS pain improved over placebo ($p < 0.001$) especially in MS ($p < 0.0042$)/Notcutt et al. [133]
Sativex	48	Brachial plexus avulsion	6 weeks in 3 two-week crossover blocks	Benefits noted in Box Scale-11 pain scores with Tetranabinex ($p = 0.002$) and Sativex ($p = 0.005$) over placebo/Berman et al. [134]
Sativex	66	Central neuropathic pain in MS	5 weeks	Numerical Rating Scale (NRS) analgesia improved over placebo ($p = 0.009$)/Rog et al. [135]
Sativex	125	Peripheral neuropathic pain	5 weeks	Improvements in NRS pain levels ($p = 0.004$), dynamic allodynia ($p = 0.042$), and punctuate allodynia ($p = 0.021$) vs. placebo/Nurmikko et al. [136]
Sativex	56	Rheumatoid arthritis	Nocturnal dosing for 5 weeks	Improvements over placebo morning pain on movement ($p = 0.044$), morning pain at rest ($p = 0.018$), DAS-28 ($p = 0.002$), and SF-MPQ pain at present ($p = 0.016$)/Blake et al. [138]
Sativex	117	Pain after spinal injury	10 days	NSD in NRS pain scores, but improved Brief Pain Inventory ($p = 0.032$), and Patients' Global Impression of Change ($p = 0.001$) (unpublished)
Sativex	177	Intractable cancer pain	2 weeks	Improvements in NRS analgesia vs. placebo ($p = 0.0142$), Tetranabinex NSD/Johnson et al. [139]
Sativex	135	Intractable lower urinary tract symptoms in MS	8 weeks	Improved bladder severity symptoms including pain over placebo ($p = 0.001$) [200]
Sativex	360	Intractable cancer pain	5 weeks/DB	CRA of lower and middle-dose cohorts improved over placebo ($p = 0.006$)/ [201]

Marinol in seven spinal cord injury patients with neuropathic pain saw two withdraw, and the remainder appreciate no greater efficacy than with diphenhydramine [81].

Nabilone, or Cesamet®, is a semisynthetic analogue of THC that is about tenfold more potent, and longer lasting [82]. It is indicated as an antiemetic in chemotherapy in the USA. Prior case reports in neuropathic pain [83] and other pain disorders [84] have been published. Sedation and dysphoria are prominent associated adverse events. An RCT of nabilone in 41 postoperative subjects dosed TID actually resulted in increased pain scores (Table 18.1) [85]. An uncontrolled study of 82 cancer patients on nabilone noted improved pain scores [86], but retention rates were limited. Nabilone improved pain ($p < 0.05$) vs. placebo in patients with mixed spasticity syndromes in a small double-blind trial (Table 18.1) [87], but was without benefits in other parameters. In a double-blind crossover comparison of nabilone to dihydrocodeine (schedule II opioid) in chronic neuropathic pain (Table 18.1) [88], both drugs produced marginal benefit, but with dihydrocodeine proving clearly superior in efficacy and modestly superior in side-effect profile. In an RCT in 40 patients of nabilone vs. placebo over 4 weeks, it showed significant decreases in VAS of pain and anxiety (Table 18.1) [89]. A more recent study of nabilone vs. amitriptyline in fibromyalgia yielded benefits on sleep, but not pain, mood, or quality of life (Table 18.1) [90]. An open-label trial of nabilone vs. gabapentin found them comparable in pain and other symptom relief in peripheral neuropathic pain [91].

Ajulemic acid (CT3), another synthetic THC analogue in development, was utilized in a phase II RCT in peripheral neuropathic pain in 21 subjects with apparent improvement (Table 18.1) [92]. Whether or not ajulemic acid is psychoactive is the subject of some controversy [93].

Evidence for Smoked or Vaporized Cannabis

Few randomized controlled clinical trials (RCTs) of pain with smoked cannabis have been undertaken to date [94–97]. One of these [96] examined cannabis effects on experimental pain in normal volunteers.

Abrams et al. [94] studied inpatient adults with painful HIV neuropathy in 25 subjects in double-blind fashion to receive either smoked cannabis as 3.56 % THC cigarettes or placebo cigarettes three times daily for 5 days (Table 18.1). The smoked cannabis group had a 34 % reduction in daily pain vs. 17 % in the placebo group ($p = 0.03$). The cannabis cohort also had a 52 % of subjects report a >30 % reduction in pain scores over the 5 days vs. 24 % in the placebo group ($p = 0.04$) (Table 18.1). The authors rated cannabis as "well tolerated" due to an absence of serious adverse events (AE)

leading to withdrawal, but all subjects were cannabis experienced. Symptoms of possible intoxication in the cannabis group including anxiety (25 %), sedation (54 %), disorientation (16 %), paranoia (13 %), confusion (17 %), dizziness (15 %), and nausea (11 %) were all statistically significantly more common than in the placebo group. Despite these findings, the authors stated that the values do not represent any serious safety concern in this short-term study. No discussion in the article addressed issues of the relative efficacy of blinding in the trial.

Wilsey et al. [95] examined neuropathic pain in 38 subjects in a double-blind crossover study comparing 7 % THC cannabis, 3.5 % THC cannabis, and placebo cigarettes via a complex cumulative dosing scheme with each dosage given once, in random order, with at least 3 day intervals separating sessions (Table 18.1). A total of 9 puffs maximum were allowed over several hours per session. Authors stated, "Psychoactive effects were minimal and well-tolerated, but neuropsychological impairment was problematic, particularly with the higher concentration of study medication." Again, only cannabis-experienced subjects were allowed entry. No withdrawals due to AE were reported, but 1 subject was removed due to elevated blood pressure. No significant differences were noted in pain relief in the two cannabis potency groups, but a significant separation of pain reduction from placebo ($p = 0.02$) was not evident until a cumulative 9 puffs at 240 min elapsed time. Pain unpleasantness was also reduced in both active treatment groups ($p < 0.01$). Subjectively, an "any drug effect" demonstrated a visual analogue scale (VAS) of 60/100 in the high-dose group, but even the low-dose group registered more of a "good drug effect" than placebo ($p < 0.001$). "Bad drug effect" was also evident. "Feeling high" and "feeling stoned" were greatest in the high-dose sessions ($p < 0.001$), while both high- and low-dose differentiated significantly from placebo ($p < 0.05$). Of greater concern, both groups rated impairment as 30/100 on VAS vs. placebo ($p = 0.003$). Sedation also demarcated both groups from placebo ($p < 0.01$), as did confusion ($p = 0.03$), and hunger ($p < 0.001$). Anxiety was not considered a prominent feature in this cannabis-experienced population. This study distinguished itself from some others in its inclusion of specific objective neuropsychological measures and demonstrated neurocognitive impairment in attention, learning, and memory, most noteworthy with 7 % THC cannabis. No commentary on blinding efficacy was included.

Ellis et al. [97] examined HIV-associated neuropathic pain in a double-blind trial of placebo vs. 1–8 % THC cannabis administered four times daily over 5 days with a 2-week washout (Table 18.1). Subjects were started at 4 % THC and then titrated upward or downward in four smoking sessions dependent upon their symptom relief and tolerance of the dose. In this study, 96 % of subjects were cannabis-experienced, and 28 out of 34 subjects completed the trial. The primary outcome measure (Descriptor Differential Scale, DDS) was improved in the active group over placebo ($p = 0.016$), with >30 % relief noted in 46 % of cannabis subjects vs. 18 % of placebo. While most adverse events (AE) were considered mild and self-limited, two subjects had to leave the trial due to toxicity. One cannabis-naïve subject was withdrawn due to "an acute cannabis-induced psychosis" at what proved to be his first actual cannabis exposure. The other subject suffered intractable cough. Pain reduction was greater in the cannabis-treated group ($p = 0.016$) among completers, as was the proportion of subjects attaining >30 % pain reduction (46 % vs. 18 %, $p = 0.043$). Blinding was assessed in this study; whereas placebo patients were inaccurate at guessing the investigational product, 93 % of those receiving cannabis guessed correctly. On safety issues, the authors stated that the frequency of some nontreatment-limiting side effects was greater for cannabis than placebo. These included concentration difficulties, fatigue, sleepiness or sedation, increased duration of sleep, reduced salivation, and thirst.

A Canadian study [98] examined single 25-mg inhalations of various cannabis potencies (0–9.4 % THC) three times daily for 5 days per cycle in 23 subjects with chronic neuropathic pain (Table 18.1). Patients were said to be cannabis-free for 1 year, but were required to have some experience of the drug. Only the highest potency demarcated from placebo on decrements in average daily pain score (5.4 vs. 6.1, $p = 0.023$). The most frequent AE in the high-dose group were headache, dry eyes, burning sensation, dizziness, numbness, and cough, but with "high" or "euphoria" reported only once in each cannabis potency group.

The current studies of smoked cannabis are noteworthy for their extremely short-term exposure and would be of uncertain relevance in a regulatory environment. The IMMPACT recommendations on chronic neuropathic pain clinical trials that are currently favored by the FDA [29] generally suggest randomized controlled clinical trials of 12-week duration as a prerequisite to demonstrate efficacy and safety. While one might assume that the degree of pain improvement demonstrated in these trials could be maintained over this longer interval, it is only reasonable to assume that cumulative adverse events would also increase to at least some degree. The combined studies represent only a total of 1,106 patient-days of cannabis exposure (Abrams: 125, Wilsey: 76, Ellis: 560, Ware 345) or 3 patient-years of experience. In contrast, over 6,000 patient-years of data have been analyzed for Sativex between clinical trials, prescription, and named-patient supplies, with vastly lower AE rates (data on file, GW Pharmaceuticals) [28, 99]. Certainly, the cognitive effects noted in California-smoked cannabis studies figure among many factors that would call the efficacy of

blinding into question for investigations employing such an approach. However, it is also important to emphasize that unwanted side effects are not unique to cannabinoids. In a prospective evaluation of specific chronic polyneuropathy syndromes and their response to pharmacological therapies, the presence of intolerable side effects did not differ in groups receiving gabapentinoids, tricyclic antidepressants, anticonvulsants, cannabinoids (including nabilone, Sativex), and topical agents [80]. Moreover, no serious adverse events were related to any of the medications.

The current studies were performed in a very select subset of patients who almost invariably have had prior experience of cannabis. Their applicability to cannabis-naïve populations is, thus, quite unclear. At best, the observed benefits might possibly accrue to some, but it is eminently likely that candidates for such therapy might refuse it on any number of grounds: not wishing to smoke, concern with respect to intoxication, etc. Sequelae of smoking in therapeutic outcomes have had little discussion in these brief RCTs [28]. Cannabis smoking poses substantial risk of chronic cough and bronchitic symptoms [100], if not obvious emphysematous degeneration [101] or increase in aerodigestive cancers [102]. Even such smoked cannabis proponents as Lester Grinspoon has acknowledged are the only well-confirmed deleterious physical effect of marihuana is harm to the pulmonary system [103]. However, population-based studies of cannabis trials have failed to show any evidence for increased risk of respiratory symptoms/chronic obstructive pulmonary disease [100] or lung cancer [102] associated with smoking cannabis.

A very detailed analysis and comparison of mainstream and sidestream smoke for cannabis vs. tobacco smoke was performed in Canada [104]. Of note, cannabis smoke contained ammonia (NH_3) at a level of 720 μg per 775 mg cigarette, a figure 20-fold higher than that found in tobacco smoke. It was hypothesized that this finding was likely attributable to nitrate fertilizers. Formaldehyde and acetaldehyde were generally lower in cannabis smoke than in tobacco, but butyraldehyde was higher. Polycyclic aromatic hydrocarbon (PAH) contents were qualitatively similar in the comparisons, but total yield was lower for cannabis mainstream smoke, but higher than tobacco for sidestream smoke. Additionally, NO, NO_x, hydrogen cyanide, and aromatic amines concentrations were 3–5 times higher in cannabis smoke than that from tobacco. Possible mutagenic and carcinogenic potential of these various compounds were mentioned. More recently, experimental analysis of cannabis smoke with resultant acetaldehyde production has posited its genotoxic potential to be attributable to reactions that produce DNA adducts [105].

Vaporizers for cannabis have been offered as a harm reduction technique that would theoretically eliminate products of combustion and associated adverse events.

The Institute of Medicine (IOM) examined cannabis issues in 1999 [106], and among their conclusions was the following (p. 4): "Recommendation 2: Clinical trials of cannabinoid drugs for symptom management should be conducted with the goal of developing rapid-onset, reliable, and safe delivery systems." One proposed technique is vaporization, whereby cannabis is heated to a temperature that volatilizes THC and other components with the goal of reducing or eliminating by-products of combustion, including potentially carcinogenic polycyclic aromatic hydrocarbons, benzene, acetaldehyde, carbon monoxide, toluene, naphthaline, phenol, toluene, hydrogen cyanide, and ammonia. Space limitations permit only a cursory review of available literature [107–115].

A pilot study of the Volcano vaporizer vs. smoking was performed in the USA in 2007 in 18 active cannabis consumers, with only 48 h of presumed abstinence [116]. NIDA 900-mg cannabis cigarettes were employed (1.7, 3.4, and 6.8 % THC) with each divided in two, so that one-half would be smoked or vaporized in a series of double-blind sessions. The Volcano vaporizer produced comparable or slightly higher THC plasma concentrations than smoking. Measured CO in exhaled vapor sessions diminished very slightly, while it increased after smoking ($p < 0.001$). Self-reported visual analogue scales of the associated high were virtually identical in vaporization vs. smoking sessions and increased with higher potency material. A contention was advanced that the absence of CO increase after vaporization can be equated to "little or no exposure to gaseous combustion toxins." Given that no measures of PAH or other components were undertaken, the assertion is questionable. It was also stated that there were no reported adverse events. Some 12 subjects preferred the Volcano, 2 chose smoking, and 2 had no preference as to technique, making the vaporizer "an acceptable system" and providing "a safer way to deliver THC."

A recent [202, 117] examined interactions of 3.2 % THC NIDA cannabis vaporized in the Volcano in conjunction with opioid treatment in a 5-day inpatient trial in 21 patients with chronic pain (Table 18.1). All subjects were prior cannabis smokers. Overall, pain scores were reduced from 39.6 to 29.1 on a VAS, a 27 % reduction, by day 5. Pain scores in subjects on morphine fell from 34.8 to 24.1, while in subjects taking oxycodone, scores dropped from 43.8 to 33.6.

The clinical studies performed with vaporizers to date have been very small pilot studies conducted over very limited timeframes (i.e., for a maximum of 5 days). Thus, these studies cannot contribute in any meaningful fashion toward possible FDA approval of vaporized cannabis as a delivery technique, device, or drug under existing policies dictated by the *Botanical Guidance* [32]. It is likewise quite unlikely that the current AE profile of smoked or vaporized cannabis would meet FDA requirements. The fact that all the vaporization trials to date have been undertaken only in cannabis-experienced subjects does not imply that results would generalize to larger patient populations. Moreover, there is certainly no reason to expect AE profiles to be better in cannabis-naïve patients. Additionally, existing standardization of cannabis product and delivery via vaporization seem far off the required marks. Although vaporizers represent an alternate delivery method devoid of the illegality associated with smoked cannabis, the presence of toxic ingredients such as PAH, ammonia, and acetaldehyde in cannabis vapor are unlikely to be acceptable to FDA in any significant amounts. Existing vaporizers still lack portability or convenience [28]. A large Internet survey revealed that only 2.2 % of cannabis users employed vaporization as their primary cannabis intake method [118]. While studies to date have established that lower temperature vaporization in the Volcano, but not necessarily other devices, can reduce the relative amounts of noxious by-products of combustion, it has yet to be demonstrated that they are totally eliminated. Until or unless this goal is achieved, along with requisite benchmarks of herbal cannabis quality, safety, and efficacy in properly designed randomized clinical trials, vaporization remains an unproven technology for therapeutic cannabinoid administration.

Evidence for Cannabis-Based Medicines

Cannador is a cannabis extract in oral capsules, with differing THC:CBD ratios [51]. Cannador was utilized in a phase III RCT of spasticity in multiple sclerosis (CAMS) (Table 18.1) [119]. While no improvement was evident in the Ashworth Scale, reduction was seen in spasm-associated pain. Both THC and Cannador improved pain scores in follow-up [120]. Cannador was also employed for postherpetic neuralgia in 65 patients, but without success (Table 18.1) [121, 122]. Slight pain reduction was observed in 30 subjects with postoperative pain (CANPOP) not receiving opiates, but psychoactive side effects were notable (Table 18.1).

Sativex® is a whole-cannabis-based extract delivered as an oromucosal spray that combines a CB_1 and CB_2 partial agonist (THC) with a cannabinoid system modulator (CBD), minor cannabinoids, and terpenoids plus ethanol and propylene glycol excipients and peppermint flavoring [51, 123]. It is approved in Canada for spasticity in MS and under a Notice of Compliance with Conditions for central neuropathic pain in multiple sclerosis and treatment of cancer pain unresponsive to opioids. Sativex is also approved in MS in the UK, Spain, and New Zealand, for spasticity in multiple sclerosis, with further approvals expected soon in some 22 countries around the world. Sativex is highly standardized and is formulated from two *Cannabis sativa* chemovars predominating in THC and CBD, respectively [124].

Each 100 µl pump-action oromucosal spray of Sativex yields 2.7 mg of THC and 2.5 mg of CBD plus additional components. Pharmacokinetic data are available [125–127]. Sativex effects begin within an interval allowing dose titration. A very favorable adverse event profile has been observed in the development program [27, 128]. Most patients stabilize at 8–10 sprays per day after 7–10 days, attaining symptomatic control without undue psychoactive sequelae. Sativex was added to optimized drug regimens in subjects with uncontrolled pain in every RCT (Table 18.1). An Investigational New Drug (IND) application to study Sativex in advanced clinical trials in the USA was approved by the FDA in January 2006 in patients with intractable cancer pain. One phase IIB dose-ranging study has already been completed [201]. Available clinical trials with Sativex have been independently assessed [129, 130].

In a phase II study of 20 patients with neurogenic symptoms [131], significant improvement was seen with both Tetranabinex (high-THC extract without CBD) and Sativex on pain, with Sativex displaying better symptom control ($p < 0.0001$), with less intoxication (Table 18.1).

In a phase II study of intractable chronic pain in 24 patients [132], Sativex again produced the best results compared to Tetranabinex ($p < 0.001$), especially in MS ($p < 0.0042$) (Table 18.1).

In a phase III study of brachial plexus avulsion ($N = 48$) [133], pain reduction with Tetranabinex and Sativex was about equal (Table 18.1).

In an RCT of 66 MS subjects, mean Numerical Rating Scale (NRS) analgesia favored Sativex over placebo (Table 18.1) [134].

In a phase III trial ($N = 125$) of peripheral neuropathic pain with allodynia [135], Sativex notably alleviated pain levels and dynamic and punctate allodynia (Table 18.1).

In a safety-extension study in 160 subjects with various symptoms of MS [136], 137 patients showed sustained improvements over a year or more in pain and other symptoms [99] without development of any tolerance requiring dose escalation or withdrawal effects in those who voluntarily discontinued treatment suddenly. Analgesia was quickly reestablished upon Sativex resumption.

In a phase II RCT in 56 rheumatoid arthritis sufferers over 5 weeks with Sativex [137], medicine was limited to only 6 evening sprays (16.2 mg THC + 15 mg CBD). By study end, morning pain on movement, morning pain at rest, DAS-28 measure of disease activity, and SF-MPQ pain all favored Sativex (Table 18.1).

In a phase III RCT in intractable cancer pain on opioids ($N = 177$), Sativex, Tetranabinex THC-predominant extract, and placebo were compared [138] demonstrating strongly statistically significant improvements in analgesia for Sativex only (Table 18.1). This suggests that the CBD component in Sativex was necessary for benefit.

In a 2-week study of spinal cord injury pain, NRS of pain was not statistically different from placebo, probably due to the short duration of the trial, but secondary endpoints were positive (Table 18.1). Additionally, an RCT of intractable lower urinary tract symptoms in MS also demonstrated pain reduction (Table 18.1).

The open-label study of various polyneuropathy patients included Sativex patients with 3 obtaining 21.56 % mean pain relief after 3 months (2/3 > 30 %), and 4 achieving 27.6 % relief after 6 months (2/4 > 30 %), comparable to conventional agents [80].

A recently completed RCT of Sativex in intractable cancer pain unresponsive to opioids over 5 weeks was performed in 360 subjects (Table 18.1). Results of a Continuous Response Analysis (CRA) showed improvements over placebo in the low-dose ($p = 0.08$) and middle-dose cohorts ($p = 0.038$) or combined ($p = 0.006$). Pain NRS improved over placebo in the low-dose ($p = 0.006$) and combined cohorts ($p = 0.019$).

Sleep has improved markedly in almost all Sativex RCTs in chronic pain based on symptom reduction, not a hypnotic effect [139].

The adverse event (AE) profile of Sativex has been quite benign with bad taste, oral stinging, dry mouth, dizziness, nausea, or fatigue most common, but not usually prompting discontinuation [128]. Most psychoactive sequelae are early and transient and have been notably lowered by more recent application of a slower, less aggressive titration schedule. While no direct comparative studies have been performed with Sativex and other agents, AE rates were comparable or greater with Marinol than with Sativex employing THC dosages some 2.5 times higher, likely due to the presence of accompanying CBD [28, 51]. Similarly, Sativex displayed a superior AE profile compared to smoked cannabis based on safety-extension studies of Sativex [28, 99], as compared to chronic use of cannabis with standardized government-supplied material in Canada for chronic pain [140] and the Netherlands for various indications [141, 142] over a period of several months or more. All AEs are more frequent with smoked cannabis, except for nausea and dizziness, both early and usually transiently reported with Sativex [27, 28, 128]. A recent meta-analysis suggested that serious AEs associated with cannabinoid-based medications did not differ from placebo and thus could not be attributable to cannabinoid use, further reinforcing the low toxicity associated with activation of cannabinoid systems.

Cannabinoid Pitfalls: Are They Surmountable?

The dangers of COX-1 and COX-2 inhibition by nonsteroidal anti-inflammatory drugs (NSAIDS) of various design (e.g., gastrointestinal ulceration and bleeding vs. coronary and cerebrovascular accidents, respectively) [143, 144] are unlikely to be mimicked by either THC or CBD, which produce no such activity at therapeutic dosages [49].

Natural cannabinoids require polar solvents and may be associated with delayed and sometimes erratic absorption after oral administration. Smoking of cannabis invariably produces rapid spikes in serum THC levels; cannabis smoking attains peak levels of serum THC above 140 ng/ml [145, 146], which, while desirable to the recreational user, has no necessity or advantage for treatment of chronic pain [28]. In contrast, comparable amounts of THC derived from oromucosal Sativex remained below 2 ng/ml with much lower propensity toward psychoactive sequelae [28, 125], with subjective intoxication levels on visual analogue scales that are indistinguishable from placebo, in the single digits out of 100 [100]. It is clear from RCTs that such psychoactivity is not a necessary accompaniment to pain control. In contrast, intoxication has continued to be prominent with oral THC [73].

In comparison to the questionable clinical trial blinding with smoked and vaporized cannabis discussed above, all indications are that such study blinding has been demonstrably effective with Sativex [147, 148] by utilizing a placebo spray with identical taste and color. Some 50 % of Sativex subjects in RCTs have had prior cannabis exposure, but results of two studies suggest that both groups exhibited comparable results in both treatment efficacy and side effect profile [134, 135].

Controversy continues to swirl around the issue of the potential dangers of cannabis use medicinally, particularly its drug abuse liability (DAL). Cannabis and cannabinoids are currently DEA schedule I substances and are forbidden in the USA (save for Marinol in schedule III and nabilone in schedule II) [73]. This is noteworthy in itself because the very same chemical compound, THC, appears simultaneously in schedule I (as THC), schedule II (as nabilone), and schedule III (as Marinol). DAL is assessed on the basis of five elements: intoxication, reinforcement, tolerance, withdrawal, and dependency plus the drug's overall observed rates of abuse and diversion. Drugs that are smoked or injected are commonly rated as more reinforcing due to more rapid delivery to the brain [149]. Sativex has intermediate onset. It is claimed that CBD in Sativex reduces the psychoactivity of THC [28]. RCT AE profiles do not indicate euphoria or other possible reinforcing psychoactive indicia as common problems with its use [99]. Similarly, acute THC effects such as tachycardia, hypothermia, orthostatic hypotension, dry mouth, ocular injection, and intraocular pressure decreases undergo prominent tachyphylaxis with regular usage [150]. Despite that observation, Sativex has not demonstrated dose tolerance to its therapeutic benefits on prolonged administration, and efficacy has been maintained for up to several years in pain conditions [99].

The existence or severity of a cannabis withdrawal syndrome remains under debate [151, 152]. In contrast to reported withdrawal sequelae in recreational users [153], 24 subjects with MS who volunteered to discontinue Sativex after a year or more suffered no withdrawal symptoms meeting Budney criteria. While symptoms such as pain recurred after some 7–10 days without Sativex, symptom control was rapidly reattained upon resumption [99].

Finally, no known abuse or diversion incidents have been reported with Sativex to date (March 2011). Formal DAL studies of Sativex vs. Marinol and placebo have been completed and demonstrate lower scores on drug liking and similar measures at comparable doses [155].

Cognitive effects of cannabis also remain at issue [155, 156], but less data are available in therapeutic applications. Studies of Sativex in neuropathic pain with allodynia have revealed no changes vs. placebo on Sativex in portions of the Halstead-Reitan Battery [135], or in central neuropathic pain in MS [134], where 80 % of tests showed no significant differences. In a recent RCT of Sativex vs. placebo in MS patients, no cognitive differences of note were observed [157]. Similarly, chronic Sativex use has not produced observable mood disorders.

Controversies have also arisen regarding the possible association of cannabis abuse and onset of psychosis [156]. However, an etiological relationship is not supported by epidemiological data [158–161], but may well be affected by dose levels and duration, if pertinent. One may speculate that lower serum levels of Sativex combined with antipsychotic properties of CBD [52, 162, 163] might attenuate such concerns. Few cases of related symptoms have been reported in SAFEX studies of Sativex.

Immune function becomes impaired in experimental animals at cannabinoid doses 50–100 times necessary to produce psychoactive effects [164]. In four patients smoking cannabis medicinally for more than 20 years, no changes were evident in leukocyte, CD4, or CD8 cell counts [155]. MS patients on Cannador demonstrated no immune changes of note [165] nor were changes evident in subjects smoking cannabis in a brief trial in HIV patients [166]. Sativex RCTs have demonstrated no hematological or immune dysfunction.

No effects of THC extract, CBD extract, or Sativex were evident on the hepatic cytochrome P450 complex [167] or on human CYP450 [168]. Similarly, while Sativex might be expected to have additive sedative effects with other drugs or alcohol, no significant drug-drug interactions of any type have been observed in the entire development program to date.

No studies have demonstrated significant problems in relation to cannabis affecting driving skills at plasma levels below 5 ng/ml of THC [169]. Four oromucosal sprays of Sativex (exceeding the average single dose employed in therapy) produced serum levels well below this threshold [28]. As with other cannabinoids in therapy, it is recommended that patients not drive nor use dangerous equipment until accustomed to the effects of the drug.

Future Directions: An Array of Biosynthetic and Phytocannabinoid Analgesics

Inhibition of Endocannabinoid Transport and Degradation: A Solution?

It is essential that any cannabinoid analgesic strike a compromise between therapeutic and adverse effects that may both be mediated via CB_1 mechanisms [34]. Mechanisms to avoid psychoactive sequelae could include peripherally active synthetic cannabinoids that do not cross the blood-brain barrier or drugs that boost AEA levels by inhibiting fatty-acid amide hydrolase (FAAH) [170] or that of 2-AG by inhibiting monoacylcerol lipase (MGL). CBD also has this effect [50] and certainly seems to increase the therapeutic index of THC [51].

In preclinical studies, drugs inhibiting endocannabinoid hydrolysis [171, 172] and peripherally acting agonists [173] all show promise for suppressing neuropathic pain. AZ11713908, a peripherally restricted mixed cannabinoid agonist, reduces mechanical allodynia with efficacy comparable to the brain penetrant mixed cannabinoid agonist WIN55,212-2 [173]. An irreversible inhibitor of the 2-AG hydrolyzing enzyme MGL suppresses nerve injury-induced mechanical allodynia through a CB_1 mechanism, although these anti-allodynic effects undergo tolerance following repeated administration [172]. URB937, a brain impermeant inhibitor of FAAH, has recently been shown to elevate anandamide outside the brain and suppress neuropathic and inflammatory pain behavior without producing tolerance or unwanted CNS side effects [171]. These observations raise the possibility that peripherally restricted endocannabinoid modulators may show therapeutic potential as analgesics with limited side-effect profiles.

The Phytocannabinoid and Terpenoid Pipeline

Additional phytocannabinoids show promise in treatment of chronic pain [123, 163, 174]. Cannabichromene (CBC), another prominent phytocannabinoid, also displays anti-inflammatory [175] and analgesic properties, though less potently than THC [176]. CBC, like CBD, is a weak inhibitor of AEA reuptake [177]. CBC is additionally a potent TRPA1 agonist [178]. Cannabigerol (CBG), another phytocannabinoid, displays weak binding at both CB_1 and CB_2 [179, 180] but is a more potent GABA reuptake inhibitor

than either THC or CBD [181]. CBG is a stronger analgesic, anti-erythema, and lipooxygenase agent than THC [182]. CBG likewise inhibits AEA uptake and is a TRPV1 agonist [177], a TRPA1 agonist, and a TRPM8 antagonist [178]. CBG is also a phospholipase A2 modulator that reduces PGE-2 release in synovial cells [183]. Tetrahydrocannabivarin, a phytocannabinoid present in southern African strains, displays weak CB_1 antagonism [184] and a variety of anticonvulsant activities [185] that might prove useful in chronic neuropathic pain treatment. THCV also reduced inflammation and attendant pain in mouse experiments [187]. Most North American [187] and European [188, 189] cannabis strains have been bred to favor THC over a virtual absence of other phytocannabinoid components, but the latter are currently available in abundance via selective breeding [124, 190].

Aromatic terpenoid components of cannabis also demonstrate pain reducing activity [123, 163]. Myrcene displays an opioid-type analgesic effect blocked by naloxone [191] and reduces inflammation via PGE-2 [192]. β-Caryophyllene displays anti-inflammatory activity on par with phenylbutazone via PGE-1 [193], but contrasts by displaying gastric cytoprotective activity [194]. Surprisingly, β-caryophyllene has proven to be a phytocannabinoid in its own right as a selective CB_2 agonist [195]. α-Pinene inhibits PGE-1 [196], and linalool acts as a local anesthetic [197].

Summary

Basic science and clinical trials support the theoretical and practical basis of cannabinoid agents as analgesics for chronic pain. Their unique pharmacological profiles with multimodality effects and generally favorable efficacy and safety profiles render cannabinoid-based medicines promising agents for adjunctive treatment, particularly for neuropathic pain. It is our expectation that the coming years will mark the advent of numerous approved cannabinoids with varying mechanisms of action and delivery techniques that should offer the clinician useful new tools for treating pain.

References

1. Di Marzo V, Bisogno T, De Petrocellis L. Endocannabinoids and related compounds: walking back and forth between plant natural products and animal physiology. Chem Biol. 2007;14(7):741–56.
2. Gaoni Y, Mechoulam R. Isolation, structure and partial synthesis of an active constituent of hashish. J Am Chem Soc. 1964;86:1646–7.
3. Pate D. Chemical ecology of cannabis. J Int Hemp Assoc. 1994;2:32–7.
4. Di Marzo V, Melck D, Bisogno T, De Petrocellis L. Endocannabinoids: endogenous cannabinoid receptor ligands with neuromodulatory action. Trends Neurosci. 1998;21(12):521–8.

5. Pacher P, Batkai S, Kunos G. The endocannabinoid system as an emerging target of pharmacotherapy. Pharmacol Rev. 2006; 58(3):389–462.

6. Cravatt BF, Giang DK, Mayfield SP, Boger DL, Lerner RA, Gilula NB. Molecular characterization of an enzyme that degrades neuromodulatory fatty-acid amides. Nature. 1996;384(6604):83–7.

7. Dinh TP, Freund TF, Piomelli D. A role for monoglyceride lipase in 2-arachidonoylglycerol inactivation. Chem Phys Lipids. 2002;121(1–2):149–58.

8. Gulyas AI, Cravatt BF, Bracey MH, et al. Segregation of two endocannabinoid-hydrolyzing enzymes into pre- and postsynaptic compartments in the rat hippocampus, cerebellum and amygdala. Eur J Neurosci. 2004;20(2):441–58.

9. Mangieri RA, Piomelli D. Enhancement of endocannabinoid signaling and the pharmacotherapy of depression. Pharmacol Res. 2007;56(5):360–6.

10. Howlett AC, Johnson MR, Melvin LS, Milne GM. Nonclassical cannabinoid analgetics inhibit adenylate cyclase: development of a cannabinoid receptor model. Mol Pharmacol. 1988;33(3): 297–302.

11. Zimmer A, Zimmer AM, Hohmann AG, Herkenham M, Bonner TI. Increased mortality, hypoactivity, and hypoalgesia in cannabinoid CB1 receptor knockout mice. Proc Natl Acad Sci USA. 1999;96(10):5780–5.

12. Wilson RI, Nicoll RA. Endogenous cannabinoids mediate retrograde signalling at hippocampal synapses. Nature. 2001; 410(6828):588–92.

13. Ibrahim MM, Porreca F, Lai J, et al. CB2 cannabinoid receptor activation produces antinociception by stimulating peripheral release of endogenous opioids. Proc Natl Acad Sci USA. 2005;102(8):3093–8.

14. Guindon J, Hohmann AG. Cannabinoid CB2 receptors: a therapeutic target for the treatment of inflammatory and neuropathic pain. Br J Pharmacol. 2008;153(2):319–34.

15. Pacher P, Mechoulam R. Is lipid signaling through cannabinoid 2 receptors part of a protective system? Prog Lipid Res. 2011; 50:193–211.

16. Racz I, Nadal X, Alferink J, et al. Interferon-gamma is a critical modulator of CB(2) cannabinoid receptor signaling during neuropathic pain. J Neurosci. 2008;28(46):12136–45.

17. Guindon J, Hohmann AG. The endocannabinoid system and pain. CNS Neurol Disord Drug Targets. 2009;8(6):403–21.

18. Fankhauser M. History of cannabis in Western medicine. In: Grotenhermen F, Russo EB, editors. Cannabis and cannabinoids: pharmacology, toxicology and therapeutic potential. Binghamton: Haworth Press; 2002. p. 37–51.

19. Russo EB. History of cannabis as medicine. In: Guy GW, Whittle BA, Robson P, editors. Medicinal uses of cannabis and cannabinoids. London: Pharmaceutical Press; 2004. p. 1–16.

20. Russo EB. History of cannabis and its preparations in saga, science and sobriquet. Chem Biodivers. 2007;4(8):2624–48.

21. Mechoulam R. The pharmacohistory of Cannabis sativa. In: Mechoulam R, editor. Cannabinoids as therapeutic agents. Boca Raton: CRC Press; 1986. p. 1–19.

22. Russo E. Cannabis treatments in obstetrics and gynecology: a historical review. J Cannabis Ther. 2002;2(3–4):5–35.

23. Russo EB. Hemp for headache: an in-depth historical and scientific review of cannabis in migraine treatment. J Cannabis Ther. 2001;1(2):21–92.

24. Russo EB. The role of cannabis and cannabinoids in pain management. In: Cole BE, Boswell M, editors. Weiner's pain management: a practical guide for clinicians. 7th ed. Boca Raton: CRC Press; 2006. p. 823–44.

25. Russo EB. Cannabis in India: ancient lore and modern medicine. In: Mechoulam R, editor. Cannabinoids as therapeutics. Basel: Birkhäuser Verlag; 2005. p. 1–22.

26. ABC News, USA Today, Stanford Medical Center Poll. Broad experience with pain sparks search for relief. 9 May 2005.

27. Russo EB. Cannabinoids in the management of difficult to treat pain. Ther Clin Risk Manag. 2008;4(1):245–59.

28. Russo EB. The solution to the medicinal cannabis problem. In: Schatman ME, editor. Ethical issues in chronic pain management. Boca Raton: Taylor & Francis; 2006. p. 165–94.

29. Dworkin RH, Turk DC, Farrar JT, et al. Core outcome measures for chronic pain clinical trials: IMMPACT recommendations. Pain. 2005;113(1–2):9–19.

30. Tyler VE. Phytomedicines in Western Europe: potential impact on herbal medicine in the United States. In: Kinghorn AD, Balandrin MF, editors. Human medicinal agents from plants (ACS symposium, No. 534). Washington, D.C.: American Chemical Society; 1993. p. 25–37.

31. Russo EB. Handbook of psychotropic herbs: a scientific analysis of herbal remedies for psychiatric conditions. Binghamton: Haworth Press; 2001.

32. Food and Drug Administration. Guidance for industry: botanical drug products. In: Services UDoHaH, editor. US Government; 2004. p. 48. http://www.fda.gov/downloads/Drugs/GuidanceCompliance RegulatoryInformation/Guidances/ucm070491.pdf.

33. Walker JM, Hohmann AG. Cannabinoid mechanisms of pain suppression. Handb Exp Pharmacol. 2005;168:509–54.

34. Rahn EJ, Hohmann AG. Cannabinoids as pharmacotherapies for neuropathic pain: from the bench to the bedside. Neurotherapeutics. 2009;6(4):713–37.

35. Richardson JD, Aanonsen L, Hargreaves KM. SR 141716A, a cannabinoid receptor antagonist, produces hyperalgesia in untreated mice. Eur J Pharmacol. 1997;319(2–3):R3–4.

36. Walker JM, Huang SM, Strangman NM, Tsou K, Sanudo-Pena MC. Pain modulation by the release of the endogenous cannabinoid anandamide. Proc Natl Acad Sci. 1999;96(21):12198–203.

37. Walker JM, Hohmann AG, Martin WJ, Strangman NM, Huang SM, Tsou K. The neurobiology of cannabinoid analgesia. Life Sci. 1999;65(6–7):665–73.

38. Martin WJ, Hohmann AG, Walker JM. Suppression of noxious stimulus-evoked activity in the ventral posterolateral nucleus of the thalamus by a cannabinoid agonist: correlation between electrophysiological and antinociceptive effects. J Neurosci. 1996; 16:6601–11.

39. Hohmann AG, Martin WJ, Tsou K, Walker JM. Inhibition of noxious stimulus-evoked activity of spinal cord dorsal horn neurons by the cannabinoid WIN 55,212-2. Life Sci. 1995;56(23–24): 2111–8.

40. Richardson JD, Aanonsen L, Hargreaves KM. Antihyperalgesic effects of spinal cannabinoids. Eur J Pharmacol. 1998;345(2): 145–53.

41. Strangman NM, Walker JM. Cannabinoid WIN 55,212-2 inhibits the activity-dependent facilitation of spinal nociceptive responses. J Neurophysiol. 1999;82(1):472–7.

42. Rahn EJ, Makriyannis A, Hohmann AG. Activation of cannabinoid CB(1) and CB(2) receptors suppresses neuropathic nociception evoked by the chemotherapeutic agent vincristine in rats. Br J Pharmacol. 2007;152:765–77.

43. Richardson JD, Kilo S, Hargreaves KM. Cannabinoids reduce hyperalgesia and inflammation via interaction with peripheral CB1 receptors. Pain. 1998;75(1):111–9.

44. Karsak M, Gaffal E, Date R, et al. Attenuation of allergic contact dermatitis through the endocannabinoid system. Science. 2007;316(5830):1494–7.

45. Luongo L, Palazzo E, Tambaro S, et al. 1-(2′,4′-Dichlorophenyl)-6-methyl-N-cyclohexylamine-1,4-dihydroindeno[1,2-c]pyrazole-3-carboxamide, a novel CB2 agonist, alleviates neuropathic pain through functional microglial changes in mice. Neurobiol Dis. 2010;37(1):177–85.

46. Hampson AJ, Grimaldi M, Axelrod J, Wink D. Cannabidiol and (-) Delta9-tetrahydrocannabinol are neuroprotective antioxidants. Proc Natl Acad Sci USA. 1998;95(14):8268–73.

47. Burstein S, Levin E, Varanelli C. Prostaglandins and cannabis. II. Inhibition of biosynthesis by the naturally occurring cannabinoids. Biochem Pharmacol. 1973;22(22):2905–10.

48. Fimiani C, Liberty T, Aquirre AJ, Amin I, Ali N, Stefano GB. Opiate, cannabinoid, and eicosanoid signaling converges on common intracellular pathways nitric oxide coupling. Prostaglandins Other Lipid Mediat. 1999;57(1):23–34.

49. Stott CG, Guy GW, Wright S, Whittle BA. The effects of cannabis extracts Tetranabinex & Nabidiolex on human cyclo-oxygenase (COX) activity. Paper presented at: Symposium on the Cannabinoids, Clearwater, June 2005.

50. Bisogno T, Hanus L, De Petrocellis L, et al. Molecular targets for cannabidiol and its synthetic analogues: effect on vanilloid VR1 receptors and on the cellular uptake and enzymatic hydrolysis of anandamide. Br J Pharmacol. 2001;134(4):845–52.

51. Russo EB, Guy GW. A tale of two cannabinoids: the therapeutic rationale for combining tetrahydrocannabinol and cannabidiol. Med Hypotheses. 2006;66(2):234–46.

52. Morgan CJ, Curran HV. Effects of cannabidiol on schizophrenia-like symptoms in people who use cannabis. Br J Psychiatry. 2008;192(4):306–7.

53. Morgan CJ, Freeman TP, Schafer GL, Curran HV. Cannabidiol attenuates the appetitive effects of delta 9-tetrahydrocannabinol in humans smoking their chosen cannabis. Neuropsychopharmacology. 2010;35(9):1879–85.

54. Morgan CJ, Schafer G, Freeman TP, Curran HV. Impact of cannabidiol on the acute memory and psychotomimetic effects of smoked cannabis: naturalistic study. Br J Psychiatry. 2010; 197(4):285–90.

55. Malfait AM, Gallily R, Sumariwalla PF, et al. The nonpsychoactive cannabis constituent cannabidiol is an oral anti-arthritic therapeutic in murine collagen-induced arthritis. Proc Natl Acad Sci USA. 2000;97(17):9561–6.

56. Carrier EJ, Auchampach JA, Hillard CJ. Inhibition of an equilibrative nucleoside transporter by cannabidiol: a mechanism of cannabinoid immunosuppression. Proc Natl Acad Sci USA. 2006; 103(20):7895–900.

57. McHugh D, Hu SS, Rimmerman N, et al. N-arachidonoyl glycine, an abundant endogenous lipid, potently drives directed cellular migration through GPR18, the putative abnormal cannabidiol receptor. BMC Neurosci. 2010;11:44.

58. Dmitrieva N, Nagabukuro H, Resuehr D, et al. Endocannabinoid involvement in endometriosis. Pain. 2010;151(3):703–10.

59. Izzo AA, Camilleri M. Emerging role of cannabinoids in gastrointestinal and liver diseases: basic and clinical aspects. Gut. 2008;57(8):1140–55.

60. Izzo AA, Sharkey KA. Cannabinoids and the gut: new developments and emerging concepts. Pharmacol Ther. 2010; 126(1):21–38.

61. Shen M, Piser TM, Seybold VS, Thayer SA. Cannabinoid receptor agonists inhibit glutamatergic synaptic transmission in rat hippocampal cultures. J Neurosci. 1996;16(14):4322–34.

62. Nicolodi M, Volpe AR, Sicuteri F. Fibromyalgia and headache. Failure of serotonergic analgesia and N-methyl-D-aspartate-mediated neuronal plasticity: their common clues. Cephalalgia. 1998;18 Suppl 21:41–4.

63. Russo EB. Clinical endocannabinoid deficiency (CECD): Can this concept explain therapeutic benefits of cannabis in migraine, fibromyalgia, irritable bowel syndrome and other treatment-resistant conditions? Neuroendocrinol Lett. 2004;25(1–2):31–9.

64. Russo E. Cannabis for migraine treatment: the once and future prescription? An historical and scientific review. Pain. 1998; 76(1–2):3–8.

65. Spadone C. Neurophysiologie du cannabis [neurophysiology of cannabis]. Encéphale. 1991;17(1):17–22.

66. Akerman S, Holland PR, Goadsby PJ. Cannabinoid (CB1) receptor activation inhibits trigeminovascular neurons. J Pharmacol Exp Ther. 2007;320(1):64–71.

67. Akerman S, Kaube H, Goadsby PJ. Anandamide is able to inhibit trigeminal neurons using an in vivo model of trigeminovascular-mediated nociception. J Pharmacol Exp Ther. 2003;309(1): 56–63.

68. Akerman S, Kaube H, Goadsby PJ. Anandamide acts as a vasodilator of dural blood vessels in vivo by activating TRPV1 receptors. Br J Pharmacol. 2004;142:1354–60.

69. Manzanares J, Corchero J, Romero J, Fernandez-Ruiz JJ, Ramos JA, Fuentes JA. Chronic administration of cannabinoids regulates proenkephalin mRNA levels in selected regions of the rat brain. Brain Res Mol Brain Res. 1998;55(1):126–32.

70. Cichewicz DL, Martin ZL, Smith FL, Welch SP. Enhancement of mu opioid antinociception by oral delta9-tetrahydrocannabinol: dose-response analysis and receptor identification. J Pharmacol Exp Ther. 1999;289(2):859–67.

71. Cichewicz DL, Welch SP. Modulation of oral morphine antinociceptive tolerance and naloxone-precipitated withdrawal signs by oral delta 9-tetrahydrocannabinol. J Pharmacol Exp Ther. 2003;305(3):812–7.

72. Cichewicz DL, McCarthy EA. Antinociceptive synergy between delta(9)-tetrahydrocannabinol and opioids after oral administration. J Pharmacol Exp Ther. 2003;304(3):1010–5.

73. Calhoun SR, Galloway GP, Smith DE. Abuse potential of dronabinol (Marinol). J Psychoactive Drugs. 1998;30(2):187–96.

74. Clermont-Gnamien S, Atlani S, Attal N, Le Mercier F, Guirimand F, Brasseur L. Utilisation thérapeutique du delta-9-tétrahydrocannabinol (dronabinol) dans les douleurs neuropathiques réfractaires. The therapeutic use of D9-tetrahydrocannabinol (dronabinol) in refractory neuropathic pain. Presse Med. 2002;31(39 Pt 1):1840–5.

75. Attal N, Brasseur L, Guirimand D, Clermond-Gnamien S, Atlami S, Bouhassira D. Are oral cannabinoids safe and effective in refractory neuropathic pain? Eur J Pain. 2004;8(2):173–7.

76. Svendsen KB, Jensen TS, Bach FW. Does the cannabinoid dronabinol reduce central pain in multiple sclerosis? Randomised double blind placebo controlled crossover trial. BMJ. 2004;329(7460):253.

77. Buggy DJ, Toogood L, Maric S, Sharpe P, Lambert DG, Rowbotham DJ. Lack of analgesic efficacy of oral delta-9-tetrahydrocannabinol in postoperative pain. Pain. 2003; 106(1–2):169–72.

78. Neff GW, O'Brien CB, Reddy KR, et al. Preliminary observation with dronabinol in patients with intractable pruritus secondary to cholestatic liver disease. Am J Gastroenterol. 2002;97(8):2117–9.

79. Narang S, Gibson D, Wasan AD, et al. Efficacy of dronabinol as an adjuvant treatment for chronic pain patients on opioid therapy. J Pain. 2008;9(3):254–64.

80. Toth C, Au S. A prospective identification of neuropathic pain in specific chronic polyneuropathy syndromes and response to pharmacological therapy. Pain. 2008;138(3):657–66.

81. Rintala DH, Fiess RN, Tan G, Holmes SA, Bruel BM. Effect of dronabinol on central neuropathic pain after spinal cord injury: a pilot study. Am J Phys Med Rehabil. 2010;89(10):840–8.

82. Lemberger L, Rubin A, Wolen R, et al. Pharmacokinetics, metabolism and drug-abuse potential of nabilone. Cancer Treat Rev. 1982;9(Suppl B):17–23.

83. Notcutt W, Price M, Chapman G. Clinical experience with nabilone for chronic pain. Pharm Sci. 1997;3:551–5.

84. Berlach DM, Shir Y, Ware MA. Experience with the synthetic cannabinoid nabilone in chronic noncancer pain. Pain Med. 2006; 7(1):25–9.

85. Beaulieu P. Effects of nabilone, a synthetic cannabinoid, on postoperative pain: Les effets de la nabilone, un cannabinoide synthetique, sur la douleur postoperatoire. Can J Anaesth. 2006;53(8):769–75.

86. Maida V. The synthetic cannabinoid nabilone improves pain and symptom management in cancer patietns. Breast Cancer Res Treat. 2007;103(Part 1):121–2.

87. Wissel J, Haydn T, Muller J, et al. Low dose treatment with the synthetic cannabinoid nabilone significantly reduces spasticity-related pain: a double-blind placebo-controlled cross-over trial. J Neurol. 2006;253(10):1337–41.

88. Frank B, Serpell MG, Hughes J, Matthews JN, Kapur D. Comparison of analgesic effects and patient tolerability of nabilone and dihydrocodeine for chronic neuropathic pain: randomised, crossover, double blind study. BMJ. 2008; 336(7637):199–201.

89. Skrabek RQ, Galimova L, Ethans K, Perry D. Nabilone for the treatment of pain in fibromyalgia. J Pain. 2008;9(2):164–73.

90. Ware MA, Fitzcharles MA, Joseph L, Shir Y. The effects of nabilone on sleep in fibromyalgia: results of a randomized controlled trial. Anesth Analg. 2010;110(2):604–10.

91. Bestard JA, Toth CC. An open-label comparison of nabilone and gabapentin as adjuvant therapy or monotherapy in the management of neuropathic pain in patients with peripheral neuropathy. Pain Pract. 2011;11:353–68. Epub 2010 Nov 18.

92. Karst M, Salim K, Burstein S, Conrad I, Hoy L, Schneider U. Analgesic effect of the synthetic cannabinoid CT-3 on chronic neuropathic pain: a randomized controlled trial. JAMA. 2003;290(13):1757–62.

93. Dyson A, Peacock M, Chen A, et al. Antihyperalgesic properties of the cannabinoid CT-3 in chronic neuropathic and inflammatory pain states in the rat. Pain. 2005;116(1–2):129–37.

94. Abrams DI, Jay CA, Shade SB, et al. Cannabis in painful HIV-associated sensory neuropathy: a randomized placebo-controlled trial. Neurology. 2007;68(7):515–21.

95. Wilsey B, Marcotte T, Tsodikov A, et al. A randomized, placebo-controlled, crossover trial of cannabis cigarettes in neuropathic pain. J Pain. 2008;9(6):506–21.

96. Wallace M, Schulteis G, Atkinson JH, et al. Dose-dependent effects of smoked cannabis on capsaicin-induced pain and hyperalgesia in healthy volunteers. Anesthesiology. 2007;107(5):785–96.

97. Ellis RJ, Toperoff W, Vaida F, et al. Smoked medicinal cannabis for neuropathic pain in HIV: a randomized, crossover clinical trial. Neuropsychopharmacology. 2009;34(3):672–80.

98. Ware MA, Wang T, Shapiro S, et al. Smoked cannabis for chronic neuropathic pain: a randomized controlled trial. CMAJ. 2010;182(14):E694–701.

99. Wade DT, Makela PM, House H, Bateman C, Robson PJ. Long-term use of a cannabis-based medicine in the treatment of spasticity and other symptoms in multiple sclerosis. Mult Scler. 2006;12:639–45.

100. Tashkin DP. Smoked marijuana as a cause of lung injury. Monaldi Arch Chest Dis. 2005;63(2):93–100.

101. Tashkin DP, Simmons MS, Sherrill DL, Coulson AH. Heavy habitual marijuana smoking does not cause an accelerated decline in FEV1 with age. Am J Respir Crit Care Med. 1997;155(1): 141–8.

102. Hashibe M, Morgenstern H, Cui Y, et al. Marijuana use and the risk of lung and upper aerodigestive tract cancers: results of a population-based case-control study. Cancer Epidemiol Biomarkers Prev. 2006;15(10):1829–34.

103. Grinspoon L, Bakalar JB. Marihuana, the forbidden medicine. Rev. and exp. edn. New Haven: Yale University Press; 1997.

104. Moir D, Rickert WS, Levasseur G, et al. A comparison of mainstream and sidestream marijuana and tobacco cigarette smoke produced under two machine smoking conditions. Chem Res Toxicol. 2008;21(2):494–502.

105. Singh R, Sandhu J, Kaur B, et al. Evaluation of the DNA damaging potential of cannabis cigarette smoke by the determination of acetaldehyde derived N2-ethyl-2′-deoxyguanosine adducts. Chem Res Toxicol. 2009;22(6):1181–8.

106. Joy JE, Watson SJ, Benson Jr JA. Marijuana and medicine: assessing the science base. Washington D.C.: Institute of Medicine; 1999.

107. Gieringer D. Marijuana waterpipe and vaporizer study. MAPS Bull. 1996;6(3):59–66.

108. Gieringer D. Cannabis "vaporization": a promising strategy for smoke harm reduction. J Cannabis Ther. 2001;1(3–4):153–70.

109. Storz M, Russo EB. An interview with Markus Storz. J Cannabis Ther. 2003;3(1):67–78.

110. Gieringer D, St. Laurent J, Goodrich S. Cannabis vaporizer combines efficient delivery of THC with effective suppression of pyrolytic compounds. J Cannabis Ther. 2004;4(1):7–27.

111. Hazekamp A, Ruhaak R, Zuurman L, van Gerven J, Verpoorte R. Evaluation of a vaporizing device (Volcano) for the pulmonary administration of tetrahydrocannabinol. J Pharm Sci. 2006;95(6): 1308–17.

112. Van der Kooy F, Pomahacova B, Verpoorte R. Cannabis smoke condensate I: the effect of different preparation methods on tetrahydrocannabinol levels. Inhal Toxicol. 2008;20(9):801–4.

113. Bloor RN, Wang TS, Spanel P, Smith D. Ammonia release from heated 'street' cannabis leaf and its potential toxic effects on cannabis users. Addiction. 2008;103(10):1671–7.

114. Zuurman L, Roy C, Schoemaker RC, et al. Effect of intrapulmonary tetrahydrocannabinol administration in humans. J Psychopharmacol (Oxford, England). 2008;22(7):707–16.

115. Pomahacova B, Van der Kooy F, Verpoorte R. Cannabis smoke condensate III: the cannabinoid content of vaporised Cannabis sativa. Inhal Toxicol. 2009;21(13):1108–12.

116. Abrams DI, Vizoso HP, Shade SB, Jay C, Kelly ME, Benowitz NL. Vaporization as a smokeless cannabis delivery system: a pilot study. Clin Pharmacol Ther. 2007;82(5):572–8.

117. Abrams DI, Couey P, Shade SB, Kelly ME, Benowitz NL. Cannabinoid-opioid interaction in chronic pain. Clinical pharmacology and therapeutics. 2011;90(6):844–51.

118. Earleywine M, Barnwell SS. Decreased respiratory symptoms in cannabis users who vaporize. Harm Reduct J. 2007;4:11.

119. Zajicek J, Fox P, Sanders H, et al. Cannabinoids for treatment of spasticity and other symptoms related to multiple sclerosis (CAMS study): multicentre randomised placebo-controlled trial. Lancet. 2003;362(9395):1517–26.

120. Zajicek JP, Sanders HP, Wright DE, et al. Cannabinoids in multiple sclerosis (CAMS) study: safety and efficacy data for 12 months follow up. J Neurol Neurosurg Psychiatry. 2005; 76(12):1664–9.

121. Ernst G, Denke C, Reif M, Schnelle M, Hagmeister H. Standardized cannabis extract in the treatment of postherpetic neuralgia: a randomized, double-blind, placebo-controlled cross-over study. Paper presented at: international association for cannabis as medicine, Leiden, 9 Sept 2005.

122. Holdcroft A, Maze M, Dore C, Tebbs S, Thompson S. A multicenter dose-escalation study of the analgesic and adverse effects of an oral cannabis extract (Cannador) for postoperative pain management. Anesthesiology. 2006;104(5):1040–6.

123. McPartland JM, Russo EB. Cannabis and cannabis extracts: greater than the sum of their parts? J Cannabis Ther. 2001;1(3–4):103–32.

124. de Meijer E. The breeding of cannabis cultivars for pharmaceutical end uses. In: Guy GW, Whittle BA, Robson P, editors. Medicinal uses of cannabis and cannabinoids. London: Pharmaceutical Press; 2004. p. 55–70.

125. Guy GW, Robson P. A phase I, double blind, three-way crossover study to assess the pharmacokinetic profile of cannabis based medicine extract (CBME) administered sublingually in variant cannabinoid ratios in normal healthy male volunteers (GWPK02125). J Cannabis Ther. 2003;3(4):121–52.

126. Karschner EL, Darwin WD, McMahon RP, et al. Subjective and physiological effects after controlled Sativex and oral THC administration. Clin Pharmacol Ther. 2011;89(3):400–7.

127. Karschner EL, Darwin WD, Goodwin RS, Wright S, Huestis MA. Plasma cannabinoid pharmacokinetics following controlled oral delta9-tetrahydrocannabinol and oromucosal cannabis extract administration. Clin Chem. 2011;57(1):66–75.

128. Russo EB, Etges T, Stott CG. Comprehensive adverse event profile of Sativex. 18th annual symposium on the cannabinoids. Vol Aviemore, Scotland: International Cannabinoid Research Society; 2008. p. 136.

129. Barnes MP. Sativex: clinical efficacy and tolerability in the treatment of symptoms of multiple sclerosis and neuropathic pain. Expert Opin Pharmacother. 2006;7(5):607–15.

130. Pérez J. Combined cannabinoid therapy via na oromucosal spray. Drugs Today. 2006;42(8):495–501.

131. Wade DT, Robson P, House H, Makela P, Aram J. A preliminary controlled study to determine whether whole-plant cannabis extracts can improve intractable neurogenic symptoms. Clin Rehabil. 2003;17:18–26.

132. Notcutt W, Price M, Miller R, et al. Initial experiences with medicinal extracts of cannabis for chronic pain: results from 34 "N of 1" studies. Anaesthesia. 2004;59:440–52.

133. Berman JS, Symonds C, Birch R. Efficacy of two cannabis based medicinal extracts for relief of central neuropathic pain from brachial plexus avulsion: results of a randomised controlled trial. Pain. 2004;112(3):299–306.

134. Rog DJ, Nurmiko T, Friede T, Young C. Randomized controlled trial of cannabis based medicine in central neuropathic pain due to multiple sclerosis. Neurology. 2005;65(6):812–9.

135. Nurmikko TJ, Serpell MG, Hoggart B, Toomey PJ, Morlion BJ, Haines D. Sativex successfully treats neuropathic pain characterised by allodynia: a randomised, double-blind, placebo-controlled clinical trial. Pain. 2007;133(1–3):210–20.

136. Wade DT, Makela P, Robson P, House H, Bateman C. Do cannabis-based medicinal extracts have general or specific effects on symptoms in multiple sclerosis? A double-blind, randomized, placebo-controlled study on 160 patients. Mult Scler. 2004; 10(4):434–41.

137. Blake DR, Robson P, Ho M, Jubb RW, McCabe CS. Preliminary assessment of the efficacy, tolerability and safety of a cannabis-based medicine (Sativex) in the treatment of pain caused by rheumatoid arthritis. Rheumatology (Oxford). 2006;45(1):50–2.

138. Johnson JR, Burnell-Nugent M, Lossignol D, Ganae-Motan ED, Potts R, Fallon MT. Multicenter, double-blind, randomized, placebo-controlled, parallel-group study of the efficacy, safety, and tolerability of THC:CBD extract and THC extract in patients with intractable cancer-related pain. J Pain Symptom Manage. 2010;39(2):167–79.

139. Russo EB, Guy GW, Robson PJ. Cannabis, pain, and sleep: lessons from therapeutic clinical trials of Sativex, a cannabis-based medicine. Chem Biodivers. 2007;4(8):1729–43.

140. Lynch ME, Young J, Clark AJ. A case series of patients using medicinal marihuana for management of chronic pain under the Canadian Marihuana Medical Access Regulations. J Pain Symptom Manage. 2006;32(5):497–501.

141. Janse AFC, Breekveldt-Postma NS, Erkens JA, Herings RMC. Medicinal gebruik van cannabis: PHARMO instituut. Institute for Drug Outcomes Research; 2004.

142. Gorter RW, Butorac M, Cobian EP, van der Sluis W. Medical use of cannabis in the Netherlands. Neurology. 2005;64(5):917–9.

143. Fitzgerald GA. Coxibs and cardiovascular disease. N Engl J Med. 2004;10:6.

144. Topol EJ. Failing the public health – rofecoxib, Merck, and the FDA. N Engl J Med. 2004;10:6.

145. Grotenhermen F. Pharmacokinetics and pharmacodynamics of cannabinoids. Clin Pharmacokinet. 2003;42(4):327–60.

146. Huestis MA, Henningfield JE, Cone EJ. Blood cannabinoids. I. Absorption of THC and formation of 11-OH-THC and THCCOOH during and after smoking marijuana. J Anal Toxicol. 1992;16(5):276–82.

147. Wright S. GWMS001 and GWMS0106: maintenance of blinding. London: GW Pharmaceuticals; 2005.

148. Clark P, Altman D. Assessment of blinding in phase III Sativex spasticity studies. GW Pharmaceuticals; 2006.

149. Samaha AN, Robinson TE. Why does the rapid delivery of drugs to the brain promote addiction? Trends Pharmacol Sci. 2005;26(2):82–7.

150. Jones RT, Benowitz N, Bachman J. Clinical studies of cannabis tolerance and dependence. Ann N Y Acad Sci. 1976;282:221–39.

151. Budney AJ, Hughes JR, Moore BA, Vandrey R. Review of the validity and significance of cannabis withdrawal syndrome. Am J Psychiatry. 2004;161(11):1967–77.

152. Smith NT. A review of the published literature into cannabis withdrawal symptoms in human users. Addiction. 2002;97(6): 621–32.

153. Solowij N, Stephens RS, Roffman RA, et al. Cognitive functioning of long-term heavy cannabis users seeking treatment. JAMA. 2002;287(9):1123–31.

154. Schoedel KA, Chen N, Hilliard A, et al. A randomized, double-blind, placebo-controlled, crossover study to evaluate the abuse potential of nabiximols oromucosal spray in subjects with a history of recreational cannabis use. Hum Psychopharmacol. 2011;26:224–36.

155. Russo EB, Mathre ML, Byrne A, et al. Chronic cannabis use in the Compassionate Use Investigational New Drug Program: an examination of benefits and adverse effects of legal clinical cannabis. J Cannabis Ther. 2002;2(1):3–57.

156. Fride E, Russo EB. Neuropsychiatry: schizophrenia, depression, and anxiety. In: Onaivi E, Sugiura T, Di Marzo V, editors. Endocannabinoids: the brain and body's marijuana and beyond. Boca Raton: Taylor & Francis; 2006. p. 371–82.

157. Aragona M, Onesti E, Tomassini V, et al. Psychopathological and cognitive effects of therapeutic cannabinoids in multiple sclerosis: a double-blind, placebo controlled, crossover study. Clin Neuropharmacol. 2009;32(1):41–7.

158. Degenhardt L, Hall W, Lynskey M. Testing hypotheses about the relationship between cannabis use and psychosis. Drug Alcohol Depend. 2003;71(1):37–48.

159. Macleod J, Davey Smith G, Hickman M. Does cannabis use cause schizophrenia? Lancet. 2006;367(9516):1055.

160. Macleod J, Hickman M. How ideology shapes the evidence and the policy: what do we know about cannabis use and what should we do? Addiction. 2010;105:1326–30.

161. Hickman M, Vickerman P, Macleod J, et al. If cannabis caused schizophrenia–how many cannabis users may need to be prevented in order to prevent one case of schizophrenia? England and Wales calculations. Addiction. 2009;104(11):1856–61.

162. Zuardi AW, Guimaraes FS. Cannabidiol as an anxiolytic and antipsychotic. In: Mathre ML, editor. Cannabis in medical practice: a legal, historical and pharmacological overview of the therapeutic use of marijuana. Jefferson: McFarland; 1997. p. 133–41.

163. Russo EB. Taming THC: potential cannabis synergy and phytocannabinoid-terpenoid entourage effects. Br J Pharmacol. 2011;163:1344–64.

164. Cabral G. Immune system. In: Grotenhermen F, Russo EB, editors. Cannabis and cannabinoids: pharmacology, toxicology and

therapeutic potential. Binghamton: Haworth Press; 2001. p. 279–87.

165. Katona S, Kaminski E, Sanders H, Zajicek J. Cannabinoid influence on cytokine profile in multiple sclerosis. Clin Exp Immunol. 2005;140(3):580–5.

166. Abrams DI, Hilton JF, Leiser RJ, et al. Short-term effects of cannabinoids in patients with HIV-1 infection. A randomized, placbo-controlled clinical trial. Ann Intern Med. 2003;139:258–66.

167. Stott CG, Guy GW, Wright S, Whittle BA. The effects of cannabis extracts Tetranabinex and Nabidiolex on human cytochrome P450-mediated metabolism. Paper presented at: Symposium on the Cannabinoids, Clearwater, 27 June 2005.

168. Stott CG, Ayerakwa L, Wright S, Guy G. Lack of human cytochrome P450 induction by Sativex. 17th annual symposium on the cannabinoids. Saint-Sauveur, Quebec: International Cannabinoid Research Society; 2007. p. 211.

169. Grotenhermen F, Leson G, Berghaus G, et al. Developing limits for driving under cannabis. Addiction. 2007;102(12):1910–7.

170. Hohmann AG, Suplita 2nd RL. Endocannabinoid mechanisms of pain modulation. AAPS J. 2006;8(4):E693–708.

171. Clapper JR, Moreno-Sanz G, Russo R, et al. Anandamide suppresses pain initiation through a peripheral endocannabinoid mechanism. Nat Neurosci. 2010;13:1265–70.

172. Schlosburg JE, Blankman JL, Long JZ, et al. Chronic monoacylglycerol lipase blockade causes functional antagonism of the endocannabinoid system. Nat Neurosci. 2010;13(9):1113–9.

173. Yu XH, Cao CQ, Martino G, et al. A peripherally restricted cannabinoid receptor agonist produces robust anti-nociceptive effects in rodent models of inflammatory and neuropathic pain. Pain. 2010;151(2):337–44.

174. Izzo AA, Borrelli F, Capasso R, Di Marzo V, Mechoulam R. Non-psychotropic plant cannabinoids: new therapeutic opportunities from an ancient herb. Trends Pharmacol Sci. 2009;30(10):515–27.

175. Wirth PW, Watson ES, ElSohly M, Turner CE, Murphy JC. Anti-inflammatory properties of cannabichromene. Life Sci. 1980;26(23):1991–5.

176. Davis WM, Hatoum NS. Neurobehavioral actions of cannabichromene and interactions with delta 9-tetrahydrocannabinol. Gen Pharmacol. 1983;14(2):247–52.

177. Ligresti A, Moriello AS, Starowicz K, et al. Antitumor activity of plant cannabinoids with emphasis on the effect of cannabidiol on human breast carcinoma. J Pharmacol Exp Ther. 2006;318(3):1375–87.

178. De Petrocellis L, Starowicz K, Moriello AS, Vivese M, Orlando P, Di Marzo V. Regulation of transient receptor potential channels of melastatin type 8 (TRPM8): effect of cAMP, cannabinoid CB(1) receptors and endovanilloids. Exp Cell Res. 2007;313(9):1911–20.

179. Gauson LA, Stevenson LA, Thomas A, Baillie GL, Ross RA, Pertwee RG. Cannabigerol behaves as a partial agonist at both CB1 and CB2 receptors. 17th annual symposium on the cannabinoids. Vol Saint-Sauveur, Quebec: International Cannabinoid Research Society; 2007, p. 206.

180. Cascio MG, Gauson LA, Stevenson LA, Ross RA, Pertwee RG. Evidence that the plant cannabinoid cannabigerol is a highly potent alpha2-adrenoceptor agonist and moderately potent 5HT1A receptor antagonist. Br J Pharmacol. 2010;159(1):129-41.

181. Banerjee SP, Snyder SH, Mechoulam R. Cannabinoids: influence on neurotransmitter uptake in rat brain synaptosomes. J Pharmacol Exp Ther. 1975;194(1):74–81.

182. Evans FJ. Cannabinoids: the separation of central from peripheral effects on a structural basis. Planta Med. 1991;57(7):S60–7.

183. Evans AT, Formukong E, Evans FJ. Activation of phospholipase A2 by cannabinoids. Lack of correlation with CNS effects. FEBS Lett. 1987;211(2):119–22.

184. Pertwee RG. The diverse CB1 and CB2 receptor pharmacology of three plant cannabinoids: delta9-tetrahydrocannabinol, cannabidiol and delta9-tetrahydrocannabivarin. Br J Pharmacol. 2008;153(2):199–215.

185. Hill AJ, Weston SE, Jones NA, et al. Delta-tetrahydrocannabivarin suppresses in vitro epileptiform and in vivo seizure activity in adult rats. Epilepsia. 2010;51(8):1522–32.

186. Bolognini D, Costa B, Maione S, et al. The plant cannabinoid delta9-tetrahydrocannabivarin can decrease signs of inflammation and inflammatory pain in mice. Br J Pharmacol. 2010;160(3):677–87.

187. Mehmedic Z, Chandra S, Slade D, et al. Potency trends of delta(9)-THC and other cannabinoids in confiscated cannabis preparations from 1993 to 2008. J Forensic Sci. 2010;55:1209–17.

188. King LA, Carpentier C, Griffiths P. Cannabis potency in Europe. Addiction. 2005;100(7):884–6.

189. Potter DJ, Clark P, Brown MB. Potency of delta 9-THC and other cannabinoids in cannabis in England in 2005: implications for psychoactivity and pharmacology. J Forensic Sci. 2008;53(1):90–4.

190. Potter D. Growth and morphology of medicinal cannabis. In: Guy GW, Whittle BA, Robson P, editors. Medicinal uses of cannabis and cannabinoids. London: Pharmaceutical Press; 2004. p. 17–54.

191. Rao VS, Menezes AM, Viana GS. Effect of myrcene on nociception in mice. J Pharm Pharmacol. 1990;42(12):877–8.

192. Lorenzetti BB, Souza GE, Sarti SJ, Santos Filho D, Ferreira SH. Myrcene mimics the peripheral analgesic activity of lemongrass tea. J Ethnopharmacol. 1991;34(1):43–8.

193. Basile AC, Sertie JA, Freitas PC, Zanini AC. Anti-inflammatory activity of oleoresin from Brazilian Copaifera. J Ethnopharmacol. 1988;22(1):101–9.

194. Tambe Y, Tsujiuchi H, Honda G, Ikeshiro Y, Tanaka S. Gastric cytoprotection of the non-steroidal anti-inflammatory sesquiterpene, beta-caryophyllene. Planta Med. 1996;62(5):469–70.

195. Gertsch J, Leonti M, Raduner S, et al. Beta-caryophyllene is a dietary cannabinoid. Proc Natl Acad Sci USA. 2008;105(26):9099–104.

197. Gil ML, Jimenez J, Ocete MA, Zarzuelo A, Cabo MM. Comparative study of different essential oils of Bupleurum gibraltaricum Lamarck. Pharmazie. 1989;44(4):284–7.

198. Re L, Barocci S, Sonnino S, et al. Linalool modifies the nicotinic receptor-ion channel kinetics at the mouse neuromuscular junction. Pharmacol Res. 2000;42(2):177–82.

199. Gregg, L.C, Jung, K.M., Spradley, J.M., Nyilas, R., Suplita II, R.L., Zimmer, A., Watanabe, M., Mackie, K., Katona, I., Piomelli, D. and Hohmann, A.G. (2012) Activation of type-5 metabotropic glutamate receptors and diacylglycerol lipase-alpha initiates 2-arachidonoylglycerol formation and endocannabinoid-mediated analgesia in vivo. The Journal of Neuroscience, in press [DOI:10.1523/JNEUROSCI.0013-12.2012].

200. Kavia R, De Ridder D, Constantinescu C, Stott C, Fowler C. Randomized controlled trial of Sativex to treat detrusor overactivity in multiple sclerosis. Mult Scler. 2010;16(11):1349–59.

201. Portenoy RK, Ganae-Motan ED, Allende S, Yanagihara R, Shaiova L, Weinstein S, et al. Nabiximols for opioid-treated cancer patients with poorly-controlled chronic pain: a randomized, placebo-controlled, graded-dose trial. J Pain. 2012;13(5):438–49.

202. Abrams DI, Couey P, Shade SB, Kelly ME, Benowitz NL. Cannabinoid-opioid interaction in chronic pain. Clinical pharmacology and therapeutics. 2011;90(6):844–51.

The Future of Pain Pharmacotherapy

19

Iwona Bonney and Daniel B. Carr

Key Points

- Improve existing analgesics' safety profiles, dosing requirements, and convenience of administration routes (e.g., using controlled-release formulations and other novel delivery systems).
- Provide multimodal analgesia including combination products to achieve it safely and with few side effects.
- Design novel, condition-specific molecules whose structure is based upon understanding of pain mechanisms, neurotransmitters, and pathways involved in nociception.

Introduction

According to the American Academy of Pain Medicine (AAPM) and the Institute of Medicine [1], pain affects more Americans than cancer, diabetes, and cardiac disease combined. Current analgesics only provide modest relief, frequently carry black box warnings, and are susceptible to abuse. The ability of current medical science to treat pain effectively is limited by an incomplete understanding of the mechanisms of pain signaling in diverse individuals across different circumstances and the high prevalence of side effects after systemic or regional administration of available analgesics. Despite increasing interest in developing new

I. Bonney, Ph.D. (✉)
Department of Anesthesiology, Tufts Medical Center and Tufts University School of Medicine, 800 Washington Street, #298, Boston, MA 02111, USA
e-mail: ibonney@tuftsmedicalcenter.org

D.B. Carr, M.D., DABPM, FFPMANZCA (Hon)
Department of Public Health, Anesthesiology, Medicine, and Molecular Physiology and Pharmacology, Tufts University School of Medicine, 136 Harrison Avenue, Boston, MA 02111, USA
e-mail: daniel.carr@tufts.edu

analgesic molecules by translating preclinical research on mechanisms of pain processing and harnessing innovative methods of drug delivery, the majority of new analgesic drug launches from 1990 to 2010 were reformulations of existing pharmaceuticals within well-established drug categories such as opioids and NSAIDs (nonsteroidal anti-inflammatory drugs). A distant second were novel drugs acting via well-known mechanisms [novel opioid molecules, norepinephrine reuptake inhibitors (NRI), serotonin-norepinephrine reuptake inhibitors (SNRI), and novel NSAIDs and coxibs]. Finally, there were those few novel molecules that acted via mechanisms not targeted by earlier approved drugs (Lyrica, Prialt, Sativex, Qutenza). At present and for the foreseeable future, drug development and discovery are likely to continue to involve these three approaches, supplemented by occasional leaps forward such as gene therapy to transfect neural cells with DNA that enables them to synthesize and secrete native or nonnative analgesic compounds. This chapter summarizes background knowledge on targets already exploited by existing analgesics including novel formulations of same, surveys other targets recently recognized as potentially worth addressing, and recounts the rapidly changing developmental status of the latter. We recognize that the fast pace of and frequent unexpected findings during clinical drug development will date many of our brief status reports, but this is unavoidable and in any event highlights the dynamic nature of translational research in analgesia. The chapter concludes with the question "Quo vadis?" ("Where are you going?") which we approach using current estimates of the number of "drugable" targets and our assessment of the progress made towards harnessing these therapeutically.

Pharmacological Background

A number of neurotransmitters of various chemical classes are released from afferent fibers, ascending and descending neurons, and interneurons upon peripheral nociceptive input.

T.R. Deer et al. (eds.), *Treatment of Chronic Pain by Medical Approaches: the AMERICAN ACADEMY of PAIN MEDICINE Textbook on Patient Management*, DOI 10.1007/978-1-4939-1818-8_19,
© American Academy of Pain Medicine 2015

Neurotransmitters display a complex pattern of colocalization, comodulation, and corelease in primary afferent fibers and central nociceptive pathways [2]. All potentially relevant to analgesic pharmacology, these include substance P, gamma-aminobutyric acid (GABA), serotonin, norepinephrine, leu- and met-enkephalin, neurotensin, acetylcholine, dynorphin, cholecystokinin (CCK), vasocative intestinal peptide (VIP), calcitonin gene-related peptide (CGRP), somatostatin, adenosine, neuropeptide Y, glutamate, and prostaglandins. Also relevant are the enzymes involved in their generation or degradation, such as nitric oxide synthase, enkephalinases, and cholinesterases.

Changes in the magnitude and patterns of neurotransmitter release, along with diminished inhibitory interneuron function [3], contribute to altered nociceptor function after tissue damage, inflammation, or nerve injury. Those conditions can alter the threshold, excitability, and transmission properties of nociceptors, contributing to hyperalgesia and spontaneous pain. Hyperalgesia may be primary (in the immediate area of tissue injury, due to sensitization of local primary afferent nociceptors by locally released inflammatory mediators) and secondary (surrounding the area of injury that is centrally mediated) [4]. Hyperalgesia often coexists with allodynia (a painful response to normally innocuous stimulus).

Immune cells are also involved in pain, as they are activated peripherally and within the central nervous system by peripheral tissue damage, inflammation, or mechanical nerve lesions [5]. Immune cells enhance nociception through the release of cytokines or (e.g., for granulocytes and monocytes) promote analgesia by secreting β-endorphin and enkephalins [6]. For example, interleukin (IL-6) induces allodynia and hyperalgesia in dorsal horn neurons, IL-1β enhances the release of substance P in spinal cord and induces cyclooxygenase (COX)-2 expression, and tissue necrosis factor α (TNFα) may facilitate postsynaptic ion currents provoked by excitatory amino acids (EAA) [7]. Opioid peptide precursors, including pro-opiomelanocortin (POMC) and proenkephalin (PENK), have been detected in immune cells. POMC was found to be expressed by leukocytes, and pre-PENK mRNA was found in T and B cells, macrophages, and mast cells [8]. Opioid peptides are released from immune cells by stress or by secretagogues (CRH and/or IL-1) to bind to and activate opioid receptors located on peripheral terminals of sensory neurons [8]. Immune cells producing opioid peptides can migrate to inflamed tissue, where the peripheral actions of opioid peptides can contribute to potent, clinically relevant analgesia. The neurotrophin family includes nerve growth factor (NGF), brain-derived neurotrophic factor (BDNF), neurotrophins-3 (NT-3), and NT-4/5. NGF has been shown to play an important role in nociceptive function in adults [9]. Upregulation of NGF after inflammatory injury to the skin leads to increased levels of substance P and CGRP. NGF can also regulate the levels of BDNF. BDNF levels in sensory neurons may be increased by exogenous administration of NGF or by endogenous NGF whose synthesis is increased after tissue injury. NGF is released from mast cells, macrophages, lymphocytes, fibroblasts, and keratinocytes following tissue injury and may contribute to the transition from acute to chronic pain, especially in inflammatory conditions. Recent studies suggest that within the spinal cord, BDNF functions as a retrograde modulator of presynaptic neurotransmitter release. BDNF rapidly and specifically enhances phosphorylation of the postsynaptic NMDA receptor, whose activation plays a pivotal role in the induction and maintenance of central sensitization [10].

Based on their involvement in nociceptive processing, the TRPV1 receptor and glycine receptor subtype α3 (GlyR α3) are viewed as promising targets for drug development. The vanilloid TRPV1 receptor is part of a family of transient receptor potential (TRP) channels densely expressed in small diameter primary afferent fibers. The TRPV1 receptor integrates noxious stimuli, including heat and acids, and endogenous pro-inflammatory substances [11]. The abnormal expression of TRPV1 in neurons that normally do not express TRPV1 has been linked to the development of inflammatory hyperalgesia and neuropathic pain [11, 12], as does the observation that TRPV1 –/– mice exhibit reduced hyperalgesia compared to wild-type mice.

Scientific Basis for Pharmacotherapy

As we shift from a biomedical to a patient-centered model, pain assessment and management have received growing attention. Individuals vary considerably in their reports of pain and their estimates of the efficacy of identical analgesics given at the same doses under seemingly identical circumstances.

Even allowing for interindividual differences, an important reality in pain care is that different mechanisms of nociception predominate in different conditions, resulting in different apparent rank efficacies of the same drugs across different models. Drugs such as NSAIDs and coxibs are anti-hyperalgesic, reducing the increased nociceptive input from damaged tissue or sensitized sensory neurons.

NSAIDs are the most widely prescribed drugs worldwide, but not all are equally effective. The potency and intrinsic efficacy of some NSAIDs is greater than others. Several of the newer NSAIDs have potency comparable to or greater than that of opioid analgesics and are therefore applied for postoperative pain management. With many NSAIDs, a higher dose provides a faster onset time, higher peak effect, and a longer duration. Most NSAIDs display a dose-response relationship for analgesia up to a certain ceiling. Patients' responses to NSAIDs vary considerably, and therapeutic failure to one drug does not preclude success with other within the same broad class. To achieve a greater analgesic response to a constant opioid dose, NSAIDs or acetaminophen analgesics are often used in combination; examples of common combinations with acetaminophen include hyodrocodone or oxycodone.

Acute moderate to severe pain generally requires an opioid analgesic to bring it under control, although pains of various etiologies and mechanisms are not equally opioid sensitive. Adjuvant drugs that boost opioid efficacy and minimize opioid side effects can be also beneficial. NSAIDs, acetaminophen, glucocorticoids, antidepressants, anxiolytic agents, and anticonvulsants have all been reported to act as analgesic adjuvants. Opioid analgesics can control nearly all types of pain. Systemic opioids induce analgesia by acting on different levels of central nervous system (spinal cord, limbic system, hypothalamus) via mu, delta, and kappa opioid receptors and in the periphery. Opioid analgesia is dose-dependent, and its side effects also increase with increasing doses. Common opioid side effects include sedation, drowsiness, dizziness, constipation, respiratory depression, nausea and vomiting, pruritus, and the development of tolerance and physical dependence.

In an effort to gain better control over acute and chronic pain, doctors involved in pain treatment often advance from single drug therapy to combination drugs [13]. The potential benefits of such multimodal therapy include improvement of analgesic efficacy through additive or synergistic interactions, reduction of side effects through dose reductions of each component, and slowing of opioid dose escalation. In combination therapies, an opioid is typically coadministered with another opioid (e.g., morphine with sufentanil or fentanyl), a local anesthetic (morphine or fentanyl and bupivacaine), clonidine, or NMDA antagonists such as ketamine [13].

A Brief Survey of Novel Analgesics

Oral delivery is the most popular route of administration due to its versatility, ease, and probably most importantly, high level of patient compliance. Providing patients with simplified, convenient oral medications that improve compliance has been a major driver of innovation in the oral drug delivery market. Oral products represent about 70 % of the value of pharmaceutical sales and 60 % of drug delivery market [14]. A review of recent Food and Drug Administration (FDA) approvals over the past years shows that new chemical entities (NCEs) have accounted for only 25 % of all products approved; the majority of approvals have been reformulations or combinations of previously approved products [15]. With a reformulation costing approximately $40 million and taking 4–5 years to develop compared to the average clinical development cost of a next-generation

product—in the region of $330 million—the potential for reformulation using oral controlled-release technologies has never been greater [16, 17]. Moreover, the entire developmental cost of an NCE has been estimated at between $1.3 and 1.7 billion [18].

Extended-release formulations deliver a portion of the total dose shortly after ingestion and the remainder over an extended time frame. Typically, oral drug delivery systems are developed as matrix or reservoir systems. Two of the most widely commercialized controlled-release technologies are the OROS (the osmotic controlled-release oral delivery system that uses osmotic pressure as the driving force to deliver drug) and SODAS (spheroidal oral drug absorption system) technologies. Avinza® (King and Pfizer) uses the proprietary SODAS® technology for morphine sulfate extended-release capsules. Avinza® is a long-acting opioid for patients with moderate to severe chronic pain who require around-the-clock pain relief for an extended period of time. Avinza® consists of two components: an immediate release component that rapidly achieves plateau morphine plasma concentrations and an extended-release component that maintains plasma concentrations throughout the 24-h dosing interval. Within the gastrointestinal tract, due to the permeability of the ammonio methacrylate copolymers of the beads, fluid enters the beads and solubilizes the drug that then diffuses out in a predetermined manner.

Other examples of extended-release oral formulations of opioid analgesics indicated for moderate to severe pain for tolerant patients requiring continuous, around-the-clock opioid therapy for extended period of time are hydromorphone hydrochloride (Exalgo®, Covidien) and oxymorphone hydrochloride (Opana® ER, Endo).

Another area of opportunity to improve opioid oral formulations is to create abuse-resistant delivery systems. At present, a record of 36 million Americans has abused prescription drugs at least once in their lifetime [19]. It is estimated that the market for abuse-resistant opioid formulations, driven by oxycodone and morphine anti-abuse formulations, will be $1.2 billion by 2017 [20]. Conversely, a concern evident in some FDA decisions not to approve abuse-resistant formulations is that it is still possible for patients to experience serious adverse events related to the opioid component of a properly taken abuse-resistant formulation that has not been tampered with.

King Pharmaceuticals Inc. and Pain Therapeutics, Inc. in 2010 resubmitted a New Drug Application (NDA) for Remoxy®. Remoxy, based on Durect's ORADUR® technology, offers a controlled-release formulation of oxycodone. The company presently markets EMBEDA™ capsules that contain pellets of morphine sulfate and naltrexone hydrochloride in a 100:4 ratio. The latter component may reduce the adverse outcomes associated with sudden ingestion of the opioid provided in this form.

Combination products of existing compounds have been developed to improve efficacy or reduce unwanted side effects. Examples include combination products of oxycodone with ibuprofen, hydrocodone with acetaminophen, or naproxen in combination with the proton pump inhibitor esomeprazole (Vimovo). Vimovo (naproxen and esomeprazole magnesium, AstraZeneca, and Pozen Inc.) has been approved by the US FDA on April 30, 2010, as a new drug combination. It is a delayed-release combination tablet for arthritis whose proton pump component decreases the risk of developing NSAID-associated gastric ulcers in patients prone to this complication.

There are a number of examples where observations of analgesic properties of medicines originally developed for other therapeutic indications led to their application for the treatment of pain. Historically, such agents include medications to treat depression or seizures.

Antiepileptic drugs (AEDs) affect various neurotransmitters, receptors, and ion channels to achieve their anticonvulsant activity that overlap with targets for controlling pain and other dysfunctions. Both conventional and newer AEDs may be used in patients suffering from migraine, essential tremor, spasticity, restless legs syndrome, and a number of psychiatric disorders (e.g., bipolar disease or schizophrenia). AEDs are widely used to treat neuropathic pain syndromes such as postherpetic neuralgia (PHN), painful diabetic neuropathy (PDN), central post-stroke pain syndrome, trigeminal neuralgia, and human immunodeficiency virus (HIV)-associated neuropathic pain.

Lyrica® (pregabalin, (S)-3-(aminomethyl)-5-methylhexanoic acid, Pfizer) is a second-generation anticonvulsant structurally similar to gabapentin. It is the S-enantiomer of racemic 3-isobutyl GABA. The binding affinity of pregabalin for the $Ca_v\alpha 2\beta 1$ subunit is six times greater than that of gabapentin, which allows pregabalin to be clinically effective at lower doses than gabapentin. Pregabalin is indicated for the treatment of neuropathic pain associated with diabetic peripheral neuropathy (DPN), PHN, and fibromyalgia and as an adjunctive therapy for adult patients with partial onset seizures. Pregabalin binds with high affinity to the alpha2-delta site (an auxiliary subunit of voltage-gated neuronal calcium channels) in the central nervous system. Results with genetically modified mice and with compounds structurally related to pregabalin (such as gabapentin) suggest that binding to the alpha2-delta subunit may be involved in pregabalin's antinociceptive and antiseizure effects in animals. In animal models of nerve damage, pregabalin has been shown to reduce calcium-dependent release of pronociceptive neurotransmitters in the spinal cord, possibly by disrupting alpha2-delta-containing calcium channel trafficking and/or reducing calcium currents. Additional preclinical evidence suggests that the antinociceptive activities of pregabalin may also be mediated through interactions with descending inhibitory noradrenergic and serotonergic pathways originating from the brainstem and descending to the spinal cord.

The L-type VGCC blocker, Topiramate (brand name Topamax) is another AED. Its off-label and investigational uses include the treatment of essential tremor, bulimia nervosa, obsessive-compulsive disorder, alcoholism, smoking cessation, idiopathic intracranial hypertension, neuropathic pain, cluster headache, and cocaine dependence.

Nucynta® (tapentadol, Ortho-McNeil-Janssen) combines two analgesic mechanisms: a mu-opioid agonist and norepinephrine reuptake inhibitor. It is indicated for the relief of moderate to severe acute pain in patients 18 years of age or older. In a recent phase III open-label study, tapentadol extended-release (ER) tablets were compared to an existing prescription pain medication, oxycodone controlled-release (CR) tablets [ClinicalTrials.gov Identifier: NCT00361504].

Tapentadol ER provided sustained relief of moderate to severe chronic knee or hip osteoarthritis pain or chronic low back pain for up to 1 year, with a lower overall incidence of gastrointestinal adverse events than oxycodone CR in patients with chronic knee or hip osteoarthritis pain or chronic low back pain [21].

Savella® (milnacipran hydrochloride) (Forest and Cypress) is a selective serotonin and norepinephrine reuptake inhibitor similar to some drugs used for the treatment for depression and other psychiatric disorders. It is FDA-approved for the treatment of fibromyalgia.

Cymbalta® (duloxetine HCL, delayed-release capsules, Lilly) is indicated for the treatment of major depressive disorder (MDD) and generalized anxiety disorder (GAD). The efficacy of Cymbalta was established, and it is now approved for the management of diabetic peripheral neuropathic pain (DNP), fibromyalgia, and chronic musculoskeletal pain.

Current active strategies for novel analgesic development target ion channels (sodium, calcium, TRP channels), enzymes, receptors (neurotrophins, cannabinoids), and cytokines involved in pain processing.

Voltage-gated sodium channels (VGSCs) are fundamental components to the induction and propagation of neuronal signals. There are at least nine different VGSC subtypes in the nervous system, the distribution of which in aggregate is widespread but distinct for various subtypes. Their expression on afferent neurons has made VGSCs attractive targets to decrease the flow of nociceptive signals to spinal cord. Nonselective inhibitors of VGSCs, such as local anesthetics, have been employed for a century, but the use and in particular the dosing of such agents is limited to undesirable and potentially lethal side effects. Thus, there has been interest in selective VGSC blockers with improved therapeutic indices, particularly $Na_v1.8$ and 1.9 channels. Promising results have been reported for the selective sodium $Na_v1.8$ channel blocker, A-803467, in animal models of both inflammatory and neuropathic pain. The effects were dose-dependent and reversible. Systemic administration of A-803467 decreased the mechanically evoked and spontaneous firing of spinal neurons in nerve-injured rats [22].

Voltage-gated calcium channels (VGCC) or their subunits are another family of molecules with therapeutic potential for chronic pain management. Based on their physiological and pharmacological properties, VGCC can be subdivided into low voltage-activated T type ($Ca_v3.1$, $Ca_v3.2$, $Ca_v3.3$) and high voltage-activated L ($Ca_v1.1$, through $Ca_v1.4$), N ($Ca_v2.2.$), P/Q ($Ca_v2.1$) and R ($Ca_v2.3$) types depending on the channel forming $Ca_v\alpha1$ subunits [23]. All five subclasses are found in the central and peripheral nervous systems [23, 24]. Most neurons, including sensory neurons and spinal dorsal horn neurons, express multiple types of VGCC. Several types of VGCC are considered potential targets for analgesics based on their distribution, biophysical/pathological roles, and plasticity under pain-inducing conditions. Blocking the N-type VGCC at the levels of spinal cord and sensory neurons results in inhibition of stimulus-evoked release of algesic peptides, such as substance P and CGRP and the excitatory neurotransmitter, glutamate. Results from animal studies indicate that N-type VGCC are more directly involved in chronic nociception. Direct blockade of N-type VGCC by cone snail peptides (ω-conotoxins isolated from the marine fish-hunting cone snail, Conus magus) inhibits neuropathic and inflammatory pain but not acute pain, in animal models. In December 2004, the FDA approved ziconotide (a synthetic version of ω-conotoxin MVIIA) for intrathecal treatment of chronic severe pain refractory to other pain medications. ω-conotonix MVIIA is a 25-amino acid peptide. The analgesic effect of ziconotide (Prialt, Elan) is more potent and longer lasting than intrathecal morphine without tolerance or cross-tolerance to morphine analgesia. Ziconotide has been used in patients with severe chronic pain, including neuropathic pain secondary to cancer or AIDS, and in patients with recalcitrant spinal cord injury pain. The use of this drug is limited due to route of administration and undesirable side effects, including sedation, dizziness, nausea, emesis, headache, urinary retention, slurred speech, double or blurry vision, confusion, memory impairment, amnesia, anxiety, ataxia, and depression.

The ongoing search for safer and more effective N-type channel blockers continues. The compound Xen2174 (Xenome), a derivative of the χ-conopeptide from cone snail Conus marmoreus, is a peptide whose therapeutic properties were improved through structure-activity analyses to optimize its potency, efficacy, safety, stability, and ease of manufacturing. It is a stable peptide with ability to noncompetitively inhibit norepinephrine transporter. A phase I, double-blind, randomized, single-IV dose escalation study on healthy volunteers demonstrated that Xen2174 was safe and well tolerated. Phase I/II studies, designed as an open-label, single IT

bolus, dose-escalating study on cancer patients suffering severe chronic pain, found it to be efficacious and well tolerated with an acceptable side-effect profile across a wide range of dose levels. A randomized, placebo-controlled, single intrathecal injection study for acute postoperative pain using the bunionectomy model is currently underway.

The unique features of $Ca_v\alpha2\beta$ subunit of calcium channel and recent findings have suggested that the $Ca_v\alpha2\beta_1$ subunit may play an important role in neuropathic pain development. The $Ca_v\alpha2\beta_1$ subunit is upregulated in the spinal dorsal horn and DRG after nerve injury in correlation with neuropathic pain behavior. The $Ca_v\alpha2\beta_1$ subunit is also the binding site for gabapentin. Both gabapentin and pregabalin are structural derivatives of the inhibitory neurotransmitter GABA, but they do not bind to $GABA_A$, $GABA_B$, or benzodiazepine receptors or alter GABA regulation. Binding of gabapentin and pregabalin to the $Ca_v\alpha2\beta_1$ subunit of VGCC results in a reduction in the calcium-dependent release of multiple neurotransmitters leading to efficacy and tolerability for neuropathic pain management.

Gabapentin is approved by FDA for postherpetic neuralgia, neuropathic pain, and partial seizures. Several studies also suggest a clinical role for restless leg syndrome, general anxiety, and general neuropathic pain. Gabapentin is used as a first-line agent to treat neuropathic pain from central (stroke, spinal cord injury) or peripheral origin (peripheral neuropathy, radiculopathy). It has a short half-life and the administration needs to be frequent. A gabapentin extended-release (ER) has been developed. Gabapentic ER was formulated using polymer-based AcuForm technology (DepoMed). When taken with a meal, the tablet is retained in stomach for up to 8 h and the drug is gradually released over 10 h in the small intestine, its optimal site of absorption. A recent randomized, double-blind, placebo-controlled study evaluated gastric-retentive gabapentin in patients with chronic pain from postherpetic neuralgia, with statistically significant reductions in pain scores in the gabapentin ER twice-daily group. However, pain scores in the once-daily gabapentin group were not reduced more than those in the placebo group [25].

A novel prodrug of gabapentin, XP13512/GSK 1838262 (Horizant and GlaxoSmithKline) was recently developed for the treatment of restless legs syndrome (RLS), PHN, PDN, and migraine prophylaxis. This drug has significant absorption in the large intestine, allowing an extended-release formulation. XP13512 improved symptoms in all patients and reduced pain associated with RLS significantly more than placebo. A later study included 222 patients with moderate to severe RLS and showed that XP13512 significantly improved the mean International RLS total score compared with placebo at week 12. The most common treatment-related adverse events included somnolence and dizziness [26].

Transient receptor potential (TRP) channels are nonselective monovalent and divalent cation channels. TRPV channels are present in small unmyelinated and myelinated (C and A delta) fibers of primary afferent neurons, dorsal root, trigeminal ganglia, the dorsal horn of the spinal cord (lamina I and II), and spinal nucleus of the trigeminal tract. The principal interest in TRP channels has focused on TRPV1 (vanilloid receptors) due to their role in nociceptive transmission, amplification, and sensitization. The search for perfect TRPV antagonist has yielded several drugs that underwent clinical trials. In phase II, clinical trials are SB-705498 (for migraine), NGD-8243/MK-2295 (for acute pain), and GRC (for acute pain); in phase I are AMG-517, AZD-1386, and ABT-102 (for chronic pain). During phase I clinical trials with AMG 517, a highly selective TRPV1 antagonist, it was found that TRPV1 blockade elicited marked, but reversible, and generally plasma concentration-dependent hyperthermia. AZD1386 was discontinued from development in 2010 due to liver enzyme elevations.

SB-705498 is a potent, selective, and orally bioavailable TRPV1 antagonist with efficacy in preclinical pain models. The compound was safe and well tolerated at single oral doses in a phase I study. A phase II trial used a randomized, placebo-controlled, single-blind crossover design to assess the effects of SB-705498 (400 mg) on heat-evoked pain and skin sensitization induced by capsaicin or UVB irradiation. Compared with placebo, SB-705498 reduced the area of capsaicin-evoked flare and raised the heat pain threshold on non-sensitized skin at the site of UVB-evoked inflammation [27].

Because they are not neural cells, microglia represent a relatively novel therapeutic target for analgesia. Activation of p38 mitogen-activated protein kinases (p38MAPK) and P2X4 in spinal cord microglia is essential for allodynia after nerve injury. The allodynia was reversed rapidly by pharmacological blockade of p38MAPK activation or inhibiting the expression of P2X4 receptors. Inhibitions of P2X4 expression, inhibiting the function of these receptors and/or p38MAPK in spinal microglia, are therefore potential therapeutic approaches. Losmapimod (GW856553X) is a selective p38MAPK inhibitor developed by GlaxoSmithKline. p38MAPK inhibition has been shown to produce antidepressant and antipsychotic effects in animal studies, with the mechanism thought to involve increased neurogenesis probably related to BDNF release. Losmapimod has completed phase II human clinical trials for the treatment of depression, although its safety and efficacy have yet to be proven in further trials.

There are several phase I study completed (a first-time-in-human randomized, single-blind placebo-controlled study to evaluate the safety, tolerability, pharmacokinetics, and pharmacodynamics of single escalating doses of GSK1482160, in male and female healthy subjects, and to make a preliminary assessment of the effect of food), phase II completed (a randomized, double-blind study to evaluate the safety and efficacy of the p38 kinase inhibitor, GW856553, in subjects with neuropathic pain from lumbosacral radiculopathy), or under way (a randomized, double-blind study to evaluate the safety and efficacy of the p38 kinase inhibitor, GW856553, in subjects with neuropathic pain from peripheral nerve injury) [28].

Tanezumab is a monoclonal antibody that inhibits the production of NGF. NGF stimulates nerve development, triggers pain, and is often present in inflamed tissues, such as arthritic joints. Treatment with tanezumab led to significant improvements in osteoarthritis knee pain in a phase II proof-of-concept study. Patients who received various doses of tanezumab had significant reductions in knee pain while walking. However, there were reports of progressively worsening osteoarthritis that emerged following completion of this study. These reports included 16 patients who had radiographic evidence of bone necrosis that required total joint replacement [29]. The investigators concluded that the efficacy profile for tanezumab was favorable but called for more safety data. In the fall of 2010, the FDA halted the tanezumab clinical development program. It was suggested that the pain relief conferred by tanezumab was so substantial that patients increased their physical activity enough to accelerate joint damage, ultimately causing them to need earlier joint replacement. The FDA also asked the company to stop phase II stage of testing of the drug to treat chronic low back and painful diabetic peripheral neuropathy; studies testing on the drug's efficacy in patients suffering from cancer pain and chronic pancreatitis are continuing.

Also, FDA in December 2010 asked Regeneron to stop testing REGN475, another fully human antibody that selectively targets NGF, fearing that acceleration of avascular necrosis of a joint may occur. Before that point, initial results from a randomized, double-blind, four-arm, placebo-controlled phase II trial in 217 patients with osteoarthritis of the knee were very promising. REGN475 demonstrated significant improvements at the two highest doses tested as compared to placebo in average walking pain scores over 8 weeks following a single intravenous infusion. Similarly, in the end of December 2010, the FDA put on hold phase II testing of fulranumab (Johnson & Johnson) over concerns that, as with other drugs in anti-NGF class, it may cause rapidly progressive osteoarthritis or osteonecrosis resulting in the need for earlier total joint replacement.

Abbott Laboratories have ongoing (but not actively recruiting participants) phase I studies of the monoclonal antibody PG110 (a randomized, double-blind, placebo-controlled, single ascending dose, phase I study to evaluate the safety, tolerability, and pharmacokinetics of PG110 (anti-NGF monoclonal antibody) in patients with pain attributed to osteoarthritis of the knee, NCT00941746) [30]. The status of the study is "ongoing, but not recruiting participants."

All but one study with Johnson & Johnson JNJ-42160443 (fulranumab) testing it in osteoarthritis pain, cancer-related pain, diabetic painful neuropathy, neuropathic pain (postherpetic neuralgia and post-traumatic neuralgia), and bladder pain have likewise been suspended. One phase II study, "a randomized, double-blind, placebo-controlled, dose-ranging, dose-loading study to evaluate the efficacy, safety, and tolerability of JNJ-42160443 as adjunctive therapy in subjects with inadequately controlled, moderate to severe, chronic low back pain" is ongoing but not recruiting participants [31].

Marijuana and cannabinoids are now available for medicinal purposes in many US states, although inconsistencies with Federal prohibitions have interfered widely with legal patient access of such agent. The main pharmacological effects of marijuana, as well as synthetic and endogenous cannabinoids, are mediated through G protein-coupled receptors (GPCRs), including CB-1 and CB-2 receptors. The CB-1 receptor is the major cannabinoid receptor in the central nervous system and has gained increasing interest as a target for drug discovery for treatment of nausea, cachexia, obesity, pain, spasticity, neurodegenerative diseases, and mood and substance abuse disorders. GW Pharmaceuticals conducted Sativex clinical trials in over 3,000 patients, including over 20 phase II and phase III trials worldwide including patients with multiple sclerosis, cancer pain, neuropathic pain, and rheumatoid arthritis. Sativex is delivered as an oromucosal spray in which each 100-µl spray contains 2.7 mg delta-9-tetrahydrocannabinol (THC) and 2.5 mg cannabidiol (CBD) extracted from farmed *Cannabis sativa* leaf and flower. Sativex includes, among its other indications, the improvement of symptoms in patients with moderate to severe spasticity due to multiple sclerosis (MS) who have not responded adequately to other anti-spasticity medication and who demonstrate clinically significant improvement in spasticity-related symptoms during an initial trial of therapy.

In 2010, GW Pharmaceuticals announced results of phase IIb dose-ranging trial evaluating the efficacy and safety of Sativex® in the treatment of pain in patients with advanced cancer, who experience inadequate analgesia during optimized chronic opioid therapy [32]. Sativex showed statistically significant differences from placebo in pain scores. In Europe, Sativex is approved in the UK and Spain as a treatment for multiple sclerosis spasticity. In Canada, Sativex is approved for the treatment for central neuropathic pain due to MS. In the USA, cancer pain represents the initial target indication for Sativex.

Sativex showed positive results in a phase II placebo-controlled trial in 56 patients with rheumatoid arthritis (RA). RA is the most common form of inflammatory arthritis and afflicts up to 3 % of the population of Western countries. In this 56 patient study, statistically significant improvements in favor of Sativex were found for pain on movement, pain at rest, quality of sleep, and DAS28 scores. The DAS28 is the present gold standard inflammation activity measure, and this result suggests an effect on the progression of the disease itself. Sativex is approved and marketed in the UK for the relief of spasticity in MS.

Sativex is approved and marketed in Canada for the relief of neuropathic pain in MS as well as for the relief of spasticity in MS. Other completed phase III clinical studies have tested the effectiveness of Sativex in peripheral neuropathic pain [33], diabetic neuropathy [34], and cancer pain [35]. There are active phase I and II studies being conducted in California of vaporized cannabis as an analgesic for PDN [36]. In Canada, an open phase III study is exploring the effect of Sativex in treatment of neuropathic pain caused by chemotherapy [37].

ILARIS (canakinumab; ACZ885; Novartis Pharmaceuticals; injection for subcutaneous use only) is an interleukin-1β monoclonal antibody initially approved in the USA in 2009 for the treatment of cryopyrin-associated periodic syndromes (CAPS), a group of rare inherited autoinflammatory conditions including familial cold autoinflammatory syndrome (FCAS) and Muckle-Wells syndrome (MWS) (initial US approval in 2009). Signs and symptoms include recurrent rash, fever/chills, joint pain, fatigue, and eye pain/redness. Currently, there are two open phase II, placebo-controlled trials in the USA and Europe assessing the ability of canakinumab to inhibit IL-1β activity for sustained time periods and thus favorably impact OA symptoms including pain, decreased function, and stiffness [38]. Another trial taking place in Ireland, Italy, and the UK assesses the safety and efficacy of ACZ885 in patients with active recurrent or chronic TNF receptor-associated periodic syndrome (TRAPS) [39].

Botox® (botulinum toxin A (BTX-A), Allergan) is currently available in approximately 75 countries for injection into muscles to treat upper limb spasticity in people 18 years and older, abnormal head position and neck pain of cervical dystonia (CD) in people 16 years and older, and certain eye muscle problems (strabismus) or eyelid spasm (blepharospasm) in people 12 years and older. As post-marketing experience has accumulated with these and other conditions such as headache, above and beyond its wide application for cosmetic purposes, clues have emerged that its beneficial effects upon pain are separable from those upon muscle contraction. French investigators have demonstrated the long-term efficacy of repeated applications of BTX-A in a small group of patients with post-traumatic or postherpetic neuralgia. These investigators are now seeking to confirm these findings in a larger randomized, placebo-controlled phase IV study [40]. Other studies are accruing patients with diabetic neuropathic foot pain, shoulder pain, male pelvic pain syndrome, back pain, and upper thoracic muscular pain.

In 2010, Pfizer Inc. acquired FoldRx and its portfolio of investigational compounds to treat diseases caused by protein misfolding, increasingly recognized as an important mechanism of many chronic degenerative diseases. The company's lead product candidate, tafamidis meglumine, is in registration as an oral, disease-modifying therapy for transthyretin (TTR) amyloid polyneuropathy (ATTR-PN), a progressively fatal genetic neurodegenerative disease, for which liver transplant is the only current treatment option. Tafamidis is a new chemical entity, first-in-class, oral, disease-modifying agent that stabilizes TTR and prevents dissociation of the tetramer, the rate-limiting step in TTR amyloidosis. Early results from FoldRx's randomized, controlled phase II/III clinical study show that once-daily oral treatment was safe and well tolerated, while halting disease progression and reducing the burden of disease after 18 months compared to placebo.

Telcagepant (formerly MK-0974, Merck) is a calcitonin gene-related peptide receptor (CRLR) antagonist under investigation for the acute treatment and prevention of migraine. Calcitonin gene-related peptide (CGRP) is an algesic peptide involved in nociceptive neurotransmission, as well as a strong vasodilator primarily found in nervous tissue. Since vasodilation in the brain is thought to be involved in the development of migraine and CGRP levels are increased during migraine attacks, this peptide was considered a potential target for new antimigraine drugs. It was equally efficacious as rizatriptan and zolmitriptan in two phase III clinical trials. A phase IIa clinical trial studying telcagepant for the prophylaxis of episodic migraine was stopped on March 26, 2009, due to significant elevations in serum transaminases. It is still possible that this safety concern may be addressed satisfactorily and, if so, that this drug will come to the market.

Alternative Delivery Routes

Intranasal and Inhalational Drug Delivery

Intranasal formulations are in wide use and are easy to administer. Potential benefits of intranasal drug delivery include rapid onset of action and improved compliance with unit dosage forms. Intranasal opioids, in the form of a dry powder or water or saline solution, are delivered using syringe, nasal spray or dropper, or nebulized inhaler. In addition to needle-free administration, the intranasal opioid route of administration (especially fentanyl) bypasses hepatic first-pass metabolism; because of the excellent perfusion of the nasal mucosa, there is rapid absorption and a prompt rise in plasma concentrations comparable to that seen with IV injection.

Intranasal morphine (Rylomine, Javelin now Hospira) is a patient-controlled nasal spray that provides rapid analgesic onset comparable to IV simply and noninvasively to control moderate to severe pain. The drug product combines morphine mesylate and chitosan, a natural polymer derived from the shells of crustaceans. Chitosan serves as a mucoadherent to facilitate and linearly dispense morphine absorption through the nasal mucosa. A single-spray unit dose delivers 7.5 mg of morphine mesylate in 0.1-ml metered dose. Early clinical trials in acute postoperative pain showed safety and efficacy comparable to those seen with equivalent doses of systemic morphine.

A similar approach to regularizing the intranasal absorption of an opioid, in this case fentanyl, has been approved in 2011 for Lazanda (Archimedes). In the case of Lazanda, fentanyl is coformulated with the pectin, which forms a gel when it contacts the nasal mucosa thus allowing the active ingredient to be delivered in a rapid but controlled manner. This drug product is indicated to treat episodes of breakthrough pain in patients with cancer.

Intranasal ketamine (Ereska, Javelin now Hospira) has been tested in metered, subanesthetic doses with the intention to offer an alternative to morphine for acute pain and potentially to treat cancer breakthrough pain in patients on chronic opioid therapy.

AeroLEF (aerosolized liposome-encapsulated fentanyl, YM BioSciences) is a proprietary formulation of free and liposome-encapsulated fentanyl intended to provide rapid and extended inhalational analgesia for patients with acute pain episodes. AeroLEF is in development for the treatment of moderate to severe pain, including cancer pain.

Fentanyl TAIFUN (Akela and Janssen) is a dry powder being developed for inhalational use to treat breakthrough pain. Following favorable results in an open-label phase II clinical trial, phase III testing is ongoing in patients with cancer pain during maintenance opioid therapy [41].

Mucoadhesive Drug Delivery

The BioErodible MucoAdhesive (BEMA) delivery system is designed to deliver either local or systemic levels of drugs across mucosal tissues. This delivery system offers rapid onset of action, avoidance of first-pass hepatic metabolism, and improved drug bioavailability compared with the oral route. The BEMA delivery system consists of a dime-sized disk with bioerodible layers that deliver drugs rapidly across a sequence of specified time intervals. One example of this technology is the BEMA Fentanyl mouth patch from BioDelivery Sciences International (Raleigh, NC), approved by FDA in 2009 as Onsolis to manage breakthrough cancer pain.

Rapinyl (Orexo and ProStrakan) is similar in concept, i.e., a fast-dissolving tablet of fentanyl under development for the treatment of breakthrough cancer pain.

Transdermal Drug Delivery

Poultices of medications, salves, and ointments have been applied since prehistory. A heat-assisted transdermal delivery system for fentanyl briefly under development in recent decades is reminiscent of the traditional Chinese practice of "cupping" in which smoldering herbs applied to the skin are covered with a glass of porcelain cup. Since the approval of Duragesic, the original "fentanyl patch" developed by Alza and Janssen in the 1980s, a steady increase of new delivery methods has taken place for both opioids (including heat-assisted transdermal delivery) and non-opioids.

Fentanyl transdermal system (Mylan Pharmaceuticals) has an innovative matrix design that, in contrast to Duragesic, employs neither metal nor a gel reservoir. Like Duragesic, it is indicated only for use in patients who are already tolerant to opioid therapy and for management of persistent, moderate to severe chronic pain that requires continuous opioid administration for an extended time and that cannot be managed by nonsteroidal analgesics, opioid combination products, or immediate release opioids.

The Flector® Patch (diclofenac epolamine topical patch) (King, now Pfizer) 1.3 % is used for the topical treatment of acute short-term pain due to minor strains, sprains, and contusions (bruises). Flector® Patch adheres to the affected area and delivers the efficacy of the NSAID diclofenac epolamine to the site of acute pain for 12 h of pain relief. Although the amount of systemic uptake of diclofenac is low compared with the traditional oral formulations, any of the typical NSAID and diclofenac adverse effects may occur. Therefore, as for all NSAIDs, it is recommended that the lowest strength of Flector be used for the shortest possible duration.

Future Directions: "Quo Vadis?"

The idea that there is single universal analgesic compound for pain treatment has been largely abandoned. Pain is a complex phenomenon with heterogeneous etiologies, mechanisms, and temporal characteristics. Consequently, treatment must be targeted not at the general symptom, pain, or its temporal properties, acute or chronic, but rather at the underlying neurobiological mechanisms. Recent comprehensive summaries of analgesic drugs under development attest to the ingenuity of scientists and clinical researchers in exploring many options for reformulation of existing molecules as well as creating new chemical entities [42]. Identification of key molecular targets involved in nociception and discovery and characterization of specific activators and inhibitors are not yet complete. Efforts to describe genetic influences upon pain, nociception, and the response to analgesics are likewise in the early stages. Still, it is relevant

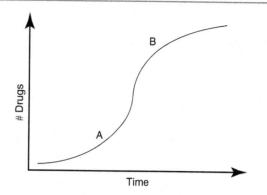

Fig. 19.1 A hypothetical graph of the number of available drugs as a function of time. The scales on the abscissa and ordinate are deliberately not specified (See text for discussion)

to the future of pain pharmacotherapy to step back and consider how far along we really are in the discovery process. The human genome, although large, is now fully sequenced and known to be finite. Together with comprehensive biological knowledge as to the range of possible drug targets (enzymes, receptors, ion channels, transporter proteins, etc.), it is now possible to estimate the total number of potential drug targets [43]. That number in turn is linked to, albeit not tightly, the total number of drugs that are likely to find a place in analgesic pharmacotherapy [44].

Figure 19.1 is the authors' attempt to convey that with increasing time, the number of available analgesic drugs will reach a plateau. One may ask what the scales should be for the abscissa and ordinate of this graph and whether we now are at point "A" or point "B." We would suggest "B" for the following reason: The relief of pain has been a continuous goal of humankind globally since prehistory [45]. Humans have swallowed, smoked, daubed on, or otherwise evaluated the analgesic properties and tolerability of nearly all substances within reach for tens of thousands of years. From this point of view, we would assert that the abscissa in Fig. 19.1 spans tens of thousands of years. It should come as no surprise that this prolonged, worldwide, high-throughput (if decentralized) screening for analgesic effectiveness has yielded agents that even today remain the foundation for analgesic pharmacotherapy: anti-inflammatories (e.g., willow bark), opioids (e.g., opium), and local anesthetics (e.g., cocaine). These drugs are supplemented by nondrug interventions first identified centuries or millennia ago such as heat, cold, splinting, and counter-stimulation with needles and/or electricity. Although the capacity of today's organized drug discovery processes dwarfs that of previous eras' empirical ad hoc observations, the former approach has proceeded for about a century while the latter has been in place for at least a hundredfold longer.

Summary/Conclusions

Despite efforts to maximize the utility of existing pain medicines, obvious shortfalls in the analgesic armamentarium persist. Analgesics based upon novel molecular and genetic mechanisms are being intensively explored to address the unmet needs of patients in pain [42]. The discovery and development of such medicines may require a surprising amount of effort and expense, however, to progress only slightly up the curve shown in Fig. 19.1. To some degree, this slowness to progress may reflect the many late-stage failures among recently developed analgesic compounds due to an unintended negative bias in the current FDA drug approval framework, such as overlooking subgroups of responders [46]. Further, on a global scale, many of the analgesic gaps between ideal and actual practice may be addressed simply by providing access to simple inexpensive agents such as anti-inflammatory drugs or opioids [47]. Nonetheless, even after taking these factors under consideration, it is safe to predict that in the wealthier nations, the search for new analgesics with an improved effect to side-effect profile and improved methods for the delivery of familiar agents will continue for some time to come.

Acknowledgment Partial support for this work was provided by the Saltonstall Fund for Pain Research.

References

1. Institute of Medicine. Relieving pain in America: a blueprint for transforming prevention, care, education and research. Washington D.C.: The National Academies Press; 2011.
2. Coggeshall RE, Carlton SM. Receptor localization in the mammalian dorsal horn and primary afferent neurons. Brain Res Rev. 1997;24:28–66.
3. Traub RJ. The spinal contribution of the induction of central sensitization. Brain Res. 1997;778:34–42.
4. Dickenson AH. Spinal cord pharmacology of pain. Br J Anaesth. 1995;75:193–200.
5. Scholz J, Woolf CJ. Can we conquer pain? Nat Neurosci. 2002;5(Suppl):1062–7.
6. Rittner HL, Brack A, Machelska H, et al. Opioid peptide-expressing leukocytes: identification, recruitment, and simultaneously increasing inhibition of inflammatory pain. Anesthesiology. 2001;95:500–8.
7. Millan MJ. The induction of pain: an integrative review. Prog Neurobiol. 1999;57:1–164.
8. Machelska H, Stein C. Immune mechanisms in pain control. Anesth Analg. 2002;95:1002–8.
9. Shu X-Q, Mendell LM. Neurotrophins and hyperalgesia. Proc Natl Acad Sci U S A. 1999;96:7693–6.
10. Thompson SWN, Bennett DLH, Kerr BJ, Bradbury EJ, McMahon SB. Brain-derived neurotrophic factor is an endogenous modulator of nociceptive responses in the spinal cord. Proc Natl Acad Sci U S A. 1999;96:7714–8.
11. Cortright DN, Szallasi A. Biochemical pharmacology of the vanilloid receptor TRPV1: an update. Eur J Biochem. 2004;271:1814–9.
12. Rashid MH, Inoune M, Kondo S, Kawashima T, Bakoshi S, Ueda H. Novel expression of vanilloid receptor 1 on capsaicin-insensitive fibers accounts for the analgesic effect of capsaicin cream in neuropathic pain. J Pharmacol Exp Ther. 2003;304:940–8.
13. Walker SM, Goudas LC, Cousins MJ, Carr DB. Combination spinal analgesic chemotherapy: a systematic review. Anesth Analg. 2002;96:674–715.
14. Colombo P, Sonvico F, Colombo G, et al. Novel platforms for oral drug delivery. Pharm Res. 2009;26(3):601–11.
15. Drug and Biologic Approval Reports. United States Food and Drug Administration. 2011. FDA Web site www.fda.gov/. Accessed 10 Jan 2011.
16. Business Insights. Lifecycle management strategies: maximizing ROI through indication expansion, reformulation and Rx-to-OTC switching. Business Insights Report. 2006.
17. Grudzinskas C, Balster RL, Gorodetzky CW, et al. Impact of formulation on the abuse liability, safety and regulation of medications: the expert panel report. Drug Alcohol Depend. 2006;83 (Supp 1):S77–82.
18. Collier R. Drug development cost estimates hard to swallow. CMAJ. 2009;180(3):279–80.
19. Associated Press. Scientists explore abuse-resistant painkillers. MSNBC Web site. 2007. Available at www.msnbc.msn.com/id/17581544/. Accessed 21 May 2009.
20. Commercial and Pipeline Insight: Opioids - Short acting and anti-abuse technologies set to fragment and grow the market. Datamonitor. March 2008. Abstract. http://www.marketresearch.com/Datamonitor-v72/Commercial-Pipeline-Insight-Opioids-Short-1728798/ Accessed 10 Feb 2011.
21. Wild JE, Grond S, Kuperwasser B, et al. Long-term safety and tolerability of tapentadol extended release for the management of chronic low back pain or osteoarthritis pain. Pain Pract. 2010;10:416–27.
22. McGaraughty S, Chu KC, Scanio MLC, Kort ME, Faltynek CR, Jarvis MF. A selective $Na_v1.8$ sodium channel blocker, A-803467 [5-(4-chlorophenyl-N-(3,5-dimethoxyphenyl)furan-2-carboxamide], attenuates spinal neuronal activity in neuropathic rats. J Pharmacol Exp Ther. 2008;324:1204–11.
23. Catterall WA. Structure and regulation of voltage-gated Ca2+ channels. Annu Rev Cell Dev Biol. 2000;16:521–55.
24. Ertel EA, Campbell KP, Harpold MM, et al. Nomenclature of voltage-gated calcium channels. Neuron. 2000;25:533–5.
25. Irving G, Jensen M, Cramer M, et al. Efficacy and tolerability of gastric-retentive gabapentin for the treatment of postherpetic neuralgia: results of double-blind, randomized, placebo-controlled clinical trial. Clin J Pain. 2009;25:185–92.
26. Kushida CA, Becker PM, Ellenbogen AL, Canafax DM, Barrett RW. Randomized, double-blind, placebo-controlled study of XP13512/GSK 1838262 in patients with RLS. Neurology. 2009;72:439–46.
27. Gunthorpe MJ, Chizh BA. Clinical development of TRPV1 antagonists: targeting a pivotal point in the pain pathway. Drug Discov Today. 2009;14(1–2):56–67.
28. A randomized, double blind study to evaluate the safety and efficacy of the p38 kinase inhibitor, GW856553, in subjects with neuropathic pain from peripheral nerve injury. GlaxoSmithKline GSK: Protocol Summaries: Compounds: Losmapimod. GSK Study ID112967. Study completed. http://www.gsk-clinicalstudyregister.com/protocol_comp_list.jsp;jsessionid=275F763F1C36638B02758F5A4C276956?compound=Losmapimod. Accessed 11 Feb 2011.
29. Lane NE, Schnitzer TJ, Birbara CA, et al. Tanezumab for the treatment of pain from osteoarthritis of the knee. N Engl J Med. 2010;363:1521–31.

30. Safety and tolerability of PG110 in patients with knee osteoarthritis pain. 2011. http://clinicaltrials.gov/ct2/show/NCT00941746. Study completed. Accessed 11 Feb 2011.

31. A dose-ranging study of the safety and effectiveness of JNJ-42160443 as add-on treatment in patients with low back pain. 2011. http://clinicaltrials.gov/ct2/show/NCT00973024. Study terminated. Accessed 11 Feb 2011.

32. A study of Sativex® for relieving persistent pain in patients with advanced cancer. 2011. http://clinicaltrials.gov/ct2/show/NCT01262651. Study currently active. Accessed 11 Feb 2011.

33. A study of Sativex® for pain relief of peripheral neuropathic pain, associated with allodynia. 2011. http://clinicaltrials.gov/ct2/show/NCT00710554. Study completed. Accessed 11 Feb 2011.

34. A study of Sativex® for pain relief due to diabetic neuropathy. 2011. http://clinicaltrials.gov/ct2/show/NCT00710424. Study completed. Accessed 11 Feb 2011.

35. Study to compare the safety and tolerability of Sativex® in patients with cancer related pain. 2011. http://clinicaltrials.gov/ct2/show/NCT00675948. Study completed. Accessed 11 Feb 2011.

36. Efficacy of inhaled cannabis in diabetic painful peripheral neuropathy. 2011. http://clinicaltrials.gov/ct2/show/NCT00781001. Study currently active. Accessed 11 Feb 2011.

37. A double blind placebo controlled crossover pilot trial of Sativex with open label extension for treatment of chemotherapy induced neuropathic pain. 2011. http://clinicaltrials.gov/ct2/show/NCT00872144. Study currently active. Accessed 11 Feb 2011.

38. A randomized, double blind, placebo and naproxen controlled, multi-center, study to determine the safety, tolerability, pharmacokinetics and effect on pain of a single intra-articular administration of canakinumab in patients with osteoarthritis in the knee. 2011. http://clinicaltrials.gov/ct2/show/NCT01160822. Study completed. Accessed 11 Feb 2011.

39. An open-label, multicenter, efficacy and safety study of 4-month canakinumab treatment with 6-month follow-up in patients with active recurrent or chronic TNF-receptor associated periodic syndrome (TRAPS). 2011. http://clinicaltrials.gov/ct2/show/NCT01242813. Study currently active. Accessed 11 Feb 2011.

40. Randomized double blind placebo controlled multicenter study of the efficacy and safety of repeated administrations of botulinum toxin type A (Botox) in the treatment of peripheral neuropathic pain. 2011. http://clinicaltrials.gov/ct2/show/NCT01251211. Study currently active. Accessed 11 Feb 2011.

41. The safety of fentanyl TAIFUN treatment after titrated dose administration and the current breakthrough pain treatment for breakthrough pain in cancer patients. 2011. http://clinicaltrials.gov/ct2/show/NCT00822614. Study currently active. Accessed 11 Feb 2011.

42. Sinatra RS, Jahr JS, Watkins-Pitchford JM, editors. The essence of analgesia and analgesics. New York: Cambridge University Press; 2011.

43. Overington JP, Al-Lazikani B, Hopkins AL. How many drug targets are there? Nat Rev Drug Discov. 2006;5:993–6.

44. Imming P, Sinning C, Meyer A. Drugs, their targets, and the nature and number of drug targets. Nat Rev Drug Discov. 2006;5:821–34.

45. Gallagher RM, Fishman SM. Pain medicine: history, emergence as a medical specialty, and evolution of the multidisciplinary approach. In: Cousins MJ, Bridenbaugh PO, Carr DB, Horlocker TT, editors. Cousins & Bridenbaugh's neural blockade in clinical anesthesia and management of pain. 4th ed. Philadelphia: Lippincott Williams & Wilkins; 2009. p. 631–43.

46. Dworkin RH, Turk DC. Accelerating the development of improved analgesic treatments: the ACTION public-private partnership. Pain Med. 2011;12:S109–17.

47. Brennan F, Carr DB, Cousins MJ. Pain management: a fundamental human right. Anesth Analg. 2007;105:205–21.

Index

9 781493 918171